WORK WITH YOUR DOCTOR
To Diagnose and Cure 27 Ailments
With Natural and Safe Methods

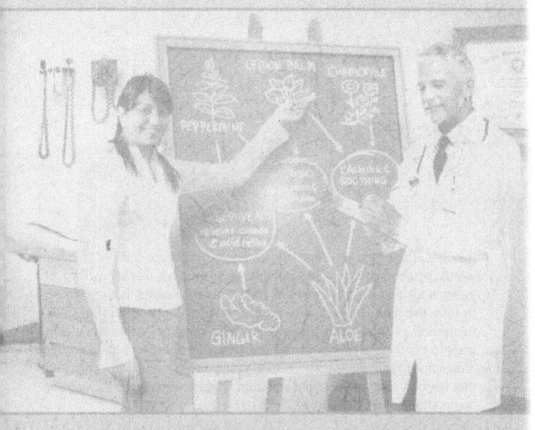

Work With Your Doctor

To Diagnose and Cure 27 Ailments
With Natural and Safe Methods

by:

Dr. Michael D. Farley, N.M.D.

Ty M. Bollinger

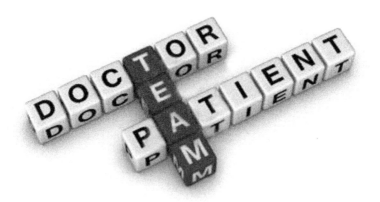

It is important that you form a partnership with your doctor. In other words, you should form a "*medical team*." There are literally millions of patients all over the USA that are looking for physicians that are willing to take the time to practice comprehensive medicine. There are also thousands of physicians that still put their patients' welfare first and want to continue learning. If you are fortunate enough to have one of these physicians, please ask them to email us the information below so that we can refer them to patients that contact us and are looking for comprehensive medical help.

Please send the physician's name, address, email, and phone number to: **referrals@medicaldreamteam.com**

FROM THE REVIEWERS

"There are a number of books on the market that list treatment options for various conditions. What is different about this book is that Dr. Farley is talking to the reader and sharing his wealth of knowledge acquired throughout 30 years of experience treating patients suffering from various ailments and conditions for which conventional medicine has been unable to find an answer. *Work With Your Doctor* is an easy book to read; in spite of this, every recommendation provided is also supported by solid research that the reader can share with his or her health care provider. This makes this wonderful book a treasure trove of 'clinical pearls' that I, as a practicing ND, have found very valuable. What I have also found extremely helpful is having the actual study abstracts printed at the end of each chapter instead of just referenced, as is usually found in most books in this category. I recommend *Work with your Doctor* to everyone who is concerned about finding help for the ailments listed and to every health care provider who is also looking 'outside the box' in an attempt to help his/her patients."

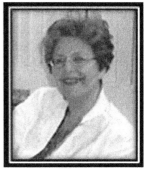

Dr. Mireille Fanous, ND

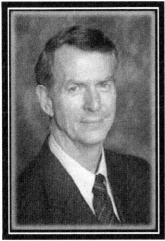

Dr. Russell Blaylock, MD
Editor of Blaylock Wellness Report
(www.blaylockwellnesscenter.com)
and Best-selling author
of "Excitotoxins:The Taste That
Kills", "Health & Nutrition Secrets
That Can Save Your Life" & "Natural
Strategies For Cancer Patients"

"*Work With Your Doctor* by Dr. Michael Farley and Ty Bollinger is an excellent introduction to under-standing modern medicine and why it is being questioned by more people than ever in its history. It is easy to read and follow and provides simple solutions to many of the problems that plague our modern society. You should keep a copy of this valuable book on your bookshelf. It is an excellent way to educate your doctor, while improving your health."

As a practicing physician in one of the oldest holistic medical clinics in the USA, I had previously not seen such concise information on common and critical diseases until I reviewed this book. *Work With Your Doctor* addresses many common and very difficult diseases and provides insight into the effective methods of treatments available along with the data to substantiate it. Every integrative practitioner, whether physician, nurse, or natural health practitioner, will benefit from the information provided in *Work With Your Doctor* by Dr. Michael Farley and Ty Bollinger. They have accurately exposed the many truths about the effectiveness of natural therapies while providing insight to the use of common treatments and their potential side effects. Seldom does a book provide information that both the patient and the doctor can use to help to treat a patient but this one does. Even I, with 35 years of clinical experience, found new and useable information to treat my patients.

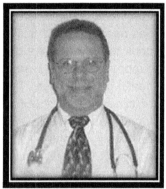

Dr. R. Ernest Cohn,
MD, NMD, DC, FACO
*Holistic Medical
Clinic of the Carolinas*

In spite of my background as a pediatric cardiologist from the Ukraine, I have often found it a challenge to communicate with medical doctors in my present career as a Naturopathic physician in British Columbia, Canada. This incredible book, *Work With Your Doctor,* has provided the common denominators, science and research, and built the bridge allowing communication and understanding between the two professions in the best interest of their patients. *Work With Your Doctor* is Dr. Farley's generous gift to patients and doctors alike in which he shares his deep knowledge of all the various aspects of conventional and natural medicine as well as his wisdom and years of clinical experience.

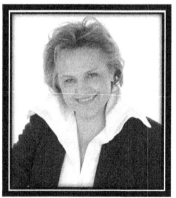

Dr. Galina Bogatch,
MD, ND

Work With Your Doctor provides the most comprehensive review on the current state of medicine in the United States, while offering a creative solution of partnership between patient and physician. While it would be natural to lash out at the current system, Ty Bollinger and Dr. Michael Farley instead offer science, studies, research and safe, natural recommendations in consideration for some of the most common physical challenges we face as a society. I truly believe that this posture alone could once again bring patient and doctor together as a team to construct solutions that are in the patient's health's best interest. This book exemplifies a spirit of harmonious collaboration instead of competition. Whether you are a doctor or patient, this book will open your eyes to a new world of possibilities. Whatever you are experiencing right now, this book gives hope that it doesn't have to stay that way. *Work With Your Doctor* contains the answers.

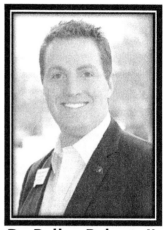

Dr. Rollan Roberts II,
DBA - *Best-selling author,
noted speaker, and
founder/CEO of
24ravens.com*

Dr. Michael Farley and Ty Bollinger and have done it again! *Work With Your Doctor* is required reading for everyone. The authors discuss a majority of the preventable diseases affecting millions and include easy to use natural solutions. Their compassion, enthusiasm, and knowledge for natural therapies just leaps off the page. The chapters on allergies, cardiovascular disease, and adrenal fatigue are excellent. The section covering the 'Top 20 Herbs' will offer the reader powerful natural resources to secure better health. You must have this book because sooner or later you will crack it open to save your life.

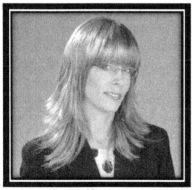

Wendy Wilson, Herbalist
*Host of syndicated radio
show "Herb Talk Live"*

Work With Your Doctor is an excellent resource for anyone concerned with their own health and the health of their loved ones. Dr. Farley's information shines as his common sense approach to healthcare covers his wide-spectrum expertise from the traditional to alternative to Native American to eastern. Couple that with Mr. Bollinger's 'outside the box' style and the result is a must have book. As a matter of fact, you'll want to get at least two copies – one for yourself and one for your doctor. Borrowing and extrapolating President Eisenhower's

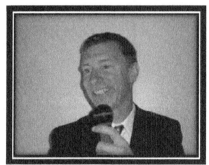

Tom Ritter
Retired rocket scientist,
health advocate, author,
and veteran talk radio host

warning of the growing 'military industrial complex,' our health freedom rights are constantly under attack from the 'pharmaceutical healthcare industrial complex.' *Work With Your Doctor* will arm you with the information you need to team up with your doctor to ensure your health and longevity. If you want to take total control of your health, this book offers the pros and cons of all options you should consider.

I have been an equine practitioner for twenty years. My practice treats horses of all disciplines with a primary focus on internal medicine. As most veterinarians, I have practiced traditional medicine. Equine veterinarians are often challenged with limitations on both diagnoses and treatment options. I have been fortunate to study with Dr. Farley and have successfully used naturalistic, alternative treatments with many of my equine patients. Whether choosing a natural remedy alone

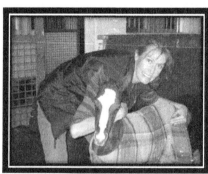

Dr. Christine F. Bridges,
DVM

or in combination with traditional medicine, it has been extremely advantageous to have these options available. As a private prac-titioner, it is both exciting and hopeful to have other options available to suc-cessfully treat horses in veterinary medicine. I thoroughly enjoyed reading this book; it is extremely beneficial and I will highly recommend it to everyone.

This book you hold in your hands is a revolutionary, groundbreaking guide containing information which has proven itself through decades of practice and research. Millions of North Americans are turning to and are in need of this comprehensive and authoritative guidance. Great health is your God given right. When we do not have the tools to make an educated decision for ourselves or our family, we allow others to orchestrate our fate. That ends here with this groundbreaking book. The intention of this book is to empower you and help you reach your full health potential and bridge the gap so that you and your doctor can make logical, intelligent decisions for you and your loved ones. By reading this book, you will awaken and restore your confidence and rid yourself of the fear of the unknown. Millions of dollars are made by keeping knowledge from you that would empower you to heal yourself and your family. Not anymore ... thanks to the brilliant work of Dr. Michael Farley and investigative researcher and author Ty Bollinger.

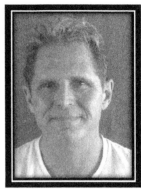

Dr. Darrell L. Wolfe,
AC, PhD
*Founder of The
Wolfe Clinic*

 Work With Your Doctor is an exceptional and completely unique book. Authors Ty Bollinger and Dr. Michael Farley go into great detail on how to treat numerous serious ailments (like Alzheimer's, Parkinsons, MS, Lupus, Cardiovascular Disease, and Diabetes) comprehensively, and encourage patients to team up with their doctors and work together. Too often, patients try the 'Lone Ranger' approach and end up in a worse place than they started because they just don't have the basic knowledge of physiology needed to properly diagnose and treat what may be ailing them. In addition, this book is unique because it contains hundreds of pages of peer-reviewed medical studies (for your doctor to review) which validate the treatments that are offered in it. The information in this book is often downright astonishing and I can't imagine anyone serious about good health not having a copy of it.

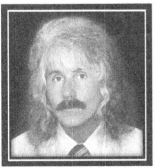

Jeff Rense
*Wordwide syndicated
talk radio host
and Editor-in-Chief
of www.Rense.com*

Work With Your Doctor is a wonderfully useful book. It is unique. Both Dr. Farley and Ty Bollinger obviously have a lot of very useful information to share with you about healing 27 different ailments – cancer, pneumonia, Alzheimer's, diabetes, acid reflux and on and on. They not only guide you about the use of natural remedies but they give you very useful information to share with your doctor. That's what makes this book unique. The authors are not trying to give you a "self-help" directory. From Dr. Farley's 30 years of experience as a practicing physician, they are educating you about how to talk to your doctor to take the best advantage of his/her ability to help you. Of course, healing requires you to take charge and they know this. But they also know that help from a doctor is frequently necessary. Get this

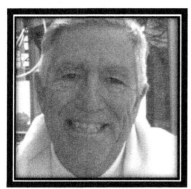

Bill Henderson
Best-selling author of
"Cure Your Cancer"
and "Cancer-Free"

book and maximize your investment in health care. One of the other things I loved about this book was the detailed explanation about the conspiracy of the Rockefeller and Carnegie money to make allopathic medicine the dominant medical option. It is one of the worst options, but the money in the early 20th century essentially gave it a monopoly and suppressed all the competitive medical options. That suppression persists 100 years later. This is the first time I've read a really detailed description about exactly how this happened. Get this book.

 As a radio talk show host for 15 years, I literally receive hundreds of books to review all wanting an interview on the radio to promote their

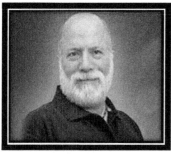

Dr. Eliezer Ben-Joseph,
ND, DSc, MD (MA)
Syndicated
talk radio host

book. It is quite refreshing to receive a book that lives up to my standards for a radio interview. The book *Work With Your Doctor* does meet my standards and more. This is the kind of reference that one will refer back to often as the information is all useful and up-to-date. For the layperson, this is one book that you will want in you library.

America is headed over a financial cliff due to an unsustainable health care system. Just like General Motors went bankrupt due to overwhelming health costs, America has $100 trillion in unfunded liabilities for Medicare and the like. Dr. Farley and Ty Bollinger have provided America with a road map out of this quandary. From documenting the humble origins of the American Medical Association, to documenting the clear advantages in the risk to benefit to cost ratio of natural medicine; these authors have assembled a bullet-proof case in favor of using a new form of medicine to make America strong and solvent again. Drugs and surgery can temporarily suppress symptoms and often at great cost in dollars and side effects. Meanwhile, there are well documented natural medicines that can prevent and reverse many common ailments. America was founded on the principles of liberty, personal accountability, and privacy. Read this book and find your own personal accountability for your health. The authors are bold and outspoken in their justified claims that natural medicine can reverse many ailments that are considered untreatable by modern allopathic medicine.

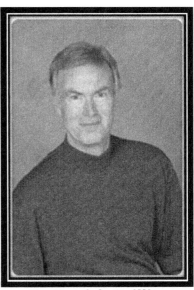

Dr. Patrick Quillin,
PhD, RD, CNS
*Best-selling author of 17
health books including
"Beating Cancer With Nutrition"*

 Have you ever thought that there was a better way to deliver health care? Do you think that the political environment misses the mark entirely? I had the same feeling. When I graduated from dental school, I was on top of the world. After all, I was a recent graduate. I knew everything there was to know about dental disease. I went to one of the best dental schools in the country. How utterly disillusioned I was when I found out that patients don't work exactly as the textbooks tell us. And the longer that I saw the same patient, the better I realized that health care is not wrapped up into a simple, short program. I've talked to some of my medical colleagues. They feel the same way.

Dr. Michael Farley and I have collaborated together for many years. Mike was looking for a dentist who might think as he does. While I initially said that I was perfectly comfortable in my implant and periodontal practice and I didn't wish to delve into the unknown, he said 'Try doing a case with me.' Reluctantly, I did. That was the beginning of some of the most fascinating work that I've done in my career. Dr. Farley and I did television together for a number of years. What impressed me most was his knowledge of the literature. It is that research that is the basis for this book. He does not look at untested solutions. He derives his solutions from the medical literature, the same literature that is available to physicians. He makes his decisions based upon that literature, his training as a naturopathic physician, and a vast array of his own experiences with his patients. As we know more about the errant conclusions and worse that pharmaceutical therapies have wrought on two generations of unsuspecting patients and their doctors, we need answers that work. We need answers that produce greater positive effects than the side-effects from medications.

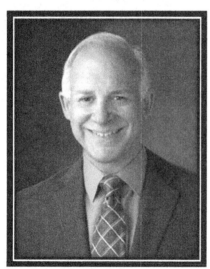

Dr. Lee N. Sheldon, DMD

We need to know the cause of the problem. And that is what Dr. Farley finds: the cause. Only then can we achieve long-term results. This book is a compilation of years of research and its application. This book is a compilation of results-oriented therapy without the need for long-term toxic chemicals. This book will help doctors and their patients find a better solution to their problems and as such a higher level quality of life. Enjoy this book. And may you enjoy greater health as a result.

Before becoming an author myself, I was appalled to learn that only 3% of all books written sell more than 1000 copies. The reason I suspect, at least for health books, is because most health books lack passion and conviction. This book by Ty Bollinger and Dr. Michael Farley will certainly not be constrained by any of these limitations.

Why? Because both authors exude a love and concern for all mankind and their common goal is to help others. *Work With Your Doctor* contains vital information necessary for all who value the autonomy of their health and bodies, presented in a manner in which all who read it will be able to digest and absorb the wealth of practical, sometimes life-changing, knowledge. As a physician for over 21 years

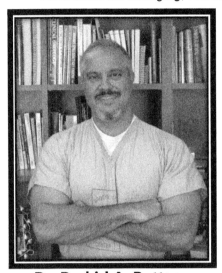

now, I have held one important premise and belief that I have preached to my patients who hail from 77 countries and practically every state in our union. That premise is that you must do everything possible to gain knowledge because as you gain knowledge, you become empowered, and once empowered, you can never become a victim of 'the system.' *Work With Your Doctor* is a one-of-a-kind book which has been meticulously researched and written in a manner which will benefit everyone who reads it, both patients and doctors alike. I highly recommend this book.

Dr. Rashid A. Buttar,
DO, FAAPM, FACAM, FAAIM
Best-selling author of "The 9 Steps to Keep the Doctor Away"

 You are about to learn not only why we are in the present state of 'dis-ease' we are in, but most importantly, how – using the most up to date and proven natural means possible – you can help your body become healthy once again. If you are ready to finally take control of your health, then read this book because Dr. Farley and Ty Bollinger have hit this one out of the park!

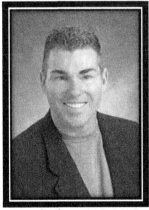

Brad King, MS, MFS
Best-selling author of the award winning "Beer Belly Blues"

WORK WITH YOUR DOCTOR

To Diagnose and Cure 27 Ailments
With Natural and Safe Methods

Published by:

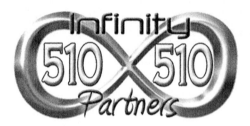

INFINITY 510² PARTNERS
HOUSTON, TX
www.Infinity510Partners.com

To order more copies of this book,
please visit the following website:

www.MedicalDreamTeam.com

Work With Your Doctor To Diagnose and Cure 27 Ailments With Natural and Safe Methods

Printed and bound in the USA.

ISBN-10: 0-9788065-5-7
ISBN-13: 978-0-9788065-5-2

The front and back cover illustrations were created by David Dees. His website is www.deesillustration.com.

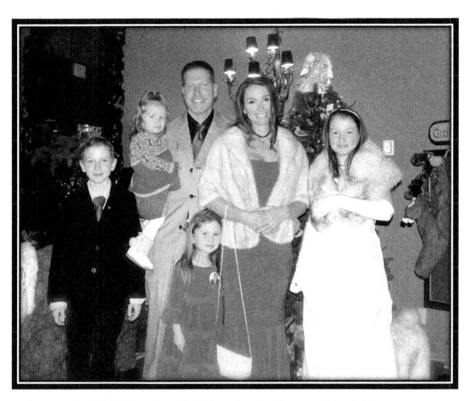

ABOVE – The Bollinger family (from left to right):
Bryce, Charity, Ty, Tabitha, Charlene, and Brianna
BELOW – Mike and Diane Farley

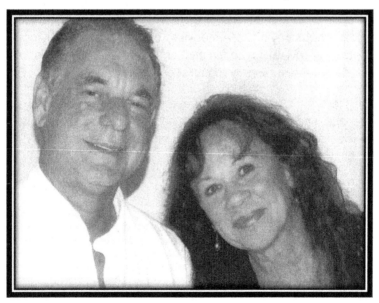

ACKNOWLEDGMENTS

From Dr. Michael Farley, NMD

First I would like to thank my wife Diane. She has worked at my side as a physician's assistant for 30 years and as a fearless patients advocate for the same length of time. I have learned as much from her as in any medical school. I must also thank her for taking over all of my "chores" and protecting my privacy so I could actually finish this book. Without her steadfast support this book would never have been written. Actually, without her constant love and support I doubt my accomplishments would have been even a fraction of what they have been. **I have been blessed with my wife and with all eight of our children that also give their unwavering backing to my work.**

Thanks to Dr. Mireille Fanous, N.D., a Canadian Naturopathic Doctor. She has been responsible for reminding me that I need to take time for myself and family and stop trying to do so much work. She actually spent hours on the phone with me in order to teach me how to be politically correct. As well, she reminded me of what I told my patients and demanded I start applying the advice to myself. She can be tough, but always with care and concern. I remember a patient I referred to her for follow up care. He told me he was more afraid of her than me, but also how much she cared for her patients and how much he respected her. I feel the same way.

Thanks to Dr. Galina Bogatch, M.D., N.D., who was trained as a cardiologist in Russia and now practices as a Naturopath in Canada. Thank you for sharing your knowledge and wisdom in order to insure a healthy life for me. She has a wealth of knowledge about cardiac healthcare and ranks as one of the most advanced cardiac specialists I know. Mireille, Galina and I now regularly have conference calls to catch up on health issues and new medical developments and also for a time to laugh together. I always look forward to those calls.

I would especially like to thank Dr. Lee Sheldon, a periodontist, in Melbourne, Florida, who has always been a steadfast friend and has given wonderful care to every patient I have sent him for help. He is the type of friend that always answers the phone, even at 3:00 A.M. if needed. I fondly remember years of exchanging emails in the middle of the night on research we were doing. It seemed with our schedule, that was the only time we had available, but he always answered.

Finally I would like to thank my co-author, Mr. Ty Bollinger. He has been the one that has pushed, prodded and made me feel that I have knowledge that needs to be shared, and is making sure that I do. In a very short time, he has also become one of those few and trusted friends that you know would do anything you asked to help. Thank you for your friendship and confidence in me Ty.

From Ty Bollinger

I want to thank my Lord and Savior, Jesus Christ, who is the "Great Physician," for giving me the knowledge and ability to research and write this book.

To my darling Charlene, you are the epitome of what a wife and mother should be, a Proverbs 31 woman, and a shining example of God's grace and love in my life. You love the truth, share the truth, and teach our children the truth, no matter who opposes you. **You are my Princess and I love you forever faithfully, infinity 510^2.** ☺

To my children (Brianna, Bryce, Tabitha, and Charity), I love you each as much as a Daddy can possibly love his children. The questions you have asked me have made this a better book, and I am proud of each one of you. **Daddy loves you!!!**I want to thank my good friend and co-author, Dr. Michael Farley, for his diligent and amazing work on this book. His knowledge of medicine and health is second to none, and I am so thankful that we were able to "team up" and work together on this book. Mike is one of the few people that I trust implicitly, and I'm honored to be able to call him my "friend."

Special thanks to KC Craichy, Dr. Paul J. LaRochelle, Dr. Russell Blaylock, Dr. Mireille Fanous, Brad King, Dr. R. Ernest Cohn, Jeff Rense, Dr. Galina Bogatch, Dr. Rollan Roberts, Wendy Wilson, Tom Ritter, Dr. Christine Bridges, Dr. Darrell Wolfe, Bill Henderson, Dr. Eliezer Ben-Joseph, Dr. Patrick Quillin, Dr. Rashid Buttar, Dr. Alan Cantwell, Dr. Lee Sheldon, and Dr. Suzanne Humphries.

TABLE OF CONTENTS

PART II - The Treatments

PART III - For Your Doctor

PART IV - Summarium

FOREWORD
K.C. Craichy

You get a call from your doctor regarding your annual testing and are asked to come to the office. There you get the dreaded news that you have cancer and they need to check you into the hospital right away and commence surgery, radiation and chemotherapy – if you are to have any hope of survival. You are filled with fear and feel you have nowhere to turn except to listen to your doctor. Is what your doctor is advising the best course of action for you? Is it really an emergency or do you have time to research your type of cancer? Are the types of further medical tests, scans and procedures being recommended safe or could they cause additional problems? Does your doctor have any understanding of legitimate alternative therapies that might be safer and more effective? The stark reality is that this kind of frightening scenario happens countless times every day in the USA and around the world and most doctors are very negative towards complementary, alternative, and nutritional therapies even though mountains of evidence exist to support them. They apparently do not have the background, understanding, or interest to learn this potentially life-saving information even though it often appears in their own medical journals. So where do we go for advice we can trust?

Fortunately, regarding cancer, there is a resource you can trust – Ty Bollinger's best-selling book, *Cancer – Step Outside the Box*. I have recommended this book to numerous people after their (or their loved one's) diagnosis of cancer to give them hope and direction. Each cancer situation is different, therefore no single therapy is best.

People have always relied on their doctors to tell them their options and even what they should do. They were a source of advice you could trust with your life. Their advice used to be known as "*doctors orders.*" Unfortunately, in this day and age of pharmaceutically dominated allopathic medicine, the vast majority of doctors' primary training is in pharmaceutical and surgical approaches to treating disease. A trip to the doctor has become a transaction – you expect to pay your co-pay and leave with a prescription or procedure, or both.

It is not the fault of the doctors, they are well-meaning people that want to help people by getting into medicine, nevertheless, it is the way they were trained and they had little (if any) choice in that training. Additionally, doctors are overworked, over paper-worked and stressed out about the possibility of medical malpractice law suits. The threat of medical liability makes doctors practice what is called the *"standard of care,"* and as long as they practice the same as their counterparts they have some degree of protection from liability, regardless of whether or not a particular drug or procedure is harming patients, or if better alternatives exist.

Thousands of medical studies are published every year validating complementary, alternative and nutritional therapies, but given the time constraints, most doctors do not read these studies and in most cases are not even aware they exist. Even if they did read these studies, they still believe they need the protection of practicing within the accepted *"standard of care."*

To make matters worse, doctors have very little time with each patient and patients come into their offices requesting, if not demanding, a certain brand of medication they saw advertised on TV, radio, or their favorite magazine and are sure that the drug will "fix" their often self-diagnosed problems. This is a vicious cycle that is sure to get worse if the "Affordable Care Act" remains the law of the land and causes doctors to leave the profession in droves.

The bottom line is that if you are going to survive, you must take full responsibility for your health, do your own research, and make your own decisions. Change your thinking about doctors from someone who gives *"doctor's orders"* to someone who is a good resource to help you answer your questions so you can make an informed decision.

Ty's passion to help others has now led him to team up with Dr. Michael Farley (and his 30 years of practicing medicine and thousands of hours of research into treating the cause of disease) and write another powerful book, the book which you now have in your hands, entitled *Work With Your Doctor To Diagnose and Cure 27 Ailments with Natural and Safe Methods*. Ty is not a doctor; he is a man who lost both his parents to "cancer treatments" and was determined to help others avoid the tragic fate his parents suffered. The truth is that being a doctor who is trained in drugs and surgery does not qualify a person to write such a book. What qualifies a person to write such a book is a passionate desire to know the truth along with a willingness to tirelessly research and write about a particular subject to help people overcome their health challenges. Ty has these qualifications and his work has been endorsed by numerous doctors, researchers, and patients.

In similar fashion to *Cancer – Step Outside the Box*, Ty says, *"the purpose of this book (Work With Your Doctor) is to offer both patients and their primary caregivers a more comprehensive approach to medicine. It is an effort to encourage them to form a 'medical team' and work together to find real solutions."*

Most likely you know at least one person whose life is affected by the diseases covered in this book. Conventional medical approaches to treating these diseases often have devastating results on one's health. There is a better way, and Ty Bollinger and Dr. Michael Farley have provided another tool to empower you (and your doctor) to make better decisions and have better outcomes.

Ultimately, all healing comes from above and is part of the very design of nature; it is the doctor's role to help the body heal itself. This book is a must-have resource for your personal library so you can be armed and ready to overcome any of these health challenges or help a loved one to do so. Great work Ty and Mike! **This one is sure to be another best-seller!**

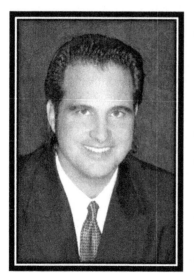

God bless you both and all who read this book!

~ KC Craichy

Founder & CEO
Living Fuel, Inc.
www.livingfuel.com

Author:
The Super Health Diet – The Last Diet You Will Ever Need!

Super Health – Seven Golden Keys to Unlock Lifelong Vitality!

Living the Seven Golden Keys!

PREFACE

Dr. Paul J. LaRochelle, MD

I knew I would be the one asked to write the preface for *Work With Your Doctor To Diagnose and Cure 27 Ailments with Natural and Safe Methods*. I certainly could say it is an honor, privilege, etc, etc, or any other number of superlatives.

In 1989, when I started a medical practice in Melbourne, Florida, I was unaware of any flaws in the medical system. Luckily, my training at McGill and interest in orthopedics allowed me to think "outside the box." I saw an immediate need for a multi-disciplinary approach for complete and proper medical care. I invited naturopaths, massage therapists, anesthesiologists interested in acupuncture, chiropractors, colonic therapists, and doctors who utilized many other unconventional methods to discuss a unified plan of medical care.

It was at one of these meetings that I first met Dr. Michael Farley. The very next week, I sent him an elderly female patient with a wrist fracture that had been treated by another orthopedic doctor who had put on a cast that was too tight and ignored the patients complaints of severe incapacitating pain. Two weeks later when I saw the patient, the cast was obviously too tight, her fingers were swollen, shiny and very painful. I immediately removed the cast which helped with some of her pain, only to find she had developed severe RSD (reflex sympathetic dystrophy). Normally, I would expect that patient would need months of extensive physiotherapy to relieve pain, swelling and to try to recover some range of motion. When I saw her a week later, her skin was normal color, not swollen, minimally tender and she had good motion of her fingers and wrist. Clearly, there was something very different going on here!

From then on, Dr. Farley helped lots of my patients and we became close friends. We continued to work on our circle of care; however, the progress was compromised by a debilitating personal accident which left me unable to work as an orthopedic surgeon. Dr. Farley got me past some of the dark days by asking advice on some of his cases; I now realize he didn't really need my help, but inadvertently was helping me get back on the right path. Over the past twelve years, he has been my mentor, opening my eyes to the powers of natural medicine, and helping me become a "true healer."

At first, I was very angry at other medical doctors and I thought, *"how come they don't get it?"* I bought all new medical school books, but none of what Dr. Farley was teaching me was in the books. I then realized that their ignorance was not their fault and that what they really know is only what they were taught. Many of my MD friends were interested in trying some of the alternative methods I had learned from Dr. Farley, but they were usually forced to stop, being told, *"that's not the standard of care"*, or *"that's not billable"*, and they were discouraged to step out of line.

At the present time, I am satisfied that my comprehensive medical training has prepared me to help any cancer patient and get their immune system back to full force. Recently, I've been involved with four patients with bladder cancers, two of whom also had concurrent prostate cancer. All were in Vietnam and had some exposure to Agent Orange. Fortunately, with a herbal combination in a liposomal base that Dr. Farley developed and by simply following the analysis of their urine, we've seen an elimination of cancer cells in the urine after 3 or 4 weeks. Atypical cells continue to be found after 6 weeks after which the urine is clear. There is no evidence of active cancer; AMAS tests are in normal ranges.

When I started reading this book I couldn't put it down. It was filled with Dr. Farley's knowledge and experience in the herbal side of his medicine combined with the passion and informative information

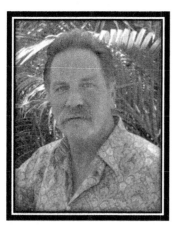

from Ty Bollinger. Dr. Farley and I have always felt frustrated that we are only able to help one person at a time. This is why the book, *Work With Your Doctor*, is so important. If we can teach other doctors so that they can become true healers, then Dr. Farley and Ty Bollinger have accomplished their goal. This book is destined to become another best-seller and change the lives of thousands of people across the globe.

~ Dr. Paul J. LaRochelle, MD

Introduction

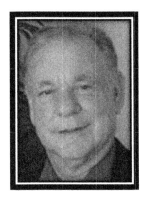 After over 30 years of practicing medicine and solving mysteries in forensic pathology, I have learned one thing. The only certain and complete truth I have found in medicine is that we need to be open to constantly learning and even if we are, we will still never know everything. I have also been blessed with a practice that allowed me the freedom to put 3 to 4 hours a day in research to try to continue learning.

I was fortunate to have been taught to always look for **cause** and not just to treat **symptoms**. This has held true from forensics to naturopathy and oriental medicine. I believe that this is the biggest difference between pharmaceutically based medicine and comprehensive medicine; we look for and treat cause and don't just treat symptoms with pharmaceuticals. Don't get me wrong, there is definitely a place for pharmaceuticals and surgery, but when they are not combined with a comprehensive approach aimed at deducing and treating the cause, then they will be less than effective and might result in deadly side effects.

The purpose of this book is to offer both patients and their primary caregivers a more comprehensive approach to medicine. It is an effort to encourage them to form a "medical team" and work together to find real solutions. This first book on the subject cannot possibly expound on all of the diseases which need to be addressed. It is my hope that learning to look at disease from a different perspective (comprehensively) will offer both physicians and patients a more holistic approach and will result in alleviating symptoms and potentially the ailment itself. At the very least, treating the cause, suggesting appropriate testing, and utilizing more non-toxic treatments may be helpful in both prolonging life and increasing the quality of life.

This book contains advice on herbal medicines as well as other supplementation for specific ailments. There are also suggested tests which may have never previously been done. It is strongly suggested that you work closely with your primary caregiver in order to benefit the most from this information. I cannot tell you how many times I have heard the words, *"my doctor doesn't listen to me,"* or *"he/she doesn't spend enough time with me."*

My answer has always been the same: in the real world of a physician's life, most have been forced into large physician groups and have to see a very large number of patients in order to meet the requirements of the group. The tests they are "allowed" to run are often the least expensive and also often offer the least usable information which is easily misinterpreted. Try to find an independent physician, or if you like the physician you are with, speak with them and ask point blank if they are willing to take the time to work with you and perhaps run a few other tests. Give them the reasons for these tests and see if they are willing to do a little extra reading. If they are willing, then stay with them. If they are not, then be brave enough to look for a physician that is willing to work with you.

Also accept the fact that, in some cases, you may have to pay for some testing and supplementation yourself if the tests and supplements are not covered by insurance. In this book, I have chosen to put your health first and ask you to accept the responsibility for doing what must be done to maximize your own health and recovery. After all, it is your life, and you are the ultimate arbiter for this most important responsibility.

Perhaps, at this point, an example of what I am discussing will help clarify the purpose of writing this book. Let's start with a very prominent problem in the USA: high blood pressure ("hypertension"). The normal treatment for hypertension (from a strictly pharmaceutical mindset) is the use of a drug to lower the blood pressure and most likely a cholesterol lowering drug as well. You will be instructed to stop smoking (if you smoke) and to eat a low fat diet and perhaps lose some weight.

In contrast to the pharmaceutical model, I will briefly present a more comprehensive approach. I always try to include studies with any recommendations that I make so forgive the extra reading. Many times physicians will require studies to verify that an alternative to pharmaceuticals is warranted or desired. If you choose, you may skip them, but I would suggest you read them to better understand both how they work and what we are trying to accomplish.

Obviously the initial problem of hypertension needs to be addressed. High blood pressure can lead to heart attacks, strokes, and other problems. The usual list of prescription drugs includes beta-blockers, calcium channel blockers, alpha-blockers, and angiotensin-converting-enzyme (ACE) inhibitors, each of which has a long list of side effects.

My personal preference for lowering blood pressure is simply a cup of hibiscus tea 1 or 2 times a day; a small bit of honey makes it a very wonderful and refreshing tea. It is healthier if you like it without the honey, but it is a bit tart, and it should be made from organic, fresh dried hibiscus flowers.

Hibiscus acts as an ACE inhibitor, and thanks to the synergy and how it performs its actions, it is much less likely (than prescription drugs) to have any detrimental side effects. It is not immediately acting and may take up to two weeks to have full effect. The higher the blood pressure the faster it seems to work. It also seems to work for the majority of people by lowering systolic pressure, diastolic pressure, and then heart rate, in that order. Hibiscus also has another benefit: it is effective and very safe at lowering cholesterol. We will get into cholesterol more deeply, and there is great debate on whether lowering cholesterol is actually beneficial. Using hibiscus is advantageous because it does not cause large (potentially harmful) drops in cholesterol, but will lower it if it is exceedingly high. (See hibiscus research on pages 245 and 246.)

And now we need to address the **cause** of the problem. Everyone has heard of hypertension and atherosclerosis (hardening of the arteries), and we've all been told by the pharmaceutical companies that this is due to high cholesterol. We are prescribed medications to lower this terrible substance and preserve our lives. But unfortunately, this is not at all factual. The real problem lies in the health of the endothelium (inner lining) of the arterial and venous walls. While it is true that cholesterol will adhere to tears or damage to the endothelial lining, it is not the cause of these lesions. In actuality, insulin causes lesions in the endothelium, so sugar (which causes insulin to be secreted) is the true culprit. The more sugar we consume, the more insulin we secrete. The more insulin we secrete, the more lesions in the endothelium we create. The more lesions we create, the more cholesterol will adhere to these lesions. If we removed all of the cholesterol from our bodies we would lose many things that we require, starting with the brain (which is made of cholesterol), hormones (which are made from cholesterol), and a functioning immune system.

Insulin also causes us to store fat, so it is completely logical that obese people have a higher incidence of heart disease. Perhaps if we dealt with medical problems honestly, rather than watching and believing complete fiction (relating to sugar and drugs) on television, we would make true progress in our health.

We will go into much more detail on treatment options for atherosclerosis later in this book, but for now, you have a brief idea of the reasons for this book and how important it is to have honest discussions with your personal primary caregiver. **Seek one that is willing to listen and work with you.**

~ Dr. Michael Farley, N.M.D.

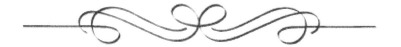

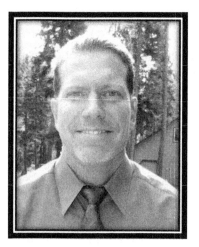

Congratulations! By reading this book, you are taking the first step toward obtaining better health. This book will open up a new world of health options and treatment protocols for whatever may be ailing you. Truth be told, this book holds the key to your future good health. However, the key doesn't do you any good unless you stick it into the keyhole in the door. In the same manner, you must also put this information to use in order to reap the benefits.

Much of this book deals with naturopathy, which Native Americans have been using for hundreds (if not thousands) of years. The word "naturopathy" comes from Greek and Latin and literally means *"nature disease."* A central belief in naturopathy is that nature has a healing power (a principle called vis *"medicatrix naturae"*). Another belief is that living organisms (including the human body) have the power to maintain (or return to) a state of balance and health and to heal themselves. Naturopaths prefer to use treatments which are the most natural and least invasive, rather than using drugs and more invasive procedures. Other key principles are "first do no harm," treat the whole person, find the cause (rather than treat the symptom), and prevention is the best cure.

Conventional ("Western") medicine is only about 200 years old and is founded on the philosophical beliefs of René Descartes (who believed the body and mind are separate) and on Sir Isaac Newton's principles of physics (which consider the universe to be a large mechanical clock where everything operates in sequential form). This machine-like perspective of medicine views the human body as a series of body parts, much like a clock. Health is considered to be the absence of disease … in other words, nothing broken at the present time. The focus of modern "sickness care" is on the symptoms of dysfunction. Doctors are trained to fix or repair broken parts through the use of drugs, radiation, surgery, or replacement of body parts.

Because conventional medicine is preoccupied with parts and symptoms and not with the entire body (and spirit) working as a whole, it typically doesn't do well with long-term systemic illnesses such as arthritis, heart disease, and hypertension. Even Hippocrates, the "father of Western medicine," espoused a holistic orientation when he taught doctors to observe their patients' life circumstances and emotional states. Socrates agreed, declaring, "Curing the soul; that is the first thing."

But this is not to say that I'm opposed to Western medicine. The fact is that Western medicine has made astonishing advances in the past two centuries. Trauma doctors regularly reattach severed limbs and successfully treat gunshot wounds, and remarkable advances have been made in countering acute problems. However, as these acute illnesses and injuries become less prevalent and life-threatening, more chronic problems (like diabetes, heart disease, and cancer) are emerging.

When Einstein introduced his theory of relativity in 1905, our way of viewing the universe changed dramatically. Einstein said that all matter is energy, energy and matter are interchangeable, and all matter is connected at the subatomic level. No single entity could be affected without all connecting parts being affected. In a very real sense, this is the proper way to view health and the human body.

I remember the egg scare a few years ago, do you? Well-orchestrated efforts convinced this entire country that eggs were the worst food ever consumed by man. It was part of a scheme by pharmaceutical companies to wage war against cholesterol. Quite conveniently, the "war on cholesterol" just happened to coincide with the development of a new class of drugs (statins) designed to lower cholesterol levels. These statin drugs have been a huge boom, generating billions of dollars of profit. You see, cholesterol has been demonized and, as a consequence, Americans have become conditioned to avoid all foods containing cholesterol.

This is a grave mistake. It's terrible to watch someone crack open an egg and toss out the yolk because it contains "too much" cholesterol. Truth be told, the yolk contains all the important nutrients. After all, the yolk is what allows the chick embryo to mature into a chicken. Cholesterol is not a health threat. It is a substance that is **essential to life** and it plays a role in the most critical body functions, including brain cell connection formation, cell integrity, muscle and tendon strength, bile and digestion, vitamin A and D metabolism, protection against infectious organisms, essential fatty acid metabolism, and the manufacture of hormones which regulate the blood levels of salt, water and calcium, and other critical metabolic processes.

Statin drugs have also been implicated in Alzheimer's Disease, cardio-myopathy, and since they target cholesterol, they actually "eat" the brain (the brain is made of cholesterol). Nobody has **ever** shown that elevated cholesterol is the **cause** of heart disease. But many doctors still regularly prescribe these dangerous drugs, while at the same time proclaiming that we should beware of herbs! Many will cite ephedrine to prove their point. If you remember, there was the "ephedrine" scare back in the early 1990s when "everyone" who used this herb was dying of heart attacks, right?

First of all, let me set a few facts straight. *Ephedra sinica* is an herb that contains small quantities of the drug ephedrine. It also contains small quantities of the drug pseudoephedrine (better known by its brand name Sudafed). I'm sure that most Americans have taken pseudoephedrine products for cold and flu symptoms. But the culprit in the "ephedrine scare" was not the *Ephedra sinica*. As a matter of fact, **all** of the offending diet or energy products contained "ephedra **extract**" or "ma huang **extract**" (the Chinese name for ephedra). This extract is essentially purified ephedrine, which is a strong stimulant that can increase heart rate, blood pressure, anxiety and sleeplessness.

The great misconception is that people are really **not** taking an "herb," but a **drug** that is extracted from an herb. The herb ephedra contains hundreds of other chemicals besides ephedrine and pseudoephedrine. One of these chemicals is known to slow down the absorption of ephedrine so that an individual will not get the high blood levels of the drug that can cause these ill effects.

Many other drugs that we use every day are extracted from herbs but are not called by their herbal name. For instance, digoxin is one of the top ten most prescribed drugs, used for heart ailments, but it is not called "purple foxglove" (the herb from which it comes). Codeine and morphine are not called "poppy" or "poppy extract." The drug tamoxifen (used to treat breast cancer) is not called "American yew."

The reason I make this point is because the whole ephedrine issue puts the use of herbs in a bad light. It gives fuel to individuals and groups who decry the use of herbs as "dangerous." What better example is there but that of the dangerous herb ephedra! I have an idea… let's call a drug a drug and an herb an herb. Drugs are dangerous, and herbs are **not**.

According to the information gathered by acclaimed researcher and scientist James Duke, PhD (former head of the USDA botanical division, author of numerous best-selling books on herbal medicine), the statistics on deaths caused by herbs compared with other causes are quite revealing:

- ❖ Herbs: 1 in 1 million
- ❖ Supplements: 1 in 1 million
- ❖ Non-steroidal anti-inflammatories (ibuprofen, acetaminophen, Aleve, etc.): 1 in 10,000
- ❖ Hospital surgery: 1 in 10,000
- ❖ Improper use of drugs: 1 in 2,000
- ❖ Angiogram: 1 in 1,000
- ❖ Alcohol: 1 in 500
- ❖ Cigarettes: 1 in 500
- ❖ Hospital caused infections: 1 in 80
- ❖ Bypass surgery: 1 in 20

Source: http://www.ars-grin.gov/duke/syllabus/module15.htm

Reading this report makes it very clear that, by comparison, the chance of being killed by herbs is pretty small. In fact, you would probably have to be pretty unlucky to kill or harm yourself with herbs, though it is not impossible. As a matter of fact, statistics from the U.S. National Poison Data System support this assertion in their 2010 annual report which showed **zero** deaths from herbs for the entire year of 2010. www.poison.org/stats/2010%20NPDS%20Annual%20Report.pdf

So my question is this: *"If herbs are allegedly as 'dangerous' as the FDA and news media claim they are, then where are the bodies?"*

The purpose of this book is to provide the reader (and his/her physician) with necessary information to develop a comprehensive approach to treat and cure over two dozen diseases and ailment. The book is divided into 3 parts: 1) "The History & The Basics," 2) "The Treatments," and 3) "For Your Doctor." Parts 1 and 2 are written in layman's terms, but part 3 contains peer-reviewed studies on each and every treatment recommended in part 2. This is for you to share with your doctor, with the goal of becoming a "team" and working together.

Remember that you must take responsibility for your own health. This means you must take the time to learn to listen to your own body, find good sources of information, and check with your physician before you change or stop any prescription medicines you are taking. Make sure that all your primary caregivers know exactly what you are doing.

~ Ty M. Bollinger

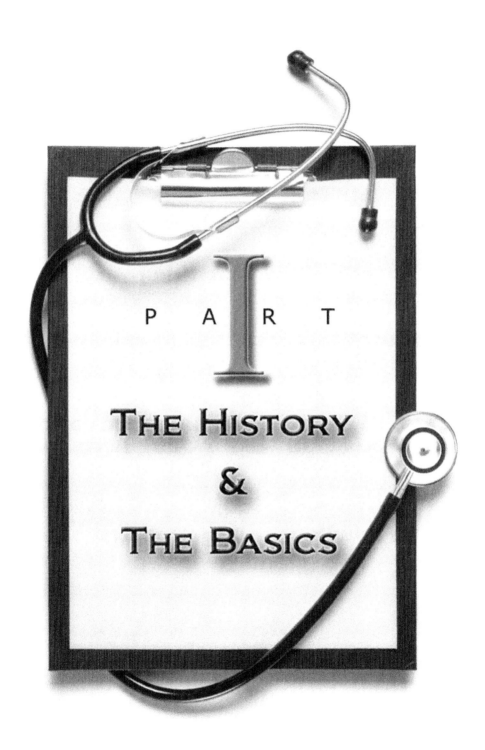

PART

I

THE HISTORY

&

THE BASICS

THE HISTORY OF MEDICINE:

100 AD: "Here, eat this root."

1680: "That root is heathen and sinful. Here, drink this tonic."

1945: "That tonic is dangerous and ineffective. Take this drug instead."

2012: "Those drugs are over-prescribed and ineffective. Here, eat this root."

HISTORY OF THE AMA

In order to understand the current state of affairs of medical practice in the USA, it's vital to understand exactly how we got here. So, let's put on our history caps and go all the way back over 100 years to the turn of the 20th century.

When Dr. George H. Simmons began in 1899 what became a 25 year reign as head of the American Medical Association (AMA), it was a weak organization with little money and little respect from the general public. The advertising revenue from its medical journal, the Journal of the American Medical Association (*JAMA*), was a paltry $34,000 per year. The AMA realized that competition was causing physicians' incomes to dwindle, as the number of medical schools had increased from around 90 (in 1880) to over 150 (in 1903). Chiropractic had just been introduced into the mainstream, homeopathy was thriving, herbalists were flourishing, all the while regular doctors were unable to profit from their medical practices.

With the state governments reluctant to create laws restricting the various healing arts, Simmons hired Joseph McCormack (the secretary of the Kentucky State Board of health) to "rouse the profession to lobby." With McCormack leading the charge, the AMA began to bolster their ranks, preaching ethics (like not competing with other physicians or publishing your prices) and decrying "quackery" (anything that competed with regular medicine).

Simmons was shrewd enough to have the AMA establish a *Council on Medical Education* in 1904. This council's stated mission was to "upgrade medical education" – a noble goal. However, the *Council on Medical Education* had actually devised a plan to rank medical schools throughout the country, but their guidelines were dubious, to say the least. For instance, just having the word "homeopathic" in the name of a medical school reduced their ranking because the AMA asserted that such schools taught "an exclusive dogma."

However, by 1910, the AMA was out of money and didn't have the funds to complete the project. The Rockefellers had joined forces with the Carnegie foundation to create an education fund, and they were approached by N. P. Colwell (secretary of the *Council on Medical*

Education) to finish the job they had started, but could no longer fund. Rockefeller and Carnegie agreed.

Simon Flexner, who was on the Board of Directors for the Rockefeller Institute, proposed that his brother, Abraham, who knew nothing about medicine, be hired for the project. Although their names are not very well known, the Flexner brothers have probably influenced the lives of more people and in a more profound way than any other brothers in the last century, with the possible exception of Wilbur and Orville Wright.

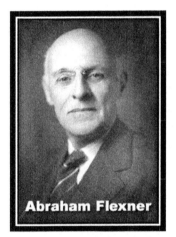

Abraham Flexner

Abraham Flexner was on the staff of the Carnegie Foundation for the Advancement of Teaching. The Rockefellers and Carnegies had traditionally worked together in the furtherance of their mutual goals, and this certainly was no exception. The Flexner brothers represented the lens that brought both the Rockefeller and the Carnegie fortunes into sharp focus on the medical profession.

Their plan was to "restructure" the AMA and "certify" medical schools based solely upon Abraham Flexner's recommendations. The AMA's head of the *Council on Medical Education* traveled with Flexner as they evaluated medical schools. Eventually, Flexner submitted a report to The Carnegie Foundation entitled "Medical Education in the United States and Canada," which is also known as the "Flexner report." Not surprisingly, the gist of the report was that it was far too easy to start a medical school and that most medical schools were not teaching "sound medicine."

The medical sociologist Paul Starr wrote in his Pulitzer Prize-winning book (The Social Transformation of American Medicine): "*The AMA Council became a national accrediting agency for medical schools, as an increasing number of states adopted its judgments of unacceptable institutions.*" Further, he noted: "*Even though no legislative body ever set up ... the AMA Council on Medical Education, their decisions came to have the force of law.*" With the AMA grading the various medical colleges, it became predictable that the homeopathic colleges, even the large and respected ones, would eventually be forced to stop teaching homeopathy or die. And that's exactly what happened.

Published in 1910, the Flexner report (quite correctly) pointed out the inadequacies of medical education at the time. No one could take exception with that. It also proposed a wide range of sweeping changes, most of which were entirely sound. No one could take exception with those, either. However, Flexner's recommendations emphatically included the strengthening of courses in pharmacology and the addition of research departments at all "qualified" medical schools.

It is what followed in the wake of the Flexner report that reveals its true purpose in the total plan. With public backing secured by the publication of the Flexner report, Carnegie and Rockefeller commenced a major upgrade in medical education by financing only those medical schools that taught what they wanted taught. In other words, they began to immediately shower hundreds of millions of dollars on those medical schools that were teaching "drug intensive" medicine.

Predictably, those schools that had the financing churned out the better doctors. In return for the financing, the schools were required to continue teaching course material that was exclusively drug oriented, with no emphasis put on natural medicine. The end result of the Flexner report was that all accredited medical schools became heavily oriented toward drugs and drug research. In 1913, Simmons and the AMA went on the offensive even more strongly by their establishment of the "Propaganda Department," which was dedicated to attacking any and all unconventional medical treatments and anyone (MD or not) who practiced them.

The purpose was to dominate the oil and chemical (pharmaceutical) markets, and the Flexner report gave both of these tycoons the "ammunition" they needed to achieve that goal. In the end, the Rockefeller/Carnegie plan was a smashing success. Those medical schools that did not conform were denied the funds and the prestige that came with those funds, and were forced out of business.

By 1925, over 10,000 herbalists were out of business. By 1940, 1500 chiropractors would be prosecuted for practicing "quackery." The 22 homeopathic medical schools that flourished in 1900 dwindled to just 2 in 1923. By 1950, all schools teaching homeopathy were closed. In the end, if a physician did not graduate from a Flexner approved medical school, he couldn't find a job.

This is why today our doctors are so heavily biased toward synthetic drug therapy and know little about nutrition.

Before you dismiss this section of the book, please understand that it is currently standard practice in the USA to simply dismiss any piece of information that punches a hole in any widely accepted explanation of a disturbing event by tagging the new explanation as a "conspiracy theory." It's time to put an end to this name-calling nonsense once and for all. It is absolutely accurate to say that conspiracies exist all around us every day of our lives and in all walks of life.

As a matter of fact, conspiracies are a very common part of life. Children conspire to play jokes on their friends, football teams conspire (in the huddle) to outmaneuver their opponents; the rich conspire with one another to get richer; governments conspire about virtually everything. As a matter of fact every single person who has ever been convicted of a crime by a jury is the subject of a conspiracy theory; only in these cases a jury has accepted the theory as truth after seeing the evidence. The fact is that any time two or more people are involved in setting private plans to do anything, you have a conspiracy. And as research has revealed, the Flexner report of 1910 was the beginning of a conspiracy to limit and eventually eliminate competition from non-pharmaceutical, non-patentable treatments for disease.

During the infamous Spanish flu epidemic of 1918-19, it has been estimated that 25 to 50 million people died worldwide. In the USA alone, 550,000 people died, which was approximately 10% of the people afflicted with the flu. Homeopathic physicians documented then more than 62,000 patients treated with homeopathy resulting in a mortality of 0.7%. For people who were sick enough to be hospitalized, conventional medicine had a mortality of 30% while with 27,000 documented hospitalized cases, homeopathy was reporting a mortality of 1.05% (*Journal of the American Institute of Homeopathy* 1921; 13:1028-43).

So, in light of the fact that the homeopathic success rate was many fold higher than the allopathic success rate, it is crystal clear that there must have been ulterior motives for closing the homeopathic hospitals, which were actually far superior than the allopathic hospitals in the treatment of the Spanish flu. This is the "icing" on the conspiracy cake.

THE STATE OF THE NATION

Due to the nature of this book, I would like to preface it with a few personal feelings and a few facts from the very reliable sources shown below.

American medicine has a great number of wonderful physicians that actually became doctors to help people. These physicians maintained their commitment in spite of medical school and have persevered through unwarranted regulations placed upon them, the constant fear of having their licenses revoked, the fear of being sued for malpractice, and large medical groups they are forced to work in. This takes an enormous amount of courage. These are the best and brightest in American medicine. They exist, and are usually low-key and very patient oriented. They spend countless hours searching literature in order to be as proficient at their craft as possible. These are the primary caregivers that are most needed and in the smallest numbers, so they must be sought out. Ask friends, ask nurses, and ask other physicians to whom they would go if they were sick. These are the doctors that will be willing to work with you and take the time to learn more of your problem and be willing to move you forward (rather than hold you back). When I (Dr. Farley) retired, my wife looked at an appointment book from the previous year, and about 70% of our clients were physicians and their families. I take that as the highest compliment I could receive.

I have been repeatedly asked why I use so few USA research abstracts. The reason is very simple: the USA is not doing the best research anymore. The current state of medical care in the USA is terrible. **The last time the World Health Organization ranked countries, the USA ranked 37th overall in total healthcare.**

The United States is ranked 50th in longevity, among all other countries. In medical care we are ranked 17th out of 17 countries with comparable lifestyles. By comparison, Canada is ranked fourth in the same medical evaluation.

The term **iatrogenic** is defined as *"induced in a patient by a physician's activity, manner, or therapy."* Iatrogenic deaths have become the third leading medical cause of death in the USA, being beaten only by cancer and cardiovascular causes. Amazingly, this ranking doesn't even take into consideration hospital deaths or delayed drug side effect deaths that occur at home or away from the hospital.

According to the most recent report, there were 783,936 iatrogenic deaths last year. ["Death By Medicine," Gary Null, PhD; Carolyn Dean MD, ND; Martin Feldman, MD; Debora Rasio, MD; and Dorothy Smith, PhD].

Below is a screenshot from the FDA's own website. Notice that it acknowledges 100,000 annual deaths due to adverse drug reactions (ADRs) and over two million serious ADRs per year. Also admitted by the FDA is that ADRs are the *"4th leading cause of death ahead of pulmonary disease, diabetes, AIDS, pneumonia, accidents and automobile deaths."*

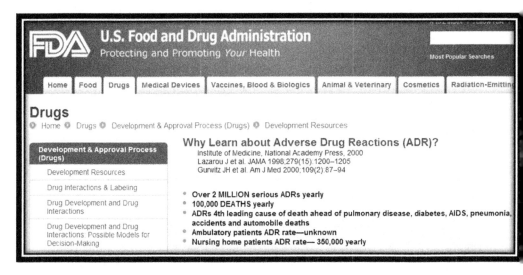

Just look at a short list of "celebrity" deaths from legal, prescription drugs: Whitney Houston, Marilyn Monroe, Elvis Presley, Kurt Cobain, Anna Nicole Smith, Chris Farley, John Belushi, Heath Ledger, and Michael Jackson. This is not an exhaustive list of celebrity deaths, of course, and some of these cases are still disputed as to the actual causes of death. When celebrities with **no lack of money or resources** fall victim, it should trigger a "red flag" and should make us question the current paradigm. **One thing is for sure:** FDA-approved prescription drugs, many of which are highly-addictive, are a primary cause of mortality in America today, and yet they continue to flood the market unabated.

Almost everyone who is aware of the "iatrogenic" problem blames the pharmaceutical companies, which is undoubtedly a legitimate claim. Due to the developed reliance on pharmaceutical research in medical schools, with the pharmaceutical company having the right to publish the findings as it interprets them, USA medical research is most definitely "tainted." Students are taught to memorize, not reason. The drug, they are taught, is always the accepted answer, regardless of the logical consequences.

Primary caregivers are in a constant quandary. They lose their license to practice or are fined (or perhaps both) if they use anything that is not FDA approved. Yet they are aware that the FDA has no credibility. When pharmaceutical representatives comprise a majority of the FDA's board and so many drugs are recalled due to causing thousands of deaths, how can they have any credibility? Yet the dilemma continues, and in all too many cases, the caregiver's hands are tied.

The system is broken. The FDA cannot be sued. Doctors have to follow their instructions or face retribution and the loss of their livelihood. And now you, the patient, must seek out the brave few that have insisted on a meaningful continuing education. These primary caregivers will probably work on a fee for service basis. In other words, they often will not accept insurance, but will insist on payment for services rendered. Whether or not Obama health care comes to full fruition, it is very wise to put money aside to have the freedom to afford healthcare from an independent physician.

You must also realize supplements, regardless of how effective they have been proven to be, will have to be paid for by you personally. You and your physician will want to make your health testing and desired care a series of personal decisions – they are far too important for paid government "appointees" or the FDA to make. If at all financially possible in these difficult times, begin a personal health insurance program, putting a small amount aside each week and leave it alone. In a short time you will have enough to at least get on the right track towards health.

I was a fee for service caregiver for almost 30 years. I remember doing, or more correctly, watching my wife (also my P.A.) do the paperwork. I quickly decided she was much more needed by patients than spending time doing paperwork. I can also honestly say that for three decades, we never turned anyone away that could not pay. We always found a way to barter so the patient placed value on the service and never felt they were taking advantage of us.

I will always remember a lung cancer patient that was carried into our office by his son. The first thing his son told us was that his father had lost everything paying for his 20% co-pay for chemotherapy. The next week, his father (the patient) was able to walk into our office, and within 6 weeks he was mowing his lawn. For many months he met our patients that were coming in from out of town at the airport. He would give them a tour of the city, suggest motels and bring them to our office. He felt wonderful about being useful again, repaying his debt, and just appreciating each and every day. We were all winners.

ALLOPATHIC VS. NATURAL MEDICINE

In the USA, the current leaning of medicine is in the treatment of diseases, **not** in the prevention of them. Patients who are suffering from chronic pain or debilitating long term illnesses are aware that "conventional" medicine does not have all the answers. In the search for alternatives to their treatment they often ask their physician (or primary caregiver) for advice on the use and efficacy of natural medicine. These patients are frustrated with their current condition and/or their lack of a speedy recovery. They often blame their doctor and feel betrayed by the existing medical structure. In all probability, the doctor is suffering from the same frustrations, including the patient's lack of recovery and his own inability to help.

Rest assured, it is **not** your doctor's fault. When asked about natural medicine (by the rare patient who has the courage to ask), the most often heard response is, "I'm not sure if that stuff is any good" or something along those lines. Patients are often discouraged from using herbals, and indeed, sometimes even vitamin and mineral supplements. The fault lies not in the doctor, but in his training.

The modern medical industry is built on the foundation of treating the symptoms of disease, while doing virtually nothing to treat the actual cause of the disease or prevent it. It reminds me of an old Chinese proverb: "*The superior doctor prevents sickness; the mediocre doctor attends to impending sickness; the inferior doctor treats actual sickness.*" However, the problem is not the doctors…**it is the system.**

The truth of the matter is that most physicians care and truly want to assist their patients in recovering from illness or pain. However, doctors work with the tools they learned in medical school. Unfortunately, medical schools are structured in a way that memorization takes the front seat while deductive reasoning falls far behind. This is due to the vast amount of data that has to be assimilated. The patient and physician both feel frustrated by the resulting medicinal approach, often referred to as "cookbook" medicine. This type of medicine is when you (the patient) describe the symptoms, the doctor recognizes those symptoms and then proceeds to prescribe the medicine and/or protocols he was taught. The reason this is dubbed "cookbook medicine" is because fewer and fewer doctors touch their patients; their hands are taking the back seat to their prescription book.

In order for students to graduate and become MD's they have no choice but to learn what has become the AMA's "medicine of today." The leaning of current medical schools is obvious when we look at a few facts. There are approximately 125 medical schools in the United States. Of those 125 schools, only 30 of them require a course in nutrition. During four years of medical school, the average training in nutrition received by U.S. physicians is 2.5 hours. When you consider the fact that the risk of death from a heart attack for the average American male is 50%, while the risk of death from a heart attack for an average American, vegetarian, male is 4%, the need for nutritional counseling for physicians is obvious. While vegetarians are not necessarily the healthiest people, this is most definitely a telling statistic.

In the USA, medical treatment has become synonymous with prescription drugs, largely due to the influence of the tremendous sales forces and political influence of the pharmaceutical industry. Also, let's not forget the fact that in this day and age people want instant health. They want and expect to be made well (or better) immediately.

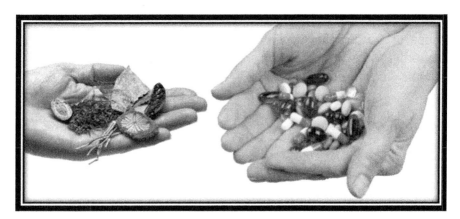

The advantages of conventional or synthetic pharmaceuticals over natural medicines, lies in the fact that they are more concentrated in specific properties which at times causes them to work faster. Another advantage for synthetic or conventional medications is that they are very consistent in concentrations and dosages, more so than many herbal companies who are quick to take advantage of an extremely fast growing market. While discussing the efficacy of drugs, it would be tremendously one-sided not to mention that there are synthetics in use today for which no herbal equivalent has yet been found.

Having said this, we will now list the advantages of herbal remedies. Herbs always contain many active constituents which often act synergistically with each other to enhance their effect. When taken in an educated manner, herbals have virtually no side effects as compared to synthetic medications. In fact, herbs tend to enhance body systems rather than deplete them. For example, the daily use of echinacea to enhance the immune system will not destroy the natural flora of the digestive tract. It will aid in fighting both viral and bacterial infections without leaving women prone to vaginal yeast infections. Unlike antibiotics, which are synthetic, the herb does not invite the development of antibiotic resistant bacteria. Herbs provide precursors for needed hormones and enzymes as well as furnish vital minerals and vitamins for the body to use. There is no question that herbs have a large place in the health care of society today.

More importantly, unlike "cookbook" medicine where doctors learn the symptoms of a patient then prescribe a drug, herbal medicine requires a more complex approach. Herbalists must know of any herbal interactions and which herbs are required to produce the desired effect. They adjust combinations to deal with several aspects of a disease process at once and treat the whole body not just a symptom. This requires not only education, but what some herbalists have dubbed a "dousing" instinct. This necessitates an intimate knowledge of plants and their products as well as a "feel" for the patient. Due to the amount of time this takes, you'll find very few herbalists or doctors of naturopathy who are able to see a new patient every fifteen minutes.

Plant and mineral-based medicines have been preventing, treating and curing disease and illnesses since mankind has been making calendars. Yet, Western Medicine would have the masses believe that because a few vaccines and some surgical procedures came along in the mid-to-late 1900's, that now only allopathic doctors should be wholly trusted with health and medicine advice, when in fact, it's just the other way around.

Staying Masculine In The Modern World

Masculinity has been going through rapid change. What it will become, we have yet to find out.

Both men and women need testosterone, estrogen, growth hormone, and many other biochemical's in different amounts, and at different times in their lives. It is a difficult and challenging time for testosterone, a hormone which is actually present in both men and women (at about one-tenth the amount as men). Testosterone has developed a very bad reputation because of overuse in sports (such as baseball, football, and even professional bicycling) and is now considered something that should be avoided at all costs. Lets take a look at some things that hurt masculinity and male hormonal health.

The effects of testosterone include greater muscle repair, anti-depression, cardiovascular benefits, and many types of repair functions that we don't want to lose, even if we are not in a relationship or otherwise sexually active. The erection power alone also requires growth hormone, estrogen, HCG, good muscle tone, good circulation, a balanced nervous system, and an available imagination. All of these can decline as we age.

It needs to be understood that hormones work as a team that maintains a balance between our brain and our body. Hormones are what turn our thoughts into body chemistry. These are the biochemical's that, to a large extent, shape our lives and control our health and happiness. When we are thinking thoughts that excite us, invigorate us, scare us, or make us sad, or happy, it is our hormones that take these thoughts and tell our bodies to produce the appropriate response, be it adrenalin, tears, an erection, or nervous sweat.

Testosterone levels in humans are in steep decline in our society due to many reasons. Both men and women need testosterone for libido, healthy hearts, and muscle tone. A common age-related decline in testosterone is to be expected once we pass through our late twenties or early thirties and will continue to fall until we meet our demise. Low levels of testosterone are undesirable for both men and women because they are associated with heart and artery diseases, cancers, chronic fatigue, depression, loss of libido, osteoporosis, lower immunity, and even death.

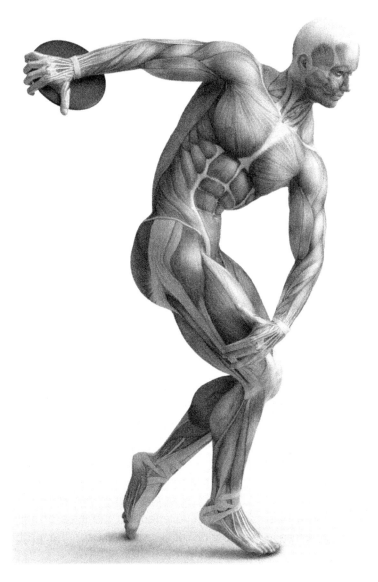

The manner in which we use hormones gets very complex; your brain (along with the pituitary gland and hypothalamus gland) monitors your hormone levels. It uses positive and negative feedback from blood levels to do this and these hormone activities are extremely complex and involve the use of many enzymes that are produced in your body.

These enzymes can be thought of as regulators and are what we use to control the balance of our hormones by activating, producing, suppressing, eliminating, or transforming our hormones.

It is the enzyme called aromatase that works in the production of estrogen and acts by catalyzing the conversion of testosterone (an androgen) to estradiol (an estrogen), which will "turn off" some of the testosterone effects, sometimes at a very unwelcome moment like when a man is with his loved one.

Testosterone levels decline along with their health benefits and resulting masculine behavior as a result of many household chemicals and environmental toxins from pesticides, plastics, and drugs which have demonstrated partial estrogen and/or anti-testosterone effects. The use of growth hormone and estrogen to make the chicken and beef we eat grow faster and more tender (and for dairy cows to produce greater amounts of milk) all add to an ever increasing amount of estrogen in our systems. They are now using hormones to increase the yield of vegetables and fruits and they are feeding us biologically engineered food in just about all the food groups. All of this is changing mankind, because of enormous amounts of estrogen now in our lives young girls are starting menstrual cycles as early as the age of 7 and developing breasts as early as 5 and 6 years of age.

For men, this has been completely de-masculating. Combine all of this added estrogen that we are now exposed to with the increased activity of the enzyme aromatase, which is killing off what testosterone we are still able to produce, and is it any surprise that men are now developing breast cancer and erectile dysfunction (which now affects 1 in 3 men)? Any other ailment that affected 1 out of 3 men would be called an epidemic, but this is rarely talked about, other than to push drugs like Viagra at us, which is one of the most sold drugs worldwide. We are aware that Viagra has had a positive effect on the lives of millions of people, but is it really necessary? It is not a fix for the problem; it merely eliminates the symptom for a few hours.

This is exactly how the pharmaceutical companies are treating other symptoms of low testosterone, depression and anxiety, in both men and women. How many of you are taking antidepressants? The pharmaceutical companies manipulate both of these symptoms into multi-billion dollar a year sales by not treating the actual problems but by temporally controlling the current symptoms. This keeps everyone coming back for more, with no end in sight.

Developing a reliance on these products is not necessary; it is possible to eliminate both of these problems by restoring the body to the proper hormonal levels that existed prior to the development of these symptoms.

Some common factors that raise levels of estrogens in men's bodies are age, a zinc deficiency, obesity, carbohydrate intolerance, insulin sensitivity, overuse of alcohol, changes in liver function, and side effects from prescription drugs.

Aromatase is most concentrated in the estrogen-producing cells in the adrenal glands, ovaries, placenta, testicles, adipose (fat) tissue, and brain. Some men have a lot of aromatase, while others have much less. Fat cells contribute a great amount of aromatase, and many nutrient deficiencies can also produce higher levels. Supreme B will help with nutritional deficiencies. Things that inhibit aromatase will preserve and stimulate more testosterone activity; this is the function of a product called De Aromatase. Learn more about both of these products at www.healthpro.dm.com.

Adequate testosterone is required by so many healthy functions that this decline in hormone levels is literally killing people before their time. More and more men and women are losing their quality of life to depression, immunity problems, fatigue, and apathy caused by inadequate levels of testosterone. Hormonal balance will affect your quality of life for as long as you live.

For men in today's modern world the challenge of holding on to their masculinity is a daunting one. We are living in a time where just about everything that you come into contact with will either lower your body's production of testosterone or increase your body's production of the enzyme aromatase, which in turn converts some of what testosterone you do have into estrogen. One must be proactive in combating this "estrogen invasion" because things are only going to get worse.

THE TRUTH ABOUT CHOLESTEROL

Ask any American what causes heart disease, and 99% of the time the answer will be "high cholesterol." You see, cholesterol has been vilified and is now regarded as a "scary scary" substance that must be lowered at all costs. However, if you speak with gerontologists that specialize in elderly medicine, you will quickly find that almost all of the most elderly patients have "high" cholesterol levels (according to the supposedly "normal" standards). But these patients are still alive and many of them are in very good health and are very active for their age.

CHOLESTEROL MYTHS:

High-fat foods and cholesterol cause atherosclerosis leading to the obstruction of blood vessels in the heart.

Lowering your cholesterol will lengthen your life

Polyunsatured oils are good for your health

All scientists and doctors support the idea that high cholesterol causes heart disease

Statin drugs are essential in controlling cholesterol levels and preventing heart disease

Believing all of these cholesterol myths, Americans decreased their intake of good fats and oils (like coconut oil, fish oil, olive oil) and started consuming more vegetable oils and margarine (a trans fat). This diet has **caused** thousands of deaths from heart disease, as have the statin drugs which supposedly prevent heart disease, but in reality have numerous deleterious effects.

Statins are considered to be "HMG-CoA reductase inhibitors", that is, they act by blocking the enzyme (HMG-CoA reductase) in your liver that is responsible for making cholesterol. There are over 900 studies proving the adverse effects of statin drugs, including anemia, cancer, chronic fatigue, acidosis, liver dysfunction, thyroid disruption, Parkinson's, Alzheimer's, and even diabetes!

Statins have been shown to increase your risk of diabetes through a few different mechanisms. The most important one is that they increase insulin resistance, which contributes to chronic inflammation (the common element of most diseases) and actually results in heart disease, which, ironically, is the primary reason for taking a cholesterol-reducing drug in the first place!

Perhaps most importantly, cholesterol is not the cause of heart disease. Your body needs cholesterol.

What Is Cholesterol?

Cholesterol is a waxy, fat-like substance that's found in all the cells of our body. It has a hormone-like structure that behaves like a fat in that it is insoluble in water and in blood. Cholesterol travels through your bloodstream in small packages called "lipoproteins" which are made of lipids (fats) on the inside and proteins on the outside.

The cholesterol percentage of each lipoprotein varies depending upon the specific type of lipoprotein. Cholesterol comprises 20% of high density lipoproteins (HDLs), 46% of lipoprotein (a), 46% of low density lipoproteins (LDLs), and 22% of very low density lipoproteins (VLDLs). If your primary caregiver is treating you for high cholesterol and does not know these facts, then you should find another primary caregiver. It is imperative for your health that your caregiver completely understands all of the ramifications of the treatment as well as the cause for cholesterol blocking your vascular system in the first place. Once again we must stress that treating the **cause** rather than a **symptom** is needed to maintain health.

What you are almost never told is that cholesterol supports many extremely important functions in the maintenance of good health. Below is a small list of cholesterol's functions.

51

Biological Functions of Cholesterol

Perhaps one of the most important functions of cholesterol is acting as an essential precursor to all of our steroid hormones, which play a crucial role in our health and without which we cannot live. Even low levels of these hormones can cause serious health problems. The fact is that when cholesterol levels fall below 160 mg/dL, cholesterol deficiency symptoms may begin to be severe enough to be noticed. One of the first problems often noticed is adrenal insufficiency, which may cause allergic reactions (that have never occurred before) to foods or plants. Sex hormones may also become detrimentally affected, thus causing the person to become hypo-gonadal or to have severe imbalances (ratios of testosterone to estradiol) and have very low DHEA levels. All of these may lead to more serious diseases, some of which may be life threatening.

Optimal serum cholesterol levels actually help to prevent some types of cerebrovascular diseases and suboptimal cholesterol levels have been associated with an increased risk of cerebrovascular diseases. Cholesterol is also an essential component of cell membranes and, helps maintain the integrity of cell membrane fluidity (which is constantly changing do to fluctuations of dietary fat consumption). Cholesterol also plays a particularly important function as a major constituent of the myelin sheath, which acts as insulation of neurons. It should be noted that cholesterol is so important to bodily functions that the cell membranes actually manufacturer it in direct response to the body's demands.

Cholesterol also creates many valuable byproducts that are required for complete digestion. These byproducts include cholic acid, chenodeoxycholic acid, and deoxycholic acid, all of which are essential components of bile, which is needed for fat digestion and their absorption into the intestines. Cholesterol plays a large role in the function of the immune system; low cholesterol levels may increase the risk of several types of cancer. Cholesterol is actually secreted by glands in the skin which help protect the skin from infections from detrimental bacteria and fungi. Cholesterol also acts as an antioxidant and possesses powerful antioxidant properties.

It has also been shown through several studies that optimal cholesterol levels are required in order to prevent aggressiveness (excessively low cholesterol levels increase the incidence of aggressiveness). It would have been interesting if the studies had analyzed sex hormone levels as well, since cholesterol is required for testosterone synthesis and it is well proven that low testosterone levels also increase aggressiveness. We realize that most physicians (and most of the public) have bought into "*'roid rage*" theory, implicating excess testosterone with rage. However, science and peer reviewed studies have proven the exact opposite to be true. Aggressiveness increases when testosterone drops below normal levels or when the ratio of testosterone to estradiol becomes low.

Cholesterol is also required to deal with stress, so you can see its importance in our Western society. Cholesterol accomplishes this task by being an essential constituent of all adrenal gland hormones. These hormones include adrenaline, cortisone, and cortisol which are released by the body in response to stress in order to counteract its effects. It should also be noted that excessive stress causes production of high quantities of endogenous cholesterol. Remember that cholesterol is the precursor in the formation of all steroid hormones.

In the presence of sunlight, the body can use the photolytic action of UV light on the cholesterol in the skin cells to make vitamin D (specifically vitamin D3), which is essential for our immune system and also maintains the balance of calcium and phosphorus for strong bones and teeth. Vitamin D3 has also been shown to protect against several cancers as well as being implicated in aiding in the prevention of Rickets, bone loss, cancers, and numerous other illnesses. For more information on vitamin D, please visit www.vitamindcouncil.org.

Perhaps most importantly, cholesterol is an essential component in the machinery that triggers the release of neurotransmitters in the brain. Mother's milk is especially rich in cholesterol and contains a special enzyme that helps the baby utilize it. Babies and children need cholesterol-rich foods throughout their growing years to ensure proper development of the brain and nervous system. Cholesterol is very concentrated in the brain, where it contributes to the functioning of "synapses" (tiny gaps between cells which allow nerves to communicate with each other). Cholesterol may also help to prevent depression, since low cholesterol (under 160 mg/dl) is associated with an increased risk of depression. Once again, remember that cholesterol is the precursor of testosterone and testosterone has been shown to be one of the most effective antidepressants for both men and women.

That is enough of cholesterols benefits. Let's take a moment to look at a symptomatic and pharmaceutical approach, rather than a truthful and comprehensive approach.   We'll start with a popular cholesterol lowering drug and take what the pharmaceutical company (Pfizer) presents and compare it to what you now know about cholesterol's numerous functions. We will use the actual words from their website.

What Should My Cholesterol Numbers Be?

The quote below was taken from www.pfizer.com/Cholesterol. Keep in mind that Pfizer sells Lipitor for lowering cholesterol levels.

> *"Your doctor knows best when it comes to your cholesterol goals, and he or she will be your partner in reaching them. National guidelines say a person's total cholesterol number should be under 200, while 220–239 is considered borderline high, and above 240 is considered high.*
>
> *National guidelines also provide direction on LDL cholesterol, part of total cholesterol and the main focus of cholesterol-lowering therapy. Having high levels of LDL cholesterol may put you at risk for heart disease. Generally, your LDL cholesterol should be below 160, if you have no other risk factors for heart disease. Managing and lowering your LDL cholesterol then helps to further reduce your risk."*

So to put these well documented facts together, in order to prevent "cholesterol deficiency symptoms" which occurs in persons whose serum LDL falls to levels below 160 mg/dL, we have to allow our liver to normally produce it. According to pharmaceutically based medicine, we have to keep our total cholesterol below 200 mg/dL. That means our total cholesterol must be maintained between 160 mg/dL and 195 mg/dL to be healthy. They would, of course, like you to perform this "miracle" by taking statin drugs. In light of the fact that statins have been definitively linked to heart attacks, does this pharmaceutical approach make any sense?

To us, a more sensible approach would be comprehensive in nature, keeping our total cholesterol levels at healthy levels, which research on low heart disease communities shows to be somewhere around 225 mg/dL. We should attempt to stop creating lesions to the arterial and venous endothelium (to which cholesterol adheres), heal and add elasticity to the arterial and venous walls, and provide adequate nutrition to both the heart and endothelium. All these efforts should be part of your overall quest to lead a healthy lifestyle.

According to recent research at Harvard, the primary causes of atherosclerosis (*hardening of the arteries which leads to heart disease*) are lesions and plaque in the arteries caused by **sugar** which causes insulin to be released. Insulin causes lesions in the endothelium of the arteries that become clogged with cholesterol. So, cholesterol gets the blame, but the real culprit is sugar. So, if you avoid sugar and simple carbs, cholesterol is not an issue.

Please see research on page 297 to share with your doctor.

TOP 20 HERBS

One problem with herbs is that few of us can afford to keep more than a small collection of them on hand. Since they are not used frequently, purchasing could be a problem, since they are likely to spoil if left in their raw form, so it is advantageous to know which ones are the most important!

This section contains a listing of the 20 most important herbs, in our opinion. These are herbs that we believe you should stock up on so you will have them on hand when you need them most. They are in alphabetical order.

Astragalus

You've probably heard of natural cold remedies like echinacea, garlic, and goldenseal. But here is a remedy that may be even better! So just what is this miracle remedy? It's an ancient Chinese herb called "*huang qi*," which means "*yellow leader*," but you probably know it by its more common name, "*astragalus*." Astragalus is a plant native to Asia, and the part of the plant used medicinally is the root, which is similar to a garlic bulb.

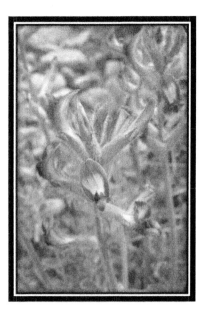

A myriad of studies show that astragalus is a powerful immune booster. However, a common misconception is that merely stimulating the immune system will be enough to "knock out cancer." Perhaps, in a few isolated cases, it will. However, the major problem with cancer is not only that the immune system has been compromised (which it has), but also that the immune response is not working. In other words, the cancer is "invisible" to the immune system and doesn't even appear on the "radar." As a result, when treating cancer, it is important to have a treatment that is both "immunomodulating" (*i.e.*, boosts the immune system) and "adaptogenic" (*i.e.*, corrects the immune response and "lights up the cancer radar").

Astragalus possesses both qualities and can also easily be made into a tincture to prolong its effective shelf life. Simply pour vodka (between 80 and 100 proof) into a dark glass bottle until it barely covers the herb. Keep it in a dark place and shake it twice daily. In 30 days, strain the mixture and you have a tincture that will be good for up to 7 years.

Berberine

Berberine is a natural alkaloid found in a wide variety of traditional herbs including goldenseal, barberry and Oregon grape. Many herbalists credit this unique alkaloid for the benefits of ancient herbal tonics used by native populations throughout the world.

Best known for its natural antibiotic activity, berberine deals a serious blow to common infectious organisms— organisms like "staph," "strep," Chlamydia, diphtheria, salmonella, cholera, diplococcus pneumoniae, pseudomonas, gonorrhea, candida, trichomonas, and many others. It's less well known that berberine has been found more effective than aspirin in relieving fever in experimental animals, and is able to stimulate some parts of the immune system. It's also a stimulant for bile secretion. It may also be made into a safe tincture using the method previously described for astragalus.

Boswellia (Frankincense)

Frankincense is an oleo gum resin from Boswellia trees, of which there are over 25 species. Arabs called the milky sap of the Boswellia tree *"al lubn"* meaning *"milk."* Al lubn became anglicized to olibanum, which is another name for frankincense. When burned, frankincense produces a brilliant flame and produces a pleasant aroma. Since frankincense encourages healthy growth and regeneration of skin cells, it is useful in treating cuts and wounds. Powder of the dried gum is a common ingredient in herbal plasters and pastes used to treat wounds, especially in Chinese medicine. A traditional recipe for an antiseptic wound powder is to mix the powdered resins of frankincense, myrrh, and dried aloe. Tree sap has antibiotic and antifungal properties which protect the tree from infections. So when humans use oleo gum resins or essential oils derived from trees, we are utilizing the molecular components of the trees immune system to boost our own. Frankincense is used for treating a variety of respiratory problems such as bronchitis and laryngitis. Steam inhalation of the essential oil, combined with other respiratory oils such as eucalyptus, is highly effective. The oleo gum resin of Indian frankincense (Boswellia serrata) contains four major pentacyclic triterpenic acids, referred to as boswellic acids. Studies have shown that boswellic acids have an anti-inflammatory action much like conventional non-steroidal anti-inflammatory drugs (NSAIDs). This being so, they have been found to be highly effective in such conditions as rheumatoid arthritis, osteoarthritis, colitis, Crohn's disease, and asthma.

When the oleo gum resin is collected exclusively for essential oil production, the fresh semi-solid material is also used. The fresh gum is chewed for strengthening the teeth and gums, to stimulate digestion, to expel congested phlegm, and to combat halitosis. Chewing of frankincense resin has the secondary benefit of cleansing the digestive system by stimulating bile flow and enzyme secretion and reducing fermentation.

Cat's Claw

Cat's claw is a plant of the Amazon rain forest which has two main species ("uncaria tomentosa" and "uncaria guianensis"). In the USA, you see mainly "uncaria tomentosa" and in Europe you will see mainly "uncaria guianensis." Commonly called "*uña* de *gato*" in Spanish and "*cat's claw*" in English, the name comes from the thorns on the plant's leaves that look like the claws of a cat. This wonder herb, according to Indian folklore, has been used to treat digestive problems, arthritis, inflammation, ulcers, and even to cure cancer. The part used medicinally is the root bark. Another of its properties is its wide spectrum antibiotic activity on numerous pathogenic organisms as well as its safety.

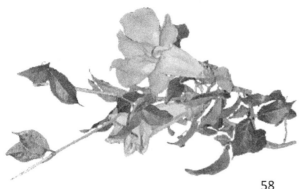

Although virtually unheard of in the USA until recently, the beneficial effects of cat's claw have been studied at research facilities in Peru, Austria, Germany, England, Hungary, and Italy since the 1970's. These studies have shown it to be an immuno-modulating herb which increases white blood cell levels and stimulates the production of natural killer cells, T-cells, and macrophages. Four alkaloids in particular boost phagocytosis (literally "cell eating") where the white blood cells attack, wrap up, and carry off the rogue cells in the body.

Cat's claw possesses amazing healing abilities and benefits to the immune system with a plethora of therapeutic applications. Dr. Julian Whitaker reports using cat's claw for its immune-stimulating effects, for cancer, to help prevent strokes and heart attacks, to reduce blood clots, and for diverticulitis and irritable bowel syndrome (IBS). Due to its anti-inflammatory properties, cat's claw has been used for rheumatoid arthritis and osteoarthritis. Compounds in cat's claw bark and roots (called "quinovic acid glycosides") block the body's production of substances called "prostaglandins" and "tumor necrosis factor" (TNF) which cause inflammation.

Cayenne (Capsaicin)

The hot fruit of the cayenne plant ("capsicum annuum") has been used as superb culinary spice for centuries. However, did you know that in addition to tickling your tongue, cayenne is perhaps the most valuable medicinal herb in the herb kingdom, not only for the entire digestive system, but also for the heart and circulatory system? Cayenne acts as a catalyst and increases the effectiveness of other herbs; the active ingredient in cayenne is called "capsaicin."

Cayenne is incredibly nourishing to the heart and has been known to stop heart attacks within 30 seconds. If you want to carry something in your first aid kit for a heart attack, carry a cayenne tincture. Even a bottle of Tabasco Sauce® might be good enough. Cayenne has traditionally 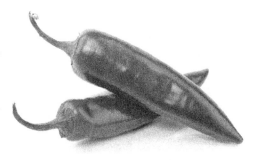 been used for overcoming fatigue and restoring energy. It is a natural stimulant without the threatening side effects (palpitations, hyper-activity or rise in blood pressure) of most other stimulating agents. Rubbed on the skin, cayenne is a potent remedy for rheumatic pains and arthritis due to what is termed a "counterirritant effect." A counterirritant is something which causes irritation to a tissue to which it is applied, thus distracting from the original irritation (such as joint pain in the case of arthritis).

Cayenne can also rebuild the tissue in the stomach and the peristaltic action in the intestines. It aids elimination and assimilation, and helps the body to create hydrochloric acid, which is so necessary for good digestion and assimilation, especially of proteins. There is also evidence to suggest that cayenne may be useful in the treatment of obesity. Results of one trial showed that consumption of 10 grams of cayenne pepper with meals helped to reduce appetite, while results of another revealed that cayenne increases the metabolism of dietary fats. Lastly, herbalists from centuries past would pour cayenne pepper directly on fresh wounds in order to sterilize and stop the bleeding.

When added to herbal formulas, it stimulates the action of other herbs. It is a preventative for heart attacks, flu, colds, indigestion, and lack of vitality. It is good for treating the spleen, pancreas, kidneys and is effective as a fomentation for rheumatism, inflammation, pleurisy, sores, and wounds. It can be rubbed on toothaches and swellings.

Chrysin

Chrysin is a bioflavonoid found in passion flower (Passiflora coerula), that promotes healthy testosterone levels and lean muscle mass by inhibiting aromatase, the enzyme that converts testosterone to estrogen. It also has the ability to bind to estradiol receptor sites and

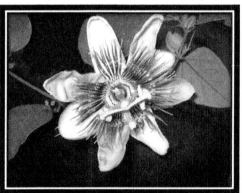

make them unable to accept estradiol. This has the affect of rendering excess free estradiol harmless. Chrysin has been used in the treatment of several estradiol receptor positive cancers as well as having been shown to cause cell death in leukemia cells while enhancing the effects of natural killer cells.

It has also been used to increase muscle growth, alleviate gout, increase sexual desire, and reduce inflammation in ulcerative colitis. The largest caveat with chrysin is that it must be combined with other specific herbs or placed in a liposome to be effective since it breaks down almost completely in the digestive tract if not protected. It should be taken either in a tested product such as De Aromatase, or placed in a liposome as previously discussed in order to have the desired effects. Considering the current and accelerating state of dropping testosterone levels and rising estradiol levels as previously discussed, we believe chrysin should definitely be an important part of your herbal supply. We both have several bottles of De Aromatase on hand to prevent unwanted hormonal shifts as well as for its numerous other benefits.

Cinnamon

Native to Japan, China, Taiwan, Vietnam, and Korea (where it was used for oils and timber), the cinnamon tree has spread to Australia, the southern USA, Caribbean, and Africa. This tree grows best in areas that are dry and disturbed, such as roadsides. The cinnamon tree ranges between twenty-five and forty feet. A quick and easy method of identifying this tree is by crushing the leaves or peeling a twig or bark. This will release oils and the scent of cinnamon.

Traditionally it has been used to stimulate the circulatory system and as an aid for treating colds, diarrhea, cramps, and spasms. It also works as an immune system enhancer and anti-inflammatory. It has several excellent components for the heart, as well as for asthma and bronchitis sufferers. Its phytochemicals contain expectorants, antiasthmatic and antihistaminic components. It contains several phytochemicals that are anticarcinogenic and some of the constituents have been shown to be helpful against the HIV virus (the soothing effect on the digestive tract might be helpful as well). Cinnamon is easily made into a tea, or may be found in capsule and tincture form.

Curcumin (Turmeric)

Turmeric (curry) is known as "the golden spice of life" and has been used in Indian cuisine for thousands of years. As a matter of fact, it is impossible to think of Indian food without turmeric. Curcumin, the active ingredient in turmeric, has several cancer-fighting properties. A recent study found that curcumin can actually repair DNA that has been damaged by radiation. This is very good news, because one cannot avoid all radiation sources. According to University of Chicago scientists, curcumin inhibits a cancer-provoking bacteria associated with gastric and colon cancer. (Magad GB, *Anticancer Research*, Nov-Dec 2002).

Yet another anti-cancer property of curcumin is that it is a powerful antioxidant. It can therefore protect our bodies from free radicals that damage DNA. This is also why turmeric (which contains curcumin) can be used for preserving foods. Tests in Germany, reported in the *Journal of Pharmacy & Pharmacology* in July 2003, found that "*all fractions of the turmeric extract preparation exhibited pronounced antioxidant activity.*" Turmeric extract tested more potent than garlic, devil's claw, and salmon oil.

Elderberry

Elderberry, which grows in Europe and North America, is a shrub or small tree which grows between ten and thirty feet high. White or yellow flowers develop into the fruit - berries that turn from green through red-brown to shiny black.

Traditionally used as an anti-hypertensive and circulatory stimulant, it's also been found to be excellent for the heart. It has hypotensives and diuretic constituents that work to lower the blood pressure and also contains capillarigenics (which increase the health of the capillaries

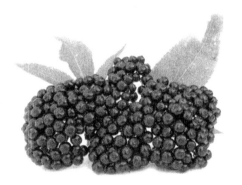

and their ability to transport blood) and cardiotonics to strengthen the heart. It is used externally as an astringent, and can be used internally as an expectorant and anti-inflammatory. Several of its phytochemicals have been shown to be cancer fighting and Kaempferol has been shown to be effective against the HIV virus. Elderberry may be taken as a syrup, tea, tincture or in capsule form.

Feverfew

Feverfew is a perennial herb native to southeastern Europe and Asia. It is naturalized widely elsewhere and oftentimes found growing on rocky slopes, walls, and waste places. The leaves have a refreshing aromatic aroma. Growing to almost three feet, the stem is covered with many daisy-like flower heads which bloom from June to August, with white ray flowers surrounding nearly flat yellow centers, growing to about one inch across.

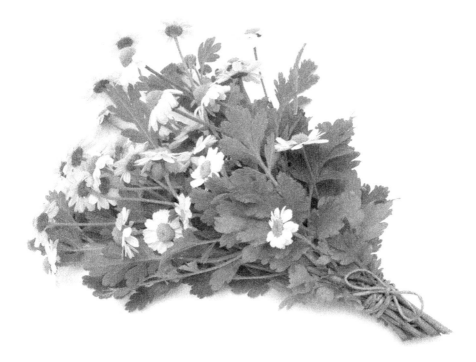

Traditionally it has been shown to work well on migraines and other headaches, arthritis, fever, and muscle tension. It is also effective in treating the discomfort of indigestion, colds and flu, and is often used to break a fever in these types of illnesses. It stimulates the appetite, uterine contractions, promotes menses and increases fluidity of lung and bronchial tube mucus. Because of its actions on the bronchial tubes it is often used with other herbal remedies for lung infections and asthma. Native Americans used it in several herbal recipes, many of which also contained wormwood, to kill and expel worms. Feverfew may be taken as powder, tincture, or capsule.

Garlic

There has been more written about the wonderful benefits of garlic than any other food source known. Its history dates back 3,500 years. Hippocrates, the father of medicine, was the first to write that garlic was an excellent medicine for eliminating tumors. Recent studies on garlic have shown that it kills insects, parasites, bad bacteria, and fungi. It also eliminates various tumors, lowers blood sugar levels, lowers harmful fats in the blood, and prevents clogging of the arteries. Researchers have also shown that allicin (the organic compound which gives garlic its aroma and flavor) acts as a very potent antioxidant.

In the 1950s, Soviet scientists found it to be equal to penicillin, yet without the harmful effects of that powerful drug. Garlic is used for all lung and respiratory ailments, and can be used as a tea or added to syrups for coughs, colds, tuberculosis, fevers, and blood diseases. Use it as a tea in an enema for worms and bowel infections. Use the fresh extract oil or eat the raw cloves.

Ginger

Aromatic, pungent and spicy, ginger adds a special flavor and zest to stir fries and many fruit and vegetable dishes. Ginger's benefits as a healing food are well-known in Asia where it is frequently called "the universal medicine." Ginger is regarded as an excellent "carminative" (a substance which promotes the elimination of intestinal gas) and "intestinal spasmolytic" (a substance which relaxes and soothes the intestinal tract).

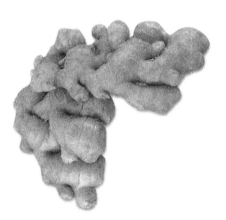

Ginger's anti-vomiting action has been shown to be very useful in reducing the nausea and vomiting of pregnancy. Ginger's effectiveness as a digestive aid is due largely to its active phytonutrient ingredients: "gingerols" and "shogaols." These substances help to neutralize stomach acids, enhance the secretion of digestive juices (stimulating the appetite), and tone the muscles of the digestive tract. But that's not all. Both gingerols and shogaols have been shown to fight cancer as well.

Gingerols are phytonutrients responsible for ginger's distinctive flavor. Scientific research has been shown that gingerols have antibacterial properties to inhibit the growth of "helicobacter pylori," involved in the development of gastric and colon cancer and suppress the growth of human colorectal cancer. Lab experiments presented by Dr. Rebecca Lui (and colleagues from the University of Michigan) at the 97th Annual Meeting of the American Association for Cancer showed that gingerols kill ovarian cancer cells by inducing apoptosis (programmed cell death) and phagocytosis (self-digestion).

Ginkgo Biloba

Ginkgo biloba is a perennial deciduous tree, native to eastern China. They grow as tall as seventy feet and live (some say) a thousand years. When male and female trees are grown together, the female produces yellow plum-like fruits in autumn which when ripe look (strangely) like little brains! The leaves are green to gold, fan-shaped, petioled, with many radiating veins and about four to five inches wide.

Traditionally it has been used to improve memory, brain function, depression, cerebral and peripheral circulation, oxygenation and blood flow. Because of its properties of increasing blood flow to the brain it is good for Alzheimer's disease, tinnitus, asthma, heart and kidney problems, as well as glucose utilization. It is also showing promise for stroke patients by aiding in their recovery and preventing blood clots. Because of this property, caution should be used if you are currently on blood thinners or aspirin.

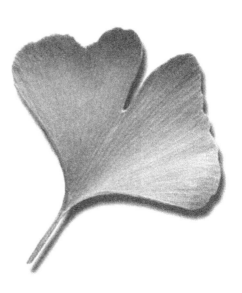

Ginkgo is also used for coughs, allergies, and asthma by acting as an expectorant, antitussive and antiasthmatic. It is also effective in the treatment of leukorrhea, spermatorrhea, bed wetting, nocturnal emission, headache, vertigo, tinnitus, coldness, arthritis, rheumatism, hearing loss, and poor peripheral circulation. The French have done excellent research in natural blood clotting, increasing arterial flow and decreasing organ transplant rejection using Gingko's remarkable attributes.

Its enhancement of peripheral circulation may be used in combinations of other herbs such as Cayenne to maximize the effects of both herbs, or in conjunction with a relaxant such as chamomile, to facilitate its relaxing effects. Ginkgo is normally taken in tincture or capsule form.

Ginseng

Ginseng is perhaps the most well-known Chinese herb and the most widely recognized plant used in traditional medicine. It should also be known that there are several types of ginseng and each has various levels of ginsenosides. The life-extending properties of ginseng were first described around 500 AD in a Chinese medical textbook by Shennong, and various forms of ginseng have been used in medicine for thousands of years.

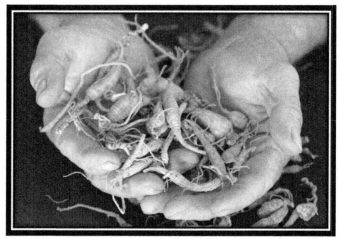

The two most common types of ginseng are *"panax ginseng"* (aka Asian, Korean or Chinese ginseng) and *"panax quinquefolius"* (aka American, Canadian, or North American ginseng). North American ginseng has the most active concentrations of ginsenosides. The word *"panax"* is derived from the Greek word *"panacea"* which means *"all healing,"* and the benefits of ginseng are recognized as such.

One other ginseng we would like to mention is tienchi ginseng, also known as "tienchi" or "yunan pao." It has many uses, but the primary reason we are mentioning it here is it has a remarkable ability to stop bleeding and inhibit infection. If you suffer from a severe cut or wound, tienchi may be poured directly into the wound to stop bleeding and help prevent infection. It is always part of our emergency aid kit.

Ginseng is commonly used as an adaptogen, meaning it normalizes physical functioning depending on what the individual needs. For example, it will lower high blood pressure, but it will raise low blood pressure. Ginseng is also effective in combating cancer, diabetes, stress, and fatigue. These effects of ginseng are mainly attributed to a group of compounds called "ginsenosides."

Other Chinese studies indicated that ginsenosides also increase protein synthesis and activity of neurotransmitters in the brain, thus ginseng is used to restore memory and enhance concentration and cognitive abilities. Additional research has shown specific effects that support the central nervous system, liver function, lung function, and circulatory system.

Green Tea

Green tea is chock-full of polyphenols, phytochemicals with potent antioxidant properties that give green tea its bitter flavor. It contains six primary polyphenols, known as catechins. Epigallocatechin gallate (EGCG) is the most active and studied of green tea's catechins. Catechins should be considered right alongside of the better-known antioxidants like vitamins E and C as potent free radical scavengers and health-supportive for this reason.

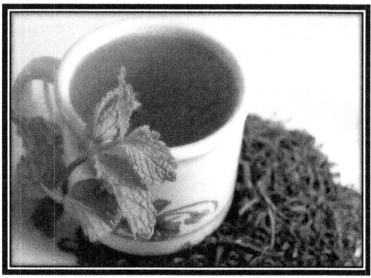

Green tea also contains alkaloids such as caffeine (although in lower quantities than black tea), which give green tea its stimulating properties. Green tea drinkers appear to have lower risk for a wide range of diseases, from simple bacterial or viral infections to chronic degenerative conditions including cardiovascular disease, cancer, stroke, periodontal disease, and osteoporosis.

Hibiscus

Hibiscus tea has been enjoyed by many for hundreds of years as relaxing refreshment as well as an herbal remedy to treat many ailments. Packed with a plethora of protective polyphenols, this rich red tea can help reduce blood pressure to a degree similar to that of prescription anti-hypertensive drugs, according to a study at Tufts University with findings published in *The Journal of Nutrition*.

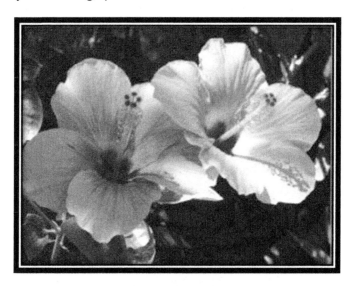

Hibiscus tea also contains an enzyme inhibitor which blocks the production of amylase (an enzyme that breaks down complex sugars and starches). This being so, drinking a cup of hibiscus tea after meals may reduce the absorption of dietary carbohydrates and will assist in weight loss. Hibiscus tea is also rich in vitamin C and can help strengthen the immune system while protecting the entire body against bacterial attacks.

Licorice Root

Indigenous to rich low-lands and river valleys of southern Europe, the Middle East, and northern China, licorice root is cultivated in many parts of the world. It is brown, wrinkled, and woody, producing an erect striated stem two to five feet in height.

Licorice root is one of the best antiulcer herbs available. Research has been wide spread and the results for ulcer sufferers are excellent. Deglycyrrhizinated licorice may stimulate the body's defense mechanisms that prevent the occurrence of ulcers by increasing the amount of mucous-secreting cells in the digestive tract. This improves the quality of mucus, lengthens intestinal cell life, and enhances microcirculation in the gastrointestinal lining. Licorice derivatives have been recommended as a standard nutritional support for ulcer sufferers in Europe. It is beneficial for ulcerative colitis, diverticulosis, colitis, gastric and duodenal ulcers as well as protecting against their development.

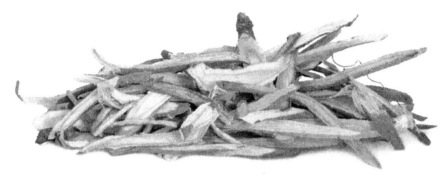

Licorice root combined with Fenugreek is extraordinary in treating ulcerative colitis, and other severe ulcerative conditions. A restoring and rejuvenative herb, it works as a general tonic for the whole body. Licorice is calming and alleviates stress, relaxes muscle pains, and decreases musculo-skeletal spasms.

Combined with other herbs which act more specifically on pain and inflammation, it is a wonderful choice for rheumatism, arthritis, and osteoarthritis. It strengthens the digestive system, improves energy and is good for hypoglycemia, bronchitis, gastritis, stress, colds, sore throats, nausea, and swelling. It is also useful in treating adrenal insufficiency and other glandular problems. Licorice root increases mucus fluidity from the lungs and bronchial tubes which results in more consistent clearing of the airways.

It also contains estrogenic phytochemicals and may benefit those who are in need of estrogen supplementation. It is the actions of these chemicals which have made licorice root a popular female tonic. Studies show that licorice root stimulates the production of interferon, which makes it very valuable as a cancer fighter and as a support herb for AIDS and HIV sufferers. Licorice may be taken as a tincture, capsule, candy, or powder form.

Psyllium

Psyllium is native to the Mediterranean region, Pakistan, and India. It is cultivated in the Northwestern region of India, which accounts for 60% of the world's production of psyllium, which grows to about eighteen inches. Its root system has a well developed tap root with few fibrous secondary roots. A large number of flowering shoots arise from the base of the plant; flowers are numerous, small, and white. The seeds are enclosed in capsules that open at maturity.

Traditionally used as a stool softener, it cleans the intestines, and prevents constipation. It is used in the treatment of colitis, ulcers and hemorrhoids.   The mucilage and aucubin in psyllium makes it an excellent laxative. Psyllium is usually taken in powder or capsule form or in combinations with other herbs for its laxative and stool softening effects.

Skullcap

Skullcap is a perennial herb native to North America which grows in rich woods, thickets, bluffs and along roadsides in wet ditches. It prefers a moist shady environment. The stems grow between one and two feet high, and the flowers are blue to lavender.

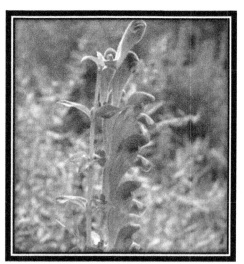

Skullcap has been used for hundreds of years by the Native Americans as a nervine. It is an excellent herb for those suffering from anxiety, skeletal muscle spasms and insomnia. It is used for more serious disorders such as hysteria, migraine headaches, epilepsy, and convulsions. It is also used to aid in drug withdrawal symptoms. This herb is often used to treat rheumatism, due to its ability to act as a mild anti-inflammatory and relax the muscle around the painful joints. Skullcap has also been found to lower blood pressure and is believed to strengthen the heart muscle. It is used for calming the gastrointestinal tract for problems such as irritable bowel syndrome, gallbladder and small intestine problems, and for some symptoms of ulcers. For a stronger sedative effect or to treat severe muscular spasms, skullcap may be combined with other herbs such as chamomile, passion flower or valerian. The Chinese use it to treat headaches, PMS, drug withdrawal, and muscular spasms.

Skullcap has been used to wean people off hard drugs. Combined with ginseng, it is good for alcoholism. Skullcap should be used as fresh as possible, otherwise its activity rather quickly dissipates.

Stinging Nettle

Common throughout North America, nettle can be found in disturbed soils, along streams, open forests, and ditches, on mountain slopes and can be found on roadsides. But because it prefers nitrogen-rich soils, its favorite habitat is garden borders.

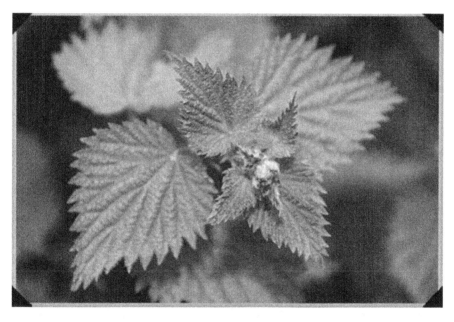

Nettle is one of the best arthritic pain relievers in the herbal kingdom. In ancient Rome, even though it was painful, the stinging nettle was rubbed over arthritic joints. It was said to stop the pain and, over time, cure the condition. Today we know that it's possible to get many of the benefits for the treatment of rheumatoid and osteoarthritic conditions, without the pain of enduring Nettle stings. Tinctures and teas are still used for treating many skin disorders such as eczema, skin eruptions, and nail fungus, but Nettle has been traditionally used to stimulate milk production.

Nettle acts as an expectorant. It contains antiasthmatic constituents which are used in the treatment of bronchitis, colds, asthma, and other lung diseases. Nettle is also used as a diuretic, general tonic, circulatory stimulant, and bowel and colon stimulant. It is beneficial for the colon, urinary disorders, allergies, leukemia, hemorrhoids, goiter, kidneys, spleen, and lungs. Nettle is also used in some worming combinations to kill and expel worms of the gastrointestinal tract. Taken internally it's a good pain reliever used primarily for rheumatism, sciatica, neuritis, lumbago, and arthritis. Its antibiotic qualities seem to work best for nephritis, cystitis, kidney and bladder infections, gravel, and other urinary tract disorders. It may be used in tea, tincture, powder or capsule form.

Now you have the basis for a fine, basic herbal cabinet! Twenty herbs is a good number to work with in keeping your basic herb supply small. If you wish, subtract some from the above list or add to it, or feel free to change it around to meet your special needs. Few of us are in a position to keep a large variety of herbs on hand.

For a complete listing of over 100 essential medicinal herbs, please visit www.survivalherbs.com and purchase *A Guide To Understanding Herbal Medicines and Surviving the Coming Pharmaceutical Monopoly*.

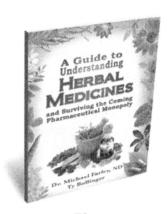

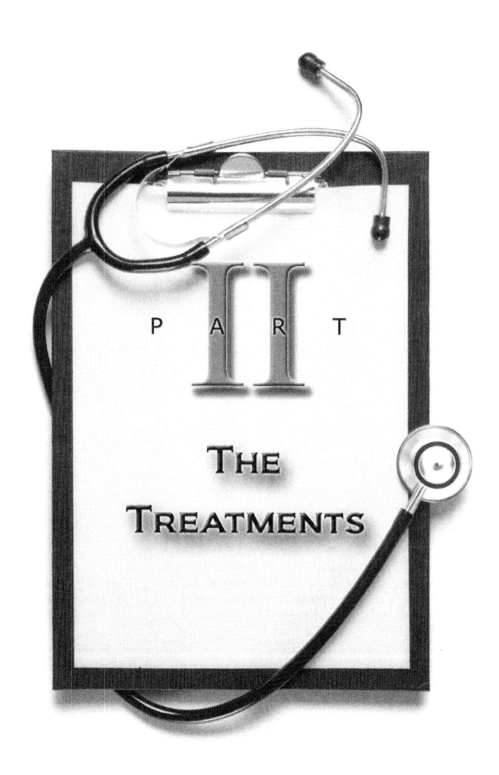

PART II

THE TREATMENTS

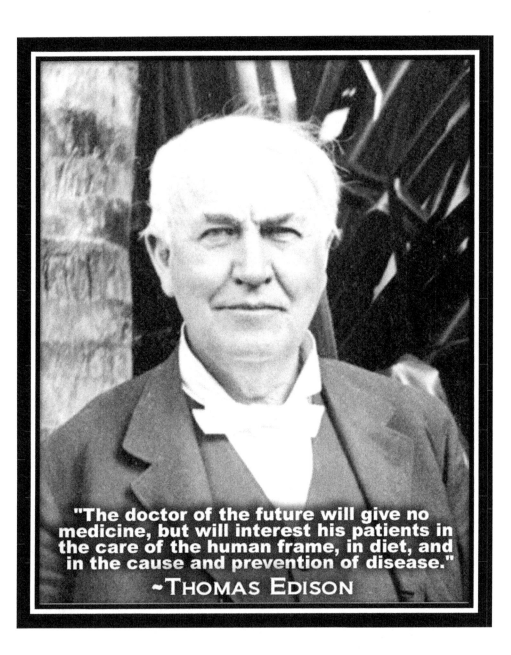

"The doctor of the future will give no medicine, but will interest his patients in the care of the human frame, in diet, and in the cause and prevention of disease."

~THOMAS EDISON

ACID REFLUX

DESCRIPTION:

Approximately 44% of the population experiences acid reflux at least once per month. The word "reflux" comes from the Medieval Latin word refluxus which comes from the Latin word refluere, meaning "to flow back, to recede". If you suffer from acid reflux, the acids from your stomach "flow back" into your esophagus, causing discomfort and pain, known as heartburn. This occurs when the pyloric valve in the lower part of the stomach fails to open. When that happens the stomach cannot empty. When the stomach still has contents we sometimes get reflux of those contents, which taste very acidic and can actually burn the esophagus. Acid reflux is the action, while heartburn is the sensation. The pain is heartburn, while the movement of acid into the esophagus from the stomach is acid reflux.

SYMPTOMS:

Asthma, chest pain, dental erosion, difficulty swallowing, heartburn, hoarseness, regurgitation, and in serious cases, actual erosion of the esophogus.

CONVENTIONAL TREATMENTS:

Commercial antacids are commonly used in the treatment of burning from acid reflux. This reduces the amount of **hydrochloric acid** (HCL) being produced or in some cases neutralize the acid already present. However it also has the consequences of stopping proper digestion of the protein in your stomach as well as making one more apt to develop food poisoning due to a lower acidic stomach environment. High stomach acid is what allows animals such as dogs to eat garbage with so few effects of food poisoning. The acid kills the bacteria.

Antacids are formulated based on the faulty presupposition that excessive HCL (**hyper**chlorhydria) is the underlying cause of heartburn and acid reflux. In fact, the opposite is very often true. Insufficient production of HCL (**hypo**chlorhydria) may be a far more common underlying cause of heartburn than excessive production of HCL. In such cases the use of pharmaceutical antacids may exacerbate the underlying cause of heartburn (by further depleting HCL). This in turn, may often lead to further problems by not allowing proper digestion of fats and other foods, leaving the body in an unhealthy state due to poor digestion and absorption of nutrients.

NATURAL TREATMENTS:

Since the pyloric valve is largely pH controlled, meaning that it will only open when the stomach has become acidic enough to do its job, many physicians have found that when acid is added to the diet,by either digestive enzymes with HCL, or the simplest and least expensive method, **organic apple cider vinegar**, the pyloric valve will open and empty the stomach leaving nothing to reflux. A tablespoon of apple cider vinegar before every meal is sufficient for the most people.

The enzymes required for digestion are the following:

- ❖ **Amylases** (which digest carbohydrates)
- ❖ **Cellulases** (which digests cellulose)
- ❖ **Lipases** (which digest dietary fats)
- ❖ **Proteases** (which digest dietary proteins)

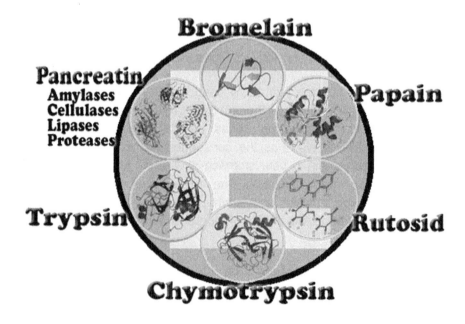

Trypsin and **chymotrypsin** are two different but related digestive enzymes produced and released by the pancreas. Both enzymes function within the intestine to help break down large protein molecules that we ingest in the foods we eat. Because these two enzymes break down proteins, they classified as proteases. **Bromelain** is a mixture of enzymes that digest protein (proteolytic) that are found in pineapples, while **papain** is an enzyme found in unripe papayas. Enteric coated, animal enzyme, plant enzyme, and rutosid combinations are the most researched systemic enzyme formulations in the world.

Disruption of these enzymes results in disruption of the digestive process, so a good **enzyme supplement** may help alleviate acid reflux. Also, **probiotics** are often helpful in restoring normal digestion. If you have ever taken a round of antibiotics and not followed with probiotics to restore the helpful digestive bacteria, that may be a cause of disrupted food digestion and acid reflux.

An interesting fact is that over 30% of people over the age of 60 are clinically diagnosed as hypochloridic, (i.e. they do not produce adequate amounts of HCL), and acid reflux rises among the elderly population.

The real key in successful treatment of acid reflux is to make sure that the pyloric valve opens at the bottom of the stomach so that all of the food taken in is passed into the small intestine where it will then have bicarbonate excreted to restore a more neutral pH for further digestion. When the pyloric valve does not open, the food in the stomach stays in the stomach, and even though it may not be acidic enough to open the pyloric valve, it is often acidic enough to cause burning of the esophageal wall. This sometimes causes mild discomfort, but in more serious cases the burning of the esophageal wall can be quite serious and painful.

Anyone suffering from acid reflux should have a **comprehensive stool analysis** to determine their gut pathology, which will give a current picture of both benificial and pathogenic bacteria and fungi, as well as what foods are not being adequately digested. Since the gut comprises about 70% of the immune system, the test becomes even more significant. Proper comprehensive stool analysis also includes a culture and sensitivity which will give your primary caregiver the most effective way of killing the pathogens and restoring the proper flora. This test, such as one offered by Genova Diagnostics can be invaluable in diagnosing the cause of the problem so that a permanent solution can be found. Their website is www.gdx.net.

In the vast majority of cases, the addition of the vinegar will add enough acidity to the stomach which opens the pyloric valve and empties the stomach so there is no longer anything to reflux. However, this is not meant for all people. Though research has shown hypochloridia, (low secretion of HCL by the stomach), to be a prominent cause of acid reflux, there are some that have a legitimate need to reduce excess stomach acid.

A few herbs and supplements may be found helpful for this condition, aside from apple cider viniger, if you are hypochloridic. **Melatonin** has shown itself to be protective of your esophogeal wall, while **limonene** lowers both the frequency and severity of attacks in many cases.

FOR YOUR DOCTOR:

See page 220 for research and studies to share with your doctor.

ADRENAL INSUFFICIENCY

(IN PROGRESSIVE AND SEVERE CASES IT IS CALLED ADDISON'S DISEASE)

DESCRIPTION:

Thomas Addison first described the essential role of the adrenal glands for human survival in 1855. Addison's disease is caused by **adrenal insufficiency** which may be caused by constant stress, pollutants or other factors which result in overworked, damaged or depleted adrenal glands.

The adrenal glands are small hormone-releasing organs located on top of each kidney. They are made up of the outer portion (the cortex) and the inner portion (the medulla).

The adrenal cortex produces three types of hormones:

1. The **glucocorticoid** hormones (such as cortisol) maintain sugar (glucose) control, suppress immune response, and help the body respond to stress and inflammation.
2. The **mineralocorticoid** hormones (such as aldosterone) regulate sodium and potassium balance.
3. The **sex hormones**, androgens (male) and estrogens (female), affect sexual development and sex drive.

The inner medulla produces catecholamines. Addison's disease results from damage to the adrenal cortex, which causes the cortex to produce less of its hormones.

The basic function of the adrenal glands are to protect the organism against acute and chronic stress. This has been popularized as the "fight-or-flight" response for the medulla and the "alarm" reaction for the cortex.

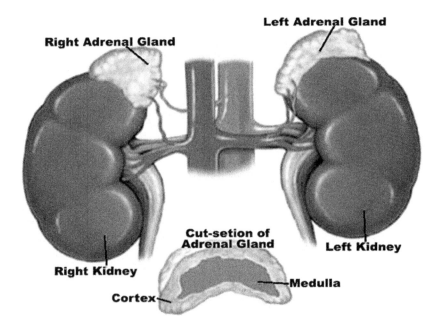

SYMPTOMS:

Changes in heart rate, changes in blood pressure, chronic diarrhea, nausea, loss of appetite, paleness, extreme fatigue, mouth lesions, salt craving, increasing allergies and allergic reactions.

CONVENTIONAL TREATMENTS:

Addison's disease is typically treated with replacement corticosteroids, which will control the symptoms, but will typically be required to be taken for life. People often receive a combination of glucocorticoids (cortisone or hydrocortisone) and mineralocorticoids (fludrocortisone). During an extreme form of adrenal insufficiency, called adrenal crisis, it may be necessary to inject hydrocortisone immediately. Supportive treatment for low blood pressure is usually needed as well.

NATURAL TREATMENTS:

There are natural herbs that will stimulate the adrenal glands to secrete cortisol and have actually been shown to rejuvenate and accelerate adrenal cells and actually reduce their destruction. One such herb is **horny goat weed**.

Licorice root has also been used with some success, but make sure that potassium is used in conjunction with it, since licorice tends to remove potassium from the system, which can cause other problems. Lastly, Americans usually do not have adequate **vitamin** and **mineral** intake, so supplementation with a high quality multivitamin/mineral is recommended. Also, it is essential to supplement for all **B vitamins** (rather than just one). They act synergistically and need to be properly balanced. An excellent B vitamin supplement is called "Supreme B" and can be purchased at www.healthpro.com.dm/supremeb.html.

Adrenal insufficiency has been extremely under diagnosed. One of the reasons is that the most common and cheap method is called an "adrenal challenge." In this test the hormone that causes cortisol to be released from the adrenals is given and the resulting cortisol is measured. The biggest problem with this test is that the adrenal glands are pulsatile and they may be capable of giving out their last bit of cortisol and meet the "normal" limits, but still be unable to repeat their secretions normally for the rest of the 24 hour cycle. Saliva tests taken throughout the day are better, but still have a long way to go. For those who are adrenally insufficient, it is advised to have your status checked periodically. If necessary, you may want to consider taking Corteff (or hydrocortisone) at "physiological" doses. In other words, if the human adrenal glands produce 20 to 30 mg of cortisol daily and yours are only capable of producing 10 mg daily, you would take 5 mg of hydrocortisone 3 times daily. This is called a physiological dose, which means what your body would normally produce, and it almost never has side effects.

It should also be noted that in times of stress, the adrenals are capable of producing more cortisol to help temporarily deal with the stress. If they are in constant stress, the adrenals will become insufficient. One way to see if this is occurring is noticing an increase in new allergy symptoms or food sensitivities. Another indication is rapidly increasing aching joints and muscles. Sometimes it will be necessary to ask your physicians to test for adrenal insufficiency instead of prescribing an antihistamine or anti-inflammatory, but it is better to learn and treat the cause rather than merely treating the symptom.

FOR YOUR DOCTOR:

See page 225 for research and studies to share with your doctor.

ALLERGIES

There is an important point we would like to make and a caution before delving into this topic. If you have an infant or young child that is consistently showing signs of allergies, the very first thing that should be done is make sure that the child is not suffering from food reactions. If they are being breast fed, it is almost never a problem, but as they grow older, or are bottle fed, the chances of food allergies increase dramatically.

Chronic earaches are one of the very common signs of food allergies and may often present as an ear infection. In the USA alone, an estimated 700,000 tubes are inserted into children's ears each ear. Inside the ear, there is a tiny physical tube, called the eustachian tube, which runs from the nasopharynx at the back of the throat all the way out to the middle ear cavity. Its purpose is to keep air flowing into the ear cavity.

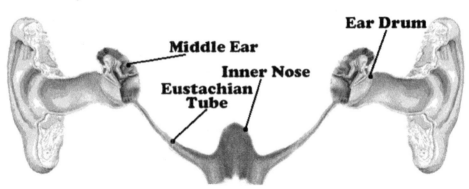

When the tube is blocked, air can no longer get into the middle ear cavity. It is this blockage that is believed by many physicians to cause a severe inflammatory reaction which causes the lining of the ear drum to become extremely painful and also causes fluid to accumulate in the middle ear cavity resulting in an increase in pain from the added pressure. If this occurs in a child, the most overlooked reason is allergy.

Allergies to dairy and gluten seem to be on the rise, or it may be that they are merely being diagnosed more frequently. The point is that at the first sign of childhood allergies, it is time to determine if they are food related. Chronic ear problems are most frequently due to cow's milk and all other dairy products. Being a good parent, many mistakenly believe that milk is the best form of calcium for their children and that it is a healthy food. Unfortunately they are wrong on both counts. Milk is no longer a safe food due to the addition of antibiotics and hormones that the milk carries, as well as the fact that the cattle are fed genetically modified grains, which to date, remain an unknown and a purposely untested safety concern.

Cow's milk does not contain nearly the bioavailable calcium that almond milk contains nor does it contain many other nutrients that almond milk contains. At the first sign of allergies in children, we suggest complete removal of all dairy products. That means **all** dairy, including yogurt, ice cream, sauces, and any other source of dairy. It may easily be replaced by almond milk and will be much healthier for the child in the long run regardless of allergies.

If milk is the culprit of the allergic reactions, if you remove it from the diet, you will know within 72 hours. It often takes only one day to see the difference. It is well worth the effort of removing all dairy products to see if it is a contributing factor to a child's allergic symptoms.

A caution to parents: do not use soy milk to replace dairy. There are three primary reasons for avoiding soy. The first is that soy causes thyroid damage to children, which is very well documented. The second is that it does not contain the vitamins, calcium and other minerals present in almond milk. The third reason is that almost all soy in the USA is genetically modified.

If removal of all dairy does not alleviate the signs of allergies, then the next most common allergen is gluten, a dietary protein which is really a combination of two proteins (gliadin and glutenin). It is the gliadin content of gluten that is responsible for most of its toxic effects. Again, the simplest method of determining if gluten is causing the problem is removing all gluten from the diet for a few days.

Celiac disease, Sjogren's syndrome, thyroiditis, type 1 diabetes, and worsening of the symptoms of autism, as well as dermatitis, and psoriasis have all been directly connected to allergies to gliadin in gluten. It is certainly worth the effort to remove it from the diet and see if it is a contributing factor. This is especially important if your child is also suffering from signs of autism.

83

The main source of gluten is wheat. Barley, oats, and rye also contain gluten to a lesser extent. It is not difficult to replace them with fresh fruits and vegetables as well as other gluten free products, and it is certainly worth the effort.

DESCRIPTION:

An allergy is an exaggerated immune reaction to substances that are generally not harmful to most people. Typically, the immune system protects the body against harmful substances, such as bacteria and viruses. It also reacts to foreign substances called allergens, which are generally harmless and in most people do not cause a problem.

However, a person with allergies has a hypersensitive immune system. When it identifies an allergen, it releases chemicals (like histamines) which fight off the allergen but also cause allergy symptoms. Common allergens include pollen, mold, insect stings, dust, pet dander, dust mites, medicines, and food.

SYMPTOMS:

Allergy symptoms may include wheezing, headaches, hives, eye irritation, coughing, runny nose, stomach cramps, vomiting, and diarrhea, amongst others.

CONVENTIONAL TREATMENTS:

Typical allergy medications include antihistamines, decongestants, allergy shots, corticosteroids, and other medicines such as leukotriene inhibitors which block the substances that trigger allergies. Emergency epinephrine shots are sometimes required.

NATURAL TREATMENTS:

There are many herbs that are very beneficial at providing relief for allergies. **Ginger, ginkgo, stinging nettle, eucalyptus**, and **ephedra** are the most commonly used herbs for this ailment.

Ginger has healing powers that work on multiple levels, so it counters a host of different allergy symptoms. Ginger is a natural antihistamine, so it relieves allergy problems centered in the sinuses. Since it also has anti-inflammatory properties, it reduces the achy feeling that may accompany allergy attacks. If your allergy attacks include digestive disorders, ginger calms the stomach. Ginger can also counteract nausea and relieve gas and bloating.

Ginkgo contains ginkgo biloba, which produces chemicals in the body that helps to prevent inflammation in the sinus area when particles enter the body.

Stinging nettle helps to prevent fevers associated with allergies as well as cough, chest congestion, runny nose, and bronchial constriction.

Eucalyptus helps you to breathe easier by opening up the lungs so that your cells get more oxygen.

Ephedra is a spice that works as an anti-inflammatory and decongestant, and has been a popular ingredient in many over the counter allergy medicines. It is an effective bronchiodilator.

For Your Doctor:

See page 227 for research and studies to share with your doctor.

ALZHEIMER'S DISEASE

DESCRIPTION:

Alzheimer's disease (AD) was discovered in 1906 by Dr. Alois Alzheimer. Sometimes referred to as "senile dementia," AD is a loss of brain function which gradually gets worse over time. It affects memory, thinking, and behavior.

There are two types of AD:

1. **Early onset AD**: Symptoms appear before age 60. This type is much less common than late onset. However, it tends to get worse quickly.
2. **Late onset AD**: This is the most common type. It occurs in people age 60 and older.

AD is an accumulation of plaque that interferes with nerve conduction and even microcirculation in the brain. This has been found to be largely induced by the accumulation of toxic metallic particles in the brain. There are six toxic metals which have been found to be causative which include aluminum, mercury, lead, cadmium, iron, and manganese.

SYMPTOMS:

Changes in personality, memory loss, difficulty speaking, difficulty performing normal tasks, getting lost on familiar routes, flat mood or mood swings, misplacing items, loss of social skills, changes in sleep patterns, difficulty reading and writing, poor judgment, paranoia, agitation, anxiety, forgetting family members and/or who you are, incontinence, difficulty swallowing, loss of the ability to love.

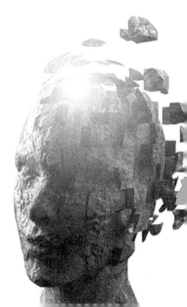

86

CONVENTIONAL TREATMENTS:

Conventional medicine offers no cure for AD. Their only efforts are to slow the progression of the disease, manage symptoms, and support family members who are having difficulty coping.

Typical prescription drugs for AD include:

* ❖ Donepezil (Aricept), Rivastigmine (Exelon), and Galantamine (Razadyne, formerly called Reminyl). Side effects include stomach upset, diarrhea, vomiting, muscle cramps, and fatigue.
* ❖ Memantine (Namenda). Possible side effects include agitation or anxiety.

Haloperidol, risperidone, and quetiapine are sometimes prescribed to control aggressive, agitated, or dangerous behaviors. However, they are typically given in very low doses due to the risk of side effects including an increased risk of death.

NATURAL TREATMENTS:

Perhaps one of the easiest and most effective aids to AD patients is modification of their diet. Many years ago, research was done and published in the *Yale Journal of Biological Medicine* that showed high protein diets exacerbated AD symptoms, and when they limited or deleted protein from their breakfast and lunch, symptoms were lessened and the amounts of medication could often be reduced. Many practitioners are failing their patients by not modifying their diets to exclude most proteins and increase complex carbohydrates, fruits and vegetables with small amounts of protein in the evening.

For optimal cognitive function, **B vitamins** are essential. Dozens of studies have linked elevations in homocysteine with increased risk of AD and other types of dementia. A hearty intake of vitamin B6, vitamin B12, and especially folic acid helps keep homocysteine in the normal range, prevents neuronal DNA damage, and reduces brain atrophy. An excellent B supplement is "Supreme B" and can be purchased at www.healthpro.com.dm/supremeb.html.

Ginkgo biloba has been shown in multiple studies to be an effective remedy for AD due to its antioxidant properties. Recommended dosage is 120 mg in the morning and 120 mg in the evening. Warning: Do not use ginkgo if you take blood-thinning medications like warfarin (Coumadin) or a class of antidepressants called monoamine oxidase inhibitors (MAOIs).

The major protein constituent of amyloid deposits in AD is the amyloid beta-peptide ("Abeta"). **St. John's Wort** contains a compound called hyperforin which has been shown to decrease amyloid deposit formation, decrease neuropathological changes and behavioral impairments, and prevent Abeta-induced neurotoxicity. What this means is that St. John's Wort, due to the hyperforin in contains, may be useful to decrease amyloid burden and toxicity in AD patients and may be an accepted therapeutic agent to fight the disease.   The therapeutic dosage of Saint John's Wort is 900 mg per day (taken as three 300 mg doses).

EDTA chelation therapy consists of I.V. drips of a synthetic amino acid, a protein, whose name is ethylene diamine tetraacetic acid, also known as EDTA. It consists of hydrogen, carbon, sodium, oxygen and nitrogen. It actually captures a metallic particle floating in the bloodstream or brain fluid, surrounds it and draws it into its center where it is trapped. The body has no use for EDTA and gets rid of it, so the EDTA molecule with the trapped metallic particle is urinated out of your system within 24 hours. This is sometimes a helpful way of detoxifying arteries and brain cells. Even the FDA affirms that chelation therapy is the best remedy for heavy-metal toxicity.

Dr. Richard Casdorph, the co-author of *Toxic Metal Syndrome*, found that when he gave chelation therapy to his patients to remove atherosclerotic plaques from the arteries, the minds of his patients began to clear up and function appropriately. He discovered that chelation therapy is effective at treating AD. Dr. Casdorph published his studies in professional journals, and many physicians around the world have adapted the Casdorph protocol for their own patients with AD.

A combination of **essential fatty acids** have also been found to help brain function and memory of AD patients. First and foremost is the omega-3 fatty acid DHA, which is most abundant in salmon, sardines, and other cold-water fish, as well as eggs from pastured hens, fish oil, cod liver oil, and cold-pressed flaxseed oil. DHA is a vital constituent of brain cell membranes. It is required for optimal cognitive function, and low levels are associated with mood and memory disturbances. We recommend 500 mg of DHA daily.

Resveratrol, a potent phytonutrient found in the skins and seeds of grapes, has also been found to be helpful. In lab studies, resveratrol promoted the breakdown of abeta-amyloid plaques, lesions found in the brains of patients with AD. It's widely believed to have therapeutic potential in the prevention and treatment of this neurodegenerative disorder. The suggested dose of resveratrol is 100 mg once or twice a day, taken with meals.

To keep your memory intact, it's also important to make sure you're getting plenty of **zinc**. Several studies recommend 30 mg of zinc along with 2 mg of **copper** daily. Finally, if you or a loved one are already facing a diagnosis of AD, try supplementing with medium chain triglycerides (MCTs), natural fatty acids that are abundant in **coconut oil**. This has also been found to be helpful in several studies.

And don't forget to be active! Both physical and mental exercises reduce the risk of AD. Regular physical activity ensures robust blood flow and delivery of oxygen and nutrients to the brain. It also reduces age-related changes. Mental activity is also important. In other words, use it or lose it.

We also suggest removing cocoa, coffee, black tea, cola, and alcohol from the diet of AD patients.

FOR YOUR DOCTOR:

See page 230 for research and studies to share with your doctor.

ASTHMA

DESCRIPTION:

Asthma is a disorder that causes the bronchial passages, or airways of the lungs to swell and become spasmodic.

SYMPTOMS:

Typical symptoms are chest tightness, coughing, wheezing, and shortness of breath. Emergency symptoms include bluish color to the lips, difficulty breathing, anxiety, rapid pulse, sweating, and confusion coupled with drowsiness.

CONVENTIONAL TREATMENTS:

Asthma patients are typically prescribed either **control drugs** (to prevent asthma attacks) and/or **quick-relief drugs** (to use during

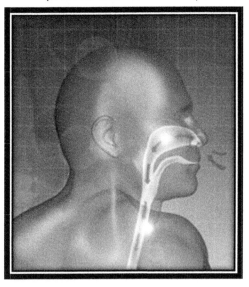

asthma attacks). Please be aware that many "rescue inhalers" that are used contain sulfites which may induce asthma. Many asthmatics are allergic to sulfites. If you're aware of this problem, ask your caregiver to prescribe Xopenex which is one of the only rescue inhalers that does not contain sulfites. Control drugs include inhaled corticosteroids and beta-agonist inhalers. Quick-relief drugs include short-acting bronchodilators (inhalers), such as Xopenex.

NATURAL TREATMENTS:

There are many herbs that offer relief for asthma sufferers. They are **aloe vera, passion fruit peel, astragalus, ginger, boswellia, mullein**, and **skullcap.**

Grind all of the herbs, measure maximum equal parts of each, place them in a large glass jar, then add just enough grain alcohol to cover the ingredients. Keep the mixture in a dark place and shake them twice daily for one month. At the end of one month, strain the liquid and then bottle it in dark glass bottles and use with honey as needed. In an emergency give 12 drops orally.

FOR YOUR DOCTOR:

See page 240 for research and studies to share with your doctor.

CANCER

DESCRIPTION:

Cancer is the uncontrolled growth of abnormal cells in the body.

SYMPTOMS:

Symptoms of cancer depend on the type and location of the cancer. Some cancers may not have any symptoms at all. In certain cancers, such as pancreatic cancer, symptoms often do not start until the disease has reached an advanced stage.

CONVENTIONAL TREATMENTS:

Typical conventional treatments for cancer are surgery, chemotherapy, and radiation.

NATURAL TREATMENTS:

For an exhaustive discussion on natural cancer treatments, please visit www.CancerTruth.net and purchase the book, *Cancer – Step Outside the Box.*

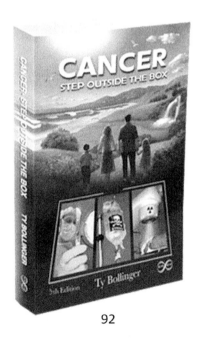

CARDIOVASCULAR DISEASE

Until recently overtaken by iatrogenic deaths (i.e. "prescription induced or physician induced"), cardiovascular disease was the number one killer in the USA. Cardiovascular disease is the occurrence of disease relating to the heart or blood vessels, including blood vessels in the brain. The term "cardiovascular disease" can encompass a variety of conditions, including **heart disease** (blockage of one or more of the main arteries that supply blood to the heart), **stroke** (sudden loss of consciousness or motion due to a rupture or clot of an artery in the brain), and **heart attacks** (when a portion of the heart muscle dies due to loss of blood supply and oxyen).

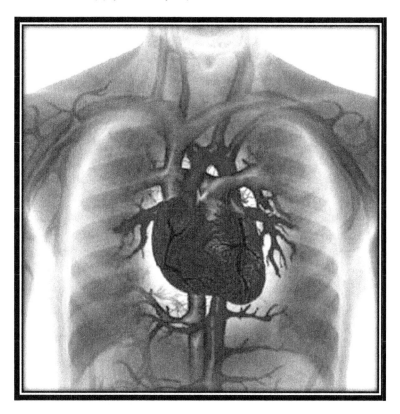

The question that we need to ask is, "***What are the causes of cardiovascular disease?***"

The answer is twofold:

1) **atheroslerosis** (plaque build-up in the arteries), which causes
2) **high blood pressure** (hypertension) which results in abnormally high pressure on the arterial walls.

This being so, in this chapter, we will focus our attention on hypertension and atherosclerosis.

1.   Hypertension

DESCRIPTION:

Hypertension is the term used to describe high blood pressure. Blood pressure is a measurement of the force against the walls of your arteries as your heart pumps blood throughout your body. There many identifiable causes for high blood pressure, which include factors like stress, alcohol, smoking, weight and lack of physical activity all seem to work together to produce this problem and must also include genetics and musculoskeletal injuries.

While everyone understands the genetic factors, few are trained in the musculoskeletal problems which can induce hypertension. Cervical injuries may cause abnormal increases in the strap muscles of the neck. If these muscles shorten and have reduced range, they have been shown to increase pressure on both the internal and external carotid arteries. This increase in arterial flow will cause increases in blood pressure and is almost always overlooked. Stretching to break down the scar tissue, as well as ranging the neck and ice packs will often reduce cervical induced hypertension.

SYMPTOMS:

Typically there are no symptoms of hypertension, though headaches and rapid heartbeat sometimes occur.

CONVENTIONAL TREATMENTS:

One or more of these blood pressure medicines are often used to treat high blood pressure: **diuretics** (water pills), **beta-blockers** (slow down the heart), **calcium channel blockers** (stop calcium from entering cells and relax blood vessels), and **ACE inhibitors** (relax blood vessels).

Recently, it has become apparent that the method used to lower blood pressure is very important. Research has shown that ACE inhibitor drugs produce added protective effects on the heart, kidneys, and brain. It seems the protective effects of these classes of drugs on these organs in patients with hypertension far exceed the protective effects produced by just lowering the blood pressure.

In the heart, these drugs reduce heart attacks (myocardial infarction), and in the brain, they reduce strokes. In the kidneys, ACE inhibitors have been shown to also reduce proteinuria (loss of protein in the urine), preserve and protect renal (kidney) function, and slow the progression of renal failure. This has been found to be particularly true in diabetics.

NATURAL TREATMENTS:

If you are an overweight male or female with hypertension, you most likely have low **testosterone** levels, or low testosterone to estradiol ratios. This is also the reason obesity is so prevealent in cardiac patients. In 2002, Dr. Roberto Fogari (and colleagues at the University of Pavia, Italy) looked at 110 men newly diagnosed with hypertension and compared them with the same number of healthy men. The researchers found that the men with high blood pressure had about 12% less circulating testosterone.

It's important to find a physician that is aware of the importance of adequate testosterone and is aware of the ramifications of low testosterone levels on blood pressure. If you have low testosterone levels, simply taking natural testosterone (by prescription) can lower blood pressure and help you feel much better. Ask your physician to run a hormone profile which must include DHEA, androstenedione, free testosterone, free estradiol, and DHT. It is equally important to realize that testosterone will convert to estradiol or DHT if aromatization is not inhibited. A natural aromatase inhibitor such as De Aromatase should always be taken with androgen supplementation.

Hibiscus is a small tree with bright red flowers that are rich in flavonoids, minerals, and other nutrients. The flowers have a fruity taste that makes hibiscus popular as both hot and cold tea. Studies have demonstrated that hibiscus acts as a diuretc and a natural ACE inhibitor, relaxing blood vessels. Several trials using hibiscus extracts have suggested that hibiscus can lower blood pressure in people with hypertension.

Garlic contains allicin, a substance which has antibacterial, antioxidant, and anti-hypertension properties. In a pilot study at Clinical Research Center of New Orleans, 9 patients with severe hypertension were given a garlic preparation containing 1.3% allicin. Sitting blood pressure fell with a significant decrease in diastolic blood pressure within 14 hours of the dose.

Olives are an integral part of the Mediterranean diet, recognized to be one of the healthiest in the world, which has given rise to the "French paradox" (the riddle of how a nation of alcohol-quaffing, croissant-munching gourmands stays healthy and slim and virtually free of heart disease). Here's why: Oil made from olives has been found to reduce blood pressure. In a study conducted on the importance of olive oil, Dr. L. Aldo Ferrara (Associate Professor at the Frederico II University of Naples in Italy) discovered that the daily use of 40 grams of olive oil reduced the dosage of blood pressure medication in hypertensive patients by about 50%.

Oregano contains the compound "carvacrol" which has been proven to be effective against blood pressure. In a study (by researchers from Eskisehir Osmangazi University in Turkey) conducted on animal subjects, carvacrol was found to reduce arterial pressure, heart rate, as well as both systolic and diastolic blood pressures.

Hawthorn has traditionally been used to treat hypertension, and so has **cinnamon**. Lastly, **coenzyme Q10** can also be very effective at lowering blood pressure as well as reducing stress on the heart muscle. CoQ10 by itself is also known as ubiquinone, which can be thought of as "non-active" CoQ10. However, many studies have shown that the "active" form of CoQ10, ubiquinol, has the ability to absorb into the bloodstream and reduce fatigue even more effectively than ubiquinone. This may be especially important for the elderly. We both personally use the ubiquinol form of CoQ10.

Personally we have found **hibiscus tea** as well as **hawthorn capsules** and **coenzyme Q10** (ubiquinol) to be extremely effective at reducing hypertension, both safely and with the additional benefits found in ACE inhibitors. A dab of honey makes the tea very tasty and the coenzyme Q10 and hawthorn work synergistically to both lower blood pressure and protect the heart. If you are currently on other medication, please be sure to discuss these additions with your primary caregiver.

FOR YOUR DOCTOR:

See page 245 for research and studies to share with your doctor.

2.   Atherosclerosis

DESCRIPTION:

While heart disease and stroke get the blame for most deaths and illnesses related to cardiovascular disease, the real culprit is actually atherosclerosis, a condition in which an artery wall thickens as a result of the accumulation of plaque. Plaque is made up of fat, cholesterol, calcium, and other substances found in the blood. Over time, plaque hardens and narrows your arteries, which then limits the flow of oxygen-rich blood to your organs and other parts of your body. Atherosclerosis can affect any artery in the body, including arteries in the heart, brain, arms, legs, pelvis, and kidneys. As a result, different diseases may develop based on which arteries are affected. Atherosclerosis is the **cause** of heart disease, stokes, and heart attacks.

I (Dr. Farley) have always approached heart disease and athero-sclerosis a bit differently than most physicians. After doing several autopsies on hospital patients that had died from cardiovascular disease, I came to the conclusion that almost all cardiovascular disease was actually **endothelial disease**, thus in order to facilitate long term recovery, the regeneration of endothelial health was of primary importance. The endothelium is the inner lining of the arterial and venous walls which (in the case of atherosclerosis) becomes inflexible and clogged.

For many years, high cholesterol has been held responsible for atherosclerosis, degenerative heart function, and heart damage resulting from reduced blood flow to the heart. This is correct in some ways, but the approach of most conventional physicians is to reduce fat and cholesterol consumption and take statins or other medications to lower cholesterol. This is a very big mistake and is an excellent example of pharmaceutical or symptom-based medicine vs. comprehensive medicine. Please see the section on "Cholesterol" in order to familiarize yourself with the absolute necessity of cholesterol for optimal health (page 50).

Now that we understand the need for cholesterol, let's discuss why it is blamed for causing atherosclerosis. When a lesion is created on the endothelial tissue of arteries and veins, cholesterol is used to fill in the lesion to protect it from further harm and to keep it from enlarging. Cholesterol actually acts as a type of "glue" and rushes to repair endothelial damage. So, in order to determine what causes atherosclerosis, we must ask, "what causes the lesions to form in the first place?" This question is relatively easily answered, but very seldom addressed in conventional medicine. It is not that it is inadequately studied; there are 4,895 peer-reviewed articles in the National Library of Medicine that prove beyond a shadow of a doubt that **insulin** is the primary cause of these lesions.

The reason insulin levels rise is quite simple: insulin rises to reduce serum sugar levels. **If we ingest too much sugar, we will produce too much insulin**. The next obvious question is always "how much sugar is OK?" The answer will surprise you. Our bodies produce about 1 teaspoon full of glucose a day, which is all that we need. The rest of the calories and energy our bodies utilize should come from complex carbohydrates, such as whole grains, as well as fruits, nuts, berries, poultry, fish and meat. Please notice that sugar coated cereal, candy, ice cream, cupcakes, and sodas are not included in a healthy diet. This is why the prevalence of atherosclerosis rates is so high. **Too much sugar = elevated insulin levels = atherosclerosis.** This is an easy equation that is absolutely true. We are addicted to sugar.

At this point, we need to discuss sugar. Over the past several months there has been a commercial running on USA television. In the commercial there is a man or a woman walking through a corn field with a child. They say that they were concerned about corn syrup but after asking their doctor they were told "sugar is sugar" and that high fructose corn syrup (HFCS) is fine. Perhaps they are allowed to lie because the government subsidizes corn. We are not sure how they can run such a dishonest commercial, but it is a **total lie.** One type of sugar is very different from another type, and the amounts of insulin released as well as the amount of time over which it is released are directly dependent on the type of sugar consumed. **HFCS is one of the worst.**

The easiest way to see the differences is by looking at a glycemic index, which is a measure of the effects of carbohydrates in food on blood sugar levels. It estimates how much each gram of available carbohydrate (total carbohydrate minus fiber) in a food raises a person's blood glucose level following consumption of the food, relative to consumption of glucose. Glucose has a glycemic index of 100, by definition, and other foods have a lower glycemic index.

An excellent bit of work entitled "Healthy Sugar Alternatives" was written by Michael Edwards and posted June 12, 2012 in Organic Lifestyle Magazine. www.organiclifestylemagazine.com/healthy-sugar-alternatives/. He took the time to make an accurate comparison of the differences in the glycemic index of various sugars and artificial sweeteners. The lower the number the less insulin that will be secreted.

Sugars & Substitutes with their Glycemic Index

		Never a Healthy Sugar Alternative
Artificial Sweeteners	N/A	All artificial chemical sweeteners are toxic and can indirectly lead to weight gain, the very reason many people consume them. They should be avoided. In fact, given a choice between high fructose corn syrup and artificial sweeteners, we recommend high fructose corn syrup by far (though it's essentially asking if you should consume poison or worse poison).
Stevia	0	**Best Healthy Sugar Alternative** Though it is 200-300 times sweeter than table sugar,

stevia is not a sugar. Unlike other popular sweeteners, it has a glycemic index rating of less than 1 and therefore does not feed candida (yeast) or cause any of the numerous other problems associated with sugar consumption. Stevia & Truvia are not the same thing.

Xylitol	7	Xylitol is a natural sugar alcohol sweetener found in the fibers of fruits and vegetables which can cause bloating, diarrhea, and flatulence with initial consumption. It's said to be safe for pregnant women, and is said to possibly treat ear infections, osteoporosis, respiratory infections, candida, and is it even helps fight cavities. In Finland, virtually all gum is sweetened w/ xylitol.
Agave Nectar	15-30	A sweet syrup made from the Blue Agave plant, Agave Nectar is obtained by the extraction and purification of "sap" from the agave plant, which is broken down by natural enzymes into the monosaccharide's (simple sugars): mainly fructose (70-75%) and dextrose (20-26%).
Fructose	17	Though fructose has a low glycemic index rating, consumption should be limited. Fructose is linked to heart disease as it raises triglycerides and cholesterol. It is devoid of nutrition.
Brown Rice Syrup	85	It is not recommended for diabetics, since its sweetness comes from maltose, which is known to cause spikes in blood sugar.

100

Raw Honey	30	**A Healthy Sugar Alternative in moderation** With antioxidants, minerals, vitamins, amino acids, enzymes, carbohydrates, and phytonutrients, raw, unprocessed honey is considered a superfood by many alternative health care practitioners and a remedy for many health ailments. Choose your honey wisely. There is nothing beneficial about processed honey.
Coconut Palm Sugar	35	Originally made from the sugary sap of the Palmyra palm , the date palm or sugar date palm (Phoenix sylvestris). It's also made from the sap of coconut palms. With a relatively low glycemic index, Coconut palm sugar is the new rage among health nuts. It's often called "coconut nectar sugar" or "coconut sugar".
Apple Juice	40	Fresh apple juice is good for you, though we recommend eating fresh raw whole apples. Concentrated apple juice (used as a sweetener) is closer to refined sugar than fresh apple juice.
Barley Malt Syrup	42	Barley malt syrup is considered to be one of the healthiest sweeteners in the natural food industry. Barley malt is made by soaking and sprouting barley to make malt, then combining it with more barley and cooking this mixture until the starch is converted to sugar. The mash is then strained and cooked down to syrup or dried into powder.
Amasake	43	This is an ancient, Oriental whole grain sweetener made from cultured brown rice. It has a thick, pudding-like

consistency. It's not easy to find, but is a great alternative to refined table sugar.

Sugar Cane Juice	43	Sugar cane juice has many nutrients and other beneficial properties and is said by some health practitioners to be almost as medicinal as raw honey.
Organic Sugar	47	Organic sugar comes from sugar cane grown without the use of chemicals or pesticides. It is usually darker than traditional white sugar because it contains some molasses. (It has not been processed to the degree white sugar is processed).
Maple Syrup	54	Maple syrup is made by boiling sap collected from natural growth maple trees during March & April. It is refined sap and is therefore processed. It has a high glycemic index, and though it is much more nutritious then refined table sugar and high fructose corn syrup, there are better choices.
Evaporated Cane Juice	55	Evaporated cane juice is often considered unrefined sugar, but juicing is a refining process, and evaporating refines further. Though better than turbinado, cane juice (un-evaporated) is a better choice as a sweetener.
Black Strap Molasses	55	White refined table sugar is sugar cane with all the nutrition taken out. Black strap molasses is all of that nutrition that was taken away. A quality organic (must be organic!) molasses provides iron, calcium, copper, magnesium, phosphorus, potassium and zinc, and is

alkalizing to the body.

Turbinado	65	Turbinado is partially processed sugar, also called raw sugar.
Raw sugar	65	Raw sugar is not actually raw sugar. It is processed, though not as refined as common white table sugar. Therefore, given a choice between raw and white, choose raw. There are many different variations of raw sugar with many different names depending on how refined it is.
Cola (and most other sodas)	70	Though cola has a lower GI ranking then some might expect, there are many other reasons to avoid any type of soda. There is nothing beneficial to the human body inside a can of soda (not to mention we should avoid drinking out of aluminum cans!).
Corn Syrup	75	Corn syrup has very little nutrition and should be avoided.
Refined, Pasteurized Honey	75	The nutrition is gone, and there is often high fructose corn syrup added to processed honey. Refined pasteurized honey is no better than white table sugar.
Refined Table Sugar	80	Conventionally grown, chemically processed, and striped of all beneficial properties, many health advocates believe that refined sugar is one of the two leading causes (high fructose corn syrup is the other) of nearly every health ailment known to man (or woman or child). Not only does it have a high GI ranking, but it also is extremely acidic to

		the body causing calcium and other mineral depletion from bones and organs (sugar is alkaline but has a very acidic effect on the body).
High Fructose Corn Syrup	87	Many health advocates believe that high fructose corn syrup and refined sugar are the two biggest contributors to health ailments in our society. High fructose corn syrup is a combination of sucrose and fructose.
Glucose (AKA Dextrose)	100	White bread was the benchmark, but for consistency glucose now holds the rating at 100.
Maltodextrin	150	Foods that have maltodextrin often say "Low Sugar" or "Complex Carbohydrate", but this sweetener should be avoided!

Now it is easy to see how dishonest the corn syrup commercial really is. It is also easy to see why the prevalence of atherosclerosis is so high in the USA and is growing with the Western diet as it expands around the world.

Though sugars play a very important role in Western food induced atherosclerosis, there are other major contributing factors. Heavy metals also play a major role and when the two are combined, the disease process will be accelerated and the complications are multiplied. A few of these heavy metals are included, such as lead, mercury, and cadmium.

SYMPTOMS:

Chest pain or discomfort (angina) is the most common symptom. It may feel heavy or like someone is squeezing your heart, with pain under your breast bone (sternum), but also in your neck, arms, stomach, or upper back. The pain usually occurs with activity or emotion, and goes away with rest. Other symptoms include shortness of breath and fatigue with activity (exertion).

Conventional Treatments:

You may be asked to take one or more medicines to treat blood pressure, diabetes, or high cholesterol levels. Treatment depends on your symptoms and how severe the disease is.

Your doctor may give you one or more medicines to treat cardiovascular disease, including:

- ❖ Diuretics to lower blood volume and therefor lower blood pressure and treat heart failure
- ❖ Beta-blockers to lower heart rate and blood pressure
- ❖ ACE inhibitors to lower blood pressure
- ❖ Aspirin to help prevent blood clots from forming in your arteries
- ❖ Calcium channel blockers to relax arteries and lower blood pressure
- ❖ Nitrates (such as nitroglycerin) to stop chest pain and improve blood flow to the heart
- ❖ Statins to lower cholesterol

Remember that you should **never** abruptly stop taking these medications. Always check with your primary caregiver first.

Natural Treatments:

In our opinion, **removing heavy metal burdens** (if they exist) is imperative as a first step. If heavy metal toxicity is not found, then you can move on to the next section, but be absolutely sure heavy metal toxicity is not part of the problem, or there will likely be no long-term improvement.

Testing for heavy metal toxicity is easy, though we don't consider a hair test to be an accurate test, since you may have been exposed to a toxic heavy metal several years ago, but have since cleared it from your system. However, it may still show up in your hair. There are other more exact ways to measure heavy metal burdens. We believe that the testing of whole blood is the most accurate method, followed by urine testing.

There are a few points to understand. Lead is stored in the bones. Very little of your body's lead will be in the blood. If you find chelation is needed, your lead levels will drop and then return as lead is pulled from the bone and goes back into circulation again. Mercury will hide in various tissues, so chelation will not have a real immediate effect. Remember that it takes time to remove toxic heavy metal burdens, so be patient.

At this point, we would like to briefly discuss **chelation** (the preferred method of heavy metal removal). By far the most proven and medically accepted method of removing toxic metals is through EDTA I.V. chelation. A properly trained physician will perform the I.V. chelation 2 to 3 times per week at his own comfort level (which will depend greatly on your response). He will probably add additional adjunctive substances to the chelation bag to both increase its effectiveness as well as to replace the needed minerals that are removed along with the heavy metals. You will need at least a day or two after each treatment in order to replenish the minerals that are lost with EDTA therapy. Make sure your caregiver has suggestions on supplemental nutritional requirements. This process may take anywhere from 15 to 45 treatments to get heavy metal levels down to the low normal range, which is where you want them to be.

Dietary change must be addressed. First of all, to the very best of your ability, you must remove all **sugars** and **simple carbohydrates** from your diet. A sweet tooth is normal; most of us crave sweets. We crave honey, molasses, maple syrup, cane sugar, and other naturally sweet food due to their value as quick energy. But we must learn to control these cravings, which is not an easy thing to do. The fact is that these sugar cravings could easily be called an "addiction" since they can be even stronger than cravings for heroin, tobacco, or opiates. That is because it is part of genetic makeup for survival. For me (Dr. Farley) personally, giving up sweets is the hardest thing I have to deal with every day. And yes, I too have these cravings.

For me, the best way is simple replacement. When I crave something that tastes sweet, I will eat a thin slice of carrot, or a few. They do taste sweet, and although they aren't sweet like a candy bar, they are sweet enough that the taste and chewing usually relieve my craving. I have also started eating more fruit, though I do not eat it in excess. Very fresh organic vegetables (such as tomatoes) are sometimes very good eaten raw. The key is to consciously place something in your mouth that is healthy whenever you have cravings for sweets. It will take a few weeks, but they will start tasting better as you go along, and your cardiovascular health will start to improve. The **less** sugar the **less** endothelium damage, the **less** chance of plaque buildup. A side benefit is you will lose fat, feel better with more energy, look and feel younger, and improve your immune function.

As a side note, we are really against genetically modified food (GMO). There are numerous health problems associated with consuming GMO foods, so if you are going to eat more healthy foods, please try to make them organic. Also please support (in any way possible) the small "mom and pop" organic family farms. They deserve our help for their diligent efforts to produce the highest quality healthy food possible.

We do not support a completely vegetarian diet, as it is very difficult to supply all of the required amino acids without supplementing with fish, fowl, and occasional other meats. Due to the increasing food allergies to beef, we are suspicious that the GMO grains they are using to "finish out" the cattle is being concentrated in their muscle and passed along to consumers. We're not certain about this, but we have found out that deer wasting syndrome (a wasting disease that causes them to lose weight and die) on the East Coast of the USA was traced back to GMO corn. However, most of the research was sponsored by the U.S. Department of Agriculture (USDA) and was never published.

If you are going to eat chicken, again, make sure it is organic, since you do not want the hormones or antibiotics that large scale operations inject into their chickens. The same rule applies to fish. Only buy wild caught fish; never farm raised, since farm raised fish (in large part) come from China where the fish are raised in contaminated water. Another problem with farm raised fish is that they have a much less varied diet, so they do not contain the nutritional value of wild fish. We realize that organic food is more expensive, but you will require less food if what you consume is more nutrient dense. And if you stop eating sweets, you'll have more money to spend on healthy food and won't be spending as much money on "medicine."

Arginine has become very well known for its major contribution in the treatment of cardiovascular disease. Among its proven traits is the ability to induce vasodilation, which means it relaxes the walls of the arteries through its ability to enhance "endothelial NO synthase" (eNOS) actions and reduce oxidative stress. Arginine has also been proven to prevent the progression of atherosclerosis in patients already inflicted with the disease, prevent free radical damage to the endothelial lining, prevent abnormal blood clotting, and reduce angina pain. We would never count on one supplement to correct this type of complex problem, but arginine is one of our top choices. If you are currently on blood pressure medication, be sure to work closely with your primary caregiver. Clinical trials that have demonstrated the value of arginine (in the treatment of angina and hypertension) have involved the use of 6,000 mg per day. Clinical trials using arginine for the treatment of congestive heart failure have involved the use of 5,600 to 12,600 mg per day. You should discuss the supplemental amount with your primary caregiver. It is an extremely safe supplement and medically monitored subjects have been given 60 grams a day without any ill effects.

Berberine has been used for several centuries for the treatment of type 2 diabetes as well as atherosclerosis and infections. Its many mechanisms are only now being investigated using scientific models, rather than empirical evidence. Science has shown that it is capable of numerous actions that are of benefit to atherosclerotic patients. It increases insulin sensitivity, thereby decreasing the amount of insulin secreted. The less insulin, the less likely new lesions will form to be filled with new plaque. This trait is especially important with diabetic patients. It has also shown itself to be able to prevent abnormal new arterial tissue to form, thereby reducing arterial blockage. Berberine has is an ability to decrease abnormal oxidative stress on the cardiovascular system, which prevents further oxidative damage. It also possesses the ability to lower both systolic and diastolic blood pressure, so be sure to work closely with your primary caregiver if you are currently on blood pressure medicine. Berberine is found in high concentrations in the herb goldenseal.

Green tea has been shown to contain many beneficial phytochemicals. One of the most thoroughly studied aspects of green tea is its polyphenol/catechin contents actions. The catechins of green tea possess many good qualities that directly relate to atherosclerosis. For

108

instance, they help prevent obesity as well as help with weight loss. This is of particular improtance since many atherosclerotic patients (due to being insulin resistant) tend to become obese. Another benefit of the catechins is that they reduce the levels of triglycerides and LDL, which means a few cups of green tea a day may be helpful. But remember, if you add sugar (or other similar sweetener), the positive benefits of the green tea may be overshadowed by the negative effects of the sweetener.

Vitamin C should also be a part of the treatment regimen. It is also easy to place in the liposomal form for much better tissue and organ absorption. Vitamin C has too many studies verifying its numerous roles to go over them all, but here are a few functions. Vitamin C has shown it offers protection of nitrous oxide from inactivation by oxygen free radicals. As previously shown, nitrous oxide allows normal dilation of blood vessels and protects the endothelium.   Low vitamin C has been shown to increase atherosclerosis by lowering HDL, raising LDL and triglycerides, and lowering the integrity of the vascular wall. Vitamin C has also been shown to offer some protection for smokers by slowing the progression of atherosclerosis and reduces the acceleration of arterial stiffness associated with atherosclerosis. This is especially true when it is combined with vitamin E. Used at higher dosages or with a liposomal delivery system, vitamin C has been shown to actually reduce some plaque formation and prevent further formation of new plaque.

Fish oil has been known for quite some time to be effective in lowering triglycerides in atherosclerosis patients. Elevated triglycerides may result not only in increased atherosclerosis, but also may increase the chances of developing (or worsening) diabetes, hypertension, pancreatitis, ischemic heart disease, male infertility and kidney failure. Other benefits of fish oil include inhibiting further atherosclerosis, preventing fatal arrhythmias, and decreasing mortality subsequent to heart attacks.

Research has shown that **lycopene** possesses many benefits for the atherosclerotic patient. Lycopene has shown itself to aid in reducing the progression of the disease, as well as preventing abnormal blood clotting, which reduces the chances of a stroke or pulmonary embolism. It is also known to concentrate in the heart and some studies have shown it reduces the chances of heart attack up to 48%.

These reasons are more than ample to justify adding lycopene to your dietary intake if you are atherosclerotic. Many studies have shown an added benefit of lowering the blood pressure as well.

Though **vitamin E** has not been shown to lower serum cholesterol levels, it has shown itself to be capable of reducing the areas of aortic lesions, as well as inhibiting plaque formation and reducing further atherosclerotic lesion formation and aortic fatty streak areas very effectively. Vitamin E has also shown the ability to increase nitrous oxide metabolite concentrations, which shows one of its mechanisms for endothelial protection. It also inhibits platelet aggregation and adhesion, which in turn prevents smooth muscle proliferation, thus preserving normal coronary dilation. Another mechanism vitamin E uses to retain more normal arterial dilation is inhibition of macrophage accumulation in the aorta. Vitamin E also reduces oxidative LDL stress and conserves intimal thickness.

Though we have listed several supplements, all have a place in a more comprehensive approach to the treatment of atherosclerosis. It is important to work closely with your primary caregiver to monitor your progress and coordinate reduction or elimination of pharmaceuticals that you may be taking that have many more side effects. There are literally hundreds of herbs and other supplements that we could have added, however we have only put those that are very well peer-reviewed and have worked well in actual practice.

FOR YOUR DOCTOR:

See page 250 for research and studies to share with your doctor.

CELIAC DISEASE

DESCRIPTION:

Celiac disease (CD), put into simple terms, is a digestive system ailment in which the jejunum of the small intestine fails to absorb and properly digest food. One of its primary characterizations is histological lesions that vary from partial to total atrophy of the small intestine's villi cells. These lesions are caused by an allergic reaction to gluten. The

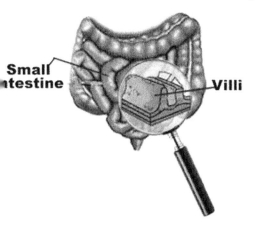

villi (small hair like structures in the small intestine) are unable to do their job of grabbing nutrients out of the gluten containing foods resulting in malabsorption of important nutrients. To compound the problem those villi, which in healthy people stand up straight, get pressed down in people with celiac rendering them useless over time and causing permanent damage to the intestines.

CD is felt to be hereditary and it is often characterized as an auto-immune disease. It is also much more prevalent than thought, or more likely, has increased, due to more frequent challenges to our digestive system by genetically modified foods and gluten sources as well as pesticides and other contaminants. At present, just less than 4% of our population is thought to be affected by CD, but the numbers are increasing with each passing day. It is interesting to note that persons of Asian and African ancestry are usually not affected by CD.

In more complex terms, CD is a health condition that some people associate with simple gluten intolerance. However, CD is felt to be a multi-system autoimmune disease in which many changes in the body occur, including direct changes in liver function, digestive tract function, and gastrointestinal dysbiosis. The term "dysbiosis" refers to the condition when good bacteria in the gut flora (required for immune system function and proper digestion) are overrun by pathogenic bacteria (which cause harm).

A specific enzyme called tissue transglutaminase (tTG) appears to be especially important in CD. Short strands of proteins, called (polypeptides) found in gliadin (one family of wheat proteins) are acted on by this enzyme, and many resulting problems associated with CD will result when tTG is not available to act on this protein.

Blood tests that are able to measure the level of autoantibodies such as anti-tissue transglutaminase (tTGA), and IgA anti-endomysium antibodies (AEA), are found to be elevated in CD patients. However, it should be noted that these tests will return a "false-negative" if a CD patient has been consuming a gluten-free diet. Measurement of antibodies to gliadin and reticulin can also be performed via blood tests, but these tests are not nearly as reliable and often give false results. CD may also have been shown to raise the risk of cancer, diabetes, dementia, depression, lupus, adrenal insufficiency, and neuropathy.

SYMPTOMS:

Anemia caused by the inability to absorb nutrients, damage to the cardiovascular system, dilated cardiomyopathy, abdominal pain and diarrhea, bloating, chronic fatigue, vomiting, constipation, itchy skin, seizures, and sometimes nosebleeds.

As you can see from the symptoms, there are several body systems affected by CD. Without proper absorption of specific nutrients which require the enzyme tissue tTGA, numerous detrimental effects occur, some of which (including cardiomyopathy and other cardiovascular damage) may be fatal.

CONVENTIONAL TREATMENTS:

According to conventional wisdom, CD has no cure. A lifelong gluten-free diet is typically recommended. Foods, beverages, and medications that contain wheat, barley, rye, and possibly oats are typically forbidden. Occasionally, corticosteroids (such as prednisone) may also be prescribed in order to lower the inflammation from the disease.

It is vital to understand that corn also contains gluten, which, as all celiac patients know, is very bad for you. Many physicians are not aware of this, as we were generally taught in school that corn was a good replacement for wheat, rye, etc. **This is not correct.** After

112

treating many CD patients and getting them to the point that they were feeling good, I noticed that many still had from a few to several short periods of symptoms every month. I would request an exact copy of their diet for a full month and soon found a direct correlation between the consumption of corn and their symptoms. I visited many medical libraries and found that research had proven not only that corn contained gluten, but that it had a direct effect on CD as well as Crohn's disease and ulcerative colitis.

CD patients need to keep their diet strict and eat only fresh organic vegetables, fruits, fish and fowl. To replace gluten laden products, we recommend small amounts of white potatoes, sweet potatoes, and long grain rice.

Experience has proved that many CD patients are adrenally insufficient and do require additional corticosteroids. However, if the disease is handled properly, low "physiological doses" of hydrocortisone are adequate and do not have the side effects of other pharmaceutical steroids. Another advantage is that hydrocortisone is exactly the same hormone that your own adrenal would produce. It has exactly the same half-life and may be given upon rising, at noon, and again in the evening to reproduce the body's own natural pulsatile secretion times. It may also be started at a low supplementation dose and then slowly built up as (and if) needed. Since we know that the normal adult secretes from 20 to 30 mg daily, it is easy to start them at 5 mg three times daily, which is called a physiological dose (i.e. a dose that is intended to support your own adrenals rather than attempt to replace them).

Natural Treatments:

There are many herbs and other supplements (such as minerals and vitamins) that, when combined, may offer relief to CD patients as well as offer protection from deficiency diseases that may occur. The first supplement we would like to suggest is **copper**. It has been found that celiac patients are deficient in copper. The normal copper dosage would be 1.2 to 2 mg per day for an adult. Most CD patients are also deficient in **zinc**, so supplemental zinc will help to counteract this deficiency. The normal dosage from zinc would be from 15 to 50 mg/day for an adult. Most CD patients are also found to be deficient in **selenium** and **carnitine** (indicating that supplemental selenium and carnitine may benefit these patients). The normal adult dosage of selenium is 200 mcg/day and the normal dosage for carnitine is 1000 to 2000 mg/day (in divided doses).

There are also several extremely important vitamins that also fail to be absorbed so that celiac patients are often very deficient in these essential elements of health. Most CD patients are found to be deficient in **vitamin A.** The normal dosage for vitamin A is 5,000 IU per day for men and 2,500 IU per day for women. We are not using maximum therapeutic doses. They are not needed if better absorption is accomplished. Women that are pregnant should not use more than 1000 IU per day. CD patients are typically deficient in **vitamin B6** as well, indicating supplemental vitamin B6 will be required for total care. The normal requirement would be about 80 mg/day for an adult. Low levels of vitamin B6 have been directly linked to depression which again is directly linked to CD. The normal replacement dosage may run from 50 to 250 mg/day. In combining these vitamins and supplements we believe that 100 mg would be more than adequate. **Vitamin B12** is also deficient in CD patients; low energy is one indication of low B12 levels. The recommended dosage for vitamin B12 is 1000 mcg/day. Please note difference between mcg (micrograms) and mg (milligrams). This is **extremely** important.

Many CD patients are also found to be deficient in **vitamin D**. Since low vitamin D levels have now been directly linked to specific cancers, these chronic low levels may be directly linked to the increased cancer rate in CD patients. This makes vitamin D supplementation of vital importance for these patients. The normal supplemental dosage would be 4000 IU of vitamin D3. Though many physicians will recommend higher doses for rickets and other bone disease, this is a very healthy dose of vitamin D that is safe for long term use. **Vitamin E** deficiency is also common with CD patients, and there are numerous problems associated with the low levels of vitamin E. Numerous studies show that neurological disorders are being linked to this deficiency. Vitamin E is absorbed through the ileum of the small intestines along with other dietary fats into the lymph and then into the blood for further storage in the liver. Since CD does not allow this pathway, it is important to not only supplement, but make sure it is *absorbed*. The optimal dosage for vitamin E is 400 to 800 IU/day. This is one reason that the use of liposomal delivery may be needed.

Many CD patients are found to be deficient in **vitamin K**, which is imperative to cardiovascular health. Vitamin K may be safely supplemented with between 1 and 10 mg/day. This definitely needs to be addressed with your primary caregiver, especially if you are taking anti-coagulant drugs. Though it seems like an endless list, all these vitamins are essential for good health and longevity, especially if you have CD.

Reduction of inflammation of the bowel is an especially important part of the comprehensive treatment of CD, as chronic inflammation places the body in a constant state of stress. **Lycopene** has shown itself to be very beneficial in reducing this chronic inflammation of the bowel. A dosage of about 20 mg/day, lycopene has been shown to be an effective adult dosage.

Pancreatic enzymes have been shown to be helpful in a large number of CD cases. They do not need (nor should they be used) in a liposome. They should be taken after each meal to assist in digestion. Oftentimes labeled as "digestive enzymes," the normal dosage is 500 to 1000 mg per meal.

The last supplements we will discuss are **probiotics.** The best choice is a "broad spectrum" probiotic, since the wider the diversity of probiotics, the better the outcome will be. Everyone carries many normal probiotics in the gastrointestinal tract, and it is difficult to maintain this diverse flora, even without CD. Antibiotics can destroy the majority of beneficial flora to the point of "dysbiosis" (discussed earlier in this section). CD patients also have a tendency to be more acidic than those not suffering from the disease, and this acidic condition makes it more difficult to keep normal healthy probiotics growing properly. Unfortunately, due to the nature of the CD, probiotics must be taken for as long as you suffer from the disease, which is typically for life. However, on the bright side, this also means that there is a way to have good health without suffering from the harmful effects of this disease. Probiotics are best taken between meals, and it is recommended to follow the directions on the box. They vary greatly in potency, and the highest quality probiotics typically require refrigeration.

At this point, many CD patients may be taking some (or most) of these supplements, yet are still suffering from some effects of the disease. If this is the case, the reason is very simple. Since absorption of these supplements is needed, and CD, by definition does not allow specific nutritional absorption, these supplements are wasted by many patients. Passing through the gastrointestinal tract without absorption is a waste, but there is a way to facilitate the absorption of these nutrients, which we will discuss next. It requires about an hour's work every week, but the increase in useful absorption and monetary savings seems well worth the effort.

MAKING A LIPOSOME

Liposomes are bilayer (double-layer), liquid-filled bubbles made from phospholipids. The bilayer structure of liposomes is nearly identical to the bilayer construction of the cell membranes that surround each of the cells in the human body. The phosphate (source of "phospho" in phospholipid) head of phospholipids is hydrophilic (it loves water), whereas the fatty-acid tails (lipids) are hydrophobic (they hate water). Researchers have discovered that these spheres can be filled with therapeutic agents and used to protect and deliver these agents into the body and even into specific cells of the body.

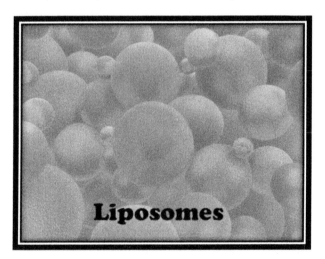

Liposomal encapsulation is a process that has made the use of natural herbal formulas much more effective. New forms of liposomes are being designed almost every day, with newer and better carrier liposomes as well as liposomes that are specific in early passage directly through the intestinal wall to directly access the blood supply, as well as some that deliver their active ingredients slowly, over a period of time.

Many believe this to be a brand new technology; however Native Americans learned long ago about the absorption and associated problems with some herbs over one thousand years ago. Many of their formulations actually required preparation with various animal tallows and sometimes also used plant extracts much like soy lecithin.

Prior to the liposome, many active components of herbal medicines, vitamins, and minerals were lost through the digestive process. In the past 20 years, advanced herbal products (such as LifeOne and Supreme B) have used liposomal delivery methods to deliver the maximum amount of actives in the herbal supplements. Liposomes also facilitate much better delivery of vitamins and minerals. However, their liposomal matrix is far more complex than will be presented in this book, due to the fact that actual complex delivery systems require several steps to produce.

Celiac disease patients are not the only ones who have trouble absorbing vitamins, minerals, and herbal active compounds. Those suffering from Crohn's disease, irritable bowel disease, as well as cancer patients, people suffering from gastrointestinal dysbiosis, or even elderly and chronically ill people will have difficulty in absorbing nutrients. For these people, the liposomal delivery system can mean the difference between getting well and remaining ill.

Brooks Bradley came up with a very simple way to make a liposomal carrier, specifically for vitamin C. Though he specifically designed it to carry vitamin C, with a few minor adjustments it may be used to carry many more constituents, such as other vitamins, minerals, and some herbal components. Here are his directions and statements.

Our vitamin C liposomal encapsulation protocol is as follows:

Using a small (2 cup) ultrasonic cleaner, like the ones sold at Harbor Freight for around $30.00, we performed the following:

1. Dissolved 3 level tablespoons of soy lecithin in 1 cup (240 ml) of distilled water.
2. Dissolved 1 level tablespoon of ascorbic acid powder (vitamin C) in half a cup (120 ml) of distilled water.

3. Pour both solutions together in the ultrasonic cleaner bowl and turned the unit on. Using a plastic straw (leaving the top of the cleaner open) gently, slowly, stirred the contents. Note: The cleaner will automatically self-stop every 2 minutes. Just push the ON button to continue. Repeat for a total of 3 series or 6 minutes   total. By that time the entire solution should be blended into a cloudy, homogeneous, milk-like mixture. The liposome is now formed.

4. This protocol furnishes about 12 grams (12,000 mg) of vitamin C product at 70% encapsulation efficiency or 8,400 mg of the liposome. This solution will keep at room temperature for 3 to 4 days. Refrigerated, it will keep much longer. So at the end, approximately 43 ml of this final solution should give you approximately 1 gram of liposomal vitamin C.

The homogenizing effect is so powerful that after 3 days at room temperature, no precipitation of solution separation appears evident. This type of sequestered vitamin c has demonstrated to be at least 5 times more effective than any other form of orally ingested vitamin c that we tested. Additionally, it appears to be even more rapid in tissue-bed availability than intravenously applications.   An astounding revelation to us!

When you are using this method, remember this is a general method and if you change amounts, you have to change all amounts, but it is important to keep ratios for the liposome the same. When you try to place all of the vitamins, minerals, and supplements in the liposomal mixture, you will find not all will become encapsulated. That is not a huge problem, because some will be encapsulated or incorporated in to the mixture, thus shaking the mixture before taking it will encapsulate the remaining ingredients.

Please remember that with comprehensive care, the problems of CD may be alleviated, and even in the worst cases, patients are frequently able to become healthy. The key is a comprehensive approach that allows the body to absorb nutrients and vitamins (that are not generally absorbed by CD patients) and to prevent dysbiosis by maintaining normal healthy gut flora.

FOR YOUR DOCTOR:

See page 286 for research and studies to share with your doctor.

DIABETES MELLITUS

DESCRIPTION:

"Diabetes" comes from Greek and it means a "siphon." Aretus the Cappadocian, a Greek physician during the second century AD, named the condition "diabainein." He said that patients who were passing too much water were like a siphon. The word became "diabetes" from the English adoption of the Latin term. In 1675, Thomas Willis added "mellitus" to the term, although it is commonly referred to simply as diabetes. The term "mel" is Latin for "honey"; the urine and blood of people with diabetes has excess glucose (sugar), and glucose is sweet like honey. Diabetes mellitus literally means "siphoning off sweet water."

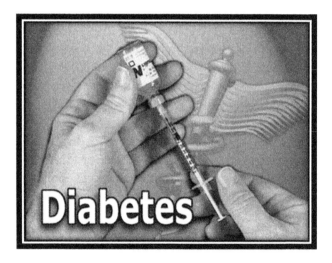

Diabetes mellitus describes a group of metabolic diseases in which the person has high blood glocose (hyperglycemia), either because insulin production is inadequate or because the cells of the body do not respond properly to insulin, or both. **Insulin** is a hormone that is produced by the pancreas which makes it possbile for cells to take in glucose. After eating, the pancreas automatically releases an adequate quantity of insulin to move the glucose present in our blood into the cells, and as soon as glucose enters the cells, the level of glucose in the blood drops. But with diabetes, the cells don't get the glucose – it remains in the blood and is eventually excreted in the urine.

There are three main types of diabetes:

1) **Type 1 diabetes** (aka juvenile diabetes, early-onset diabetes, or insulin dependent diabetes) occurs when the body does not produce insulin. Approximately 10% of diabetics have type 1 diabetes, which lasts the whole lifetime of the person and has to be managed carefully with insulin that is adequate to move the glucose into the cells. Also required is a diet of complex carbohydrates, proteins, and adequate fluid which will help to limit the up and down spikes of glucose levels. Typical foods are vegetables, fish, poultry, other meats, and fruits (in limited amounts). What is seldom explained to these patients is that proteins also induce and require insulin for proper processing and cellular uptake, so caution should also be used when ingesting concentrated proteins.

2) **Type 2 diabetes** (aka adult-onset diabetes) occurs when the body does not produce enough insulin for proper function, or the cells in the body do not react to insulin (insulin resistance). Adult onset is actually a misnomer, due to the fact that we are seeing an increase of childhood type 2 diabetes due to poor diet, poor education, and abysmal school food programs (such as allowing soda machines in the schools). Approximately 90% of all cases of diabetes worldwide are of this type, and it has grown and spread along with our Western diet. This is a progressive disease that starts with poor dietary habits that include the intake of too much sugar and simple carbohydrates. As high volumes of simple sugars are ingested, insulin is excreted by the pancreas to move the glucose into the blood cells. As this occurs, the cellular receptors to insulin become desensitized to insulin, so more insulin is needed. This insulin receptor desensitization leads to both higher serum glucose levels and higher insulin levels. As discussed previously in this book, insulin causes lesions to form in the endothelium of the blood vessels which lead to plaque formation in the blood vessels lining. This restricts normal blood flow and results in dramatic increases in heart disease and stroke, hypertension, blindness and eye problems, kidney disease, nervous system disease, amputations, dental disease, complications of pregnancy and other severe conditions, including depression, depressed immune system, coma, and diminished endurance (especially among the elderly).

3) **Gestational diabetes** affects females during pregnancy. Some women have very high levels of glucose in their blood, and their bodies are unable to produce enough insulin to transport all of the glucose into their cells, resulting in progressively rising levels of glucose. This is usually controlled by a strict diet. Gestational diabetes must be controlled or severe complications may result. As the estrogen levels rise during pregnancy, the body tries to store fat, and cravings often take the place of good judgment when choosing food.   Exercise is also recommended for gestational diabetes and is very helpful. Consult with your trusted primary caregiver to get reliable information on a recommended exercise routine.

As of the writing of this book, the most recent statistics indicate that almost 26 million Americans (adults and children) are afflicted with diabetes.

SYMPTOMS:

The characteristic symptoms are excessive urination (polyuria), excessive thirst (polydipsia), glucose in the urine (glucosuria), unexplained weight loss, and a poor diet (which may result in weight gain and lethargy).

CONVENTIONAL TREATMENTS:

As stated before, **type 1 diabetes** lasts a life time and there is no known cure. Patients are treated with regular insulin injections, as well as a special diet and exercise. This is not to say that following the instructions for type 2 diabetes will not help. We have seen numerous patients dramatically reduce required insulin amounts by following the same regime.

The *National Institute of Diabetes and Digestive and Kidney Diseases* states that **type 2 diabetes** usually lasts a lifetime; however, with knowledgeable and strict diet control and a regular exercise, it is typically manageable. As we discussed earlier in this book, sugar addiction is very hard to break, however, once you break the addiction, you will be a great deal healthier and will live longer. Simple sugars, artificial sugar substitutes, and simple carbohydrate intake are the greatest cause for the USA ranking so low on the worldwide longevity scale. Parents also need to realize that cereals with added sugars, undiluted fruit juices (such as apple juice), and white potatoes and white rice all contribute hugely to your child developing obesity, insulin resistance, and type 2 diabetes. If you wish what is best for your child, insist on outdoor activities with good exercise and decrease computer and TV time. Feed them healthy fruits, vegetables, unprocessed meats, and poultry and eliminate all simple sugars from their diets, so they grow up with a sense of appreciation of these tastes rather than a simple craving for sweetness.

We are hearing more and more about gastric bypass surgery as a treatment for type 2 diabetes. It has always seemed a foolish surgery to me (Dr. Farley) and one that can easily be avoided with self-control of food intake as well as proper hormone management. And though we are told it is a safe surgery, what we are not told is that it is almost always a "ticking time bomb." The last autopsy I assisted on was on a woman that had died of cancer and had previously had gastric bypass surgery. I was asked to assist at the request of a physician friend that was friends with the deceased woman. As the autopsy progressed, I was commenting to the medical examiner about the obvious changes to her physiology that were evident during the procedure. These changes indicated a great deal of abnormal scar tissue as well as obvious signs of vitamin and mineral deficiencies. Atherosclerosis was also evident, as well as cardiac hypertrophy. I commented to the medical examiner about these changes and told him that I had found the same changes on other gastric bypass and lap band procedures. He stated he had been finding the same thing as well as premature deaths. He asked if I would be willing to co-author a paper on the subject, but unfortunately I was far too busy at the time to help him and the paper was never written. I have oftentimes regretted this decision since gastric bypass has become such a popular surgery.

To be blunt, lap band and gastric bypass are unwarranted surgeries intended to replace the commitment to change your lifestyle by changing your diet and eating smaller portions and exercising. As a result of these surgeries, physicians oftentimes fail to find other contributing factors, such as excess estradiol to testosterone ratio. Low testosterone contributes a great deal to type 2 diabetes and insulin resistance, but is very seldom looked at prior to other treatments. Estradiol increases body fat and fat cells produce estradiol; this is a vicious circle that will lead to obesity as well as increase the chance of developing type 2 diabetes. I have heard woman after women tell me they were down to absurdly low caloric intake, yet they could still not lose weight. This was invariably linked to excessively high estradiol levels. Obesity is a major contributing factor to type 2 diabetes.

NATURAL TREATMENTS:

We strongly recommend a **hormone profile** to anyone suffering from type 2 diabetes. It is imperative that this be done for comprehensive care. The patient will suffer much unneeded frustration if their estradiol levels are higher than normal or testosterone levels are depressed. **This is true for both males and females.** Remember that this will need to be discussed with your primary caregiver. The hormone profile must be a **complete** hormone profile that includes DHEA (very often low in type 2 diabetics), androstenedione, free testosterone, free estradiol, estrone, estriol, pregnenolone, and DHT. When the term "free" is used, it simply means that is unbound by sex hormone binding globulin (SHBG), thus it is available for the body to use.

It has been well established that testosterone levels in males have been dropping an average of 1% per year for the past several years. Though research is almost non-existent, there is every reason to believe that the same is true for females. This is largely due to hormones found in meats, as well as pollution from pesticides that contain high amounts of synthetic estrogen and other pollutants that have estrogenic effects. High estrogen levels in women are becoming more and more prevalent. This shuts down testosterone production through a mechanism known as negative feedback. The endocrine functions by keeping specific ratios and if these ratios are destroyed by contamination from pollutants, then it halts the production of hormones that occur prior to estradiol, specifically DHEA and testosterone.

There are also several safe and proven effective natural treatments that may be very beneficial for you to use in your quest to prevent type 2 diabetes and insulin resistance as well as reduce obesity (if that is part of the problem).

Psyllium is a type of complex fiber known as "hemicellulose mucilage." It is actually a mixed polysaccharide, composed of xylan, xylose, arabinose, galacturonic acid, and rhamnose. In simple terms it acts as a very good fiber that is relatively inexpensive and possesses several beneficial effects. Psyllium has been proven to lower serum glucose levels, triglyceride levels, lipid levels, and also to lower insulin response. It has also been shown to be helpful with type 1 diabetes and should be considered a safe and effective adjunct therapy. Both authors (and our wives) take psyllium on a daily basis. The normal recommended dosage is 6 to 10 grams a day; it is easiest taken as psyllium husk capsules, although ground whole psyllium is best and actually has a nice nutty like flavor.

Lycium is a Chinese herb that has been used for hundreds of years. The parts of the plant that are used are the bark and fruit. Despite the fact that it is frequently used in many cancer therapies, its primary function is lowering serum glucose levels. Lycium works by increasing insulin sensitivity, and in so doing, reducing the amount of insulin that needs to be secreted in order to effectively lower glucose levels. Remember, the less insulin in the circulation, the better it is for the cardiovascular system.

Cinnamon has a unique ability to act in the same manner as insulin. In other words it is able to allow passage of glucose from the blood stream into cells for their use. This is extremely helpful in lowering insulin levels and blood glucose levels. The most obvious advantage is that it is capable of doing this without the harmful effects of insulin on the endothelium. Cinnamon also has the advantage of lowering blood lipid (fat) levels, which may offer great additional benefit for type 2 diabetics. The biggest problem with cinnamon is that based on clinical trials, the recommended daily dosage for lowering elevated blood sugar, cholesterol, and triglycerides levels is 1 to 6 grams per day, which is a relatively large dose. However, when split up into three daily doses, it is certainly manageable and inexpensive.

Coenzyme Q10 has shown beneficial effects for three major reasons: 1) it aids the mitochondria of pancreas cells and allows them to more effectively produce insulin, 2) it aids in giving the heart energy, and – most importantly – 3) it has been shown to protect the endothelium, thereby aiding in the prevention of atherosclerosis which so often accompanies type 2 diabetes.

If you have progressed to the point where these changes are not enough, or you are working with your practitioner to get off of insulin injections, we would suggest that you speak with your primary caregiver about the use of **Metformin**, which increases the sensitivity of the muscles to insulin and glucose. In other words, it counteracts insulin resistance and lowers blood sugar levels by facilitating the transport of glucose into muscle cells. Some research has shown Metformin may also help to actually prevent the onset of type 2 diabetes and may help to prevent atherosclerosis. It has been on the market for quite some time and is considered a relatively safe drug, and is much preferred to insulin.

Vitamin A acts as an antioxidant and helps convert beta-carotene efficiently, which reduces the risk of blindness in diabetics. High doses of **vitamin C** have been shown to prevent sorbitol accumulation and glycosylation (the enzymatic process that attaches sugar to other molecules) of proteins, both of which are important factors in the development of diabetic complications, such as cataracts. Studies have shown that a low **vitamin E** concentration was associated with a 3.9 times greater risk of developing diabetes. This makes sense because vitamin E reduces oxidative stress, thus improving membrane physical characteristics and related activities in glucose transport as well as promoting healing of diabetes-related lesions. **Magnesium** helps in the metabolism of glycogen and works closely with **vitamin B6** to help the metabolic process within the cell. It is interesting to note that certain nutrients like **vitamins B1**, **B2**, **B12**, **pantothenic acid**, **vitamin C**, **protein** and **potassium** (along with small frequent meals containing some carbohydrates) can actually stimulate production of insulin within the body in a healthy manner. In other words, small amounts of the right foods and proper vitamins stimulate the body to produce small adequate amounts of insulin, without inducing excessively high insulin levels (hyperinsulinemia).

Many diabetic patients experience painful neuropathy and fungal infections in their feet. We offer no references but will provide a very simple and inexpensive method of treatment that has had remarkable help in numerous patients: **soak your feet in distilled apple cider vinegar 30 minutes a day**. Use just enough to cover your ankles. The vinegar may be reused 2 to 3 times before fresh distilled vinegar is required. Give it several days and see if it helps you.

FOR YOUR DOCTOR:

See page 308 for research and studies to share with your doctor.

EARACHES

DESCRIPTION:

An earache can be a sharp, dull, or burning pain in one or both ears. There are three major types of earaches and infections: 1) **Otitis externa**, 2) **Otitis interna**, and 3) **Otitis media**. ["Ot" = ear + "itis" = inflammation]. The difference is where in the ear the problem is occurring.

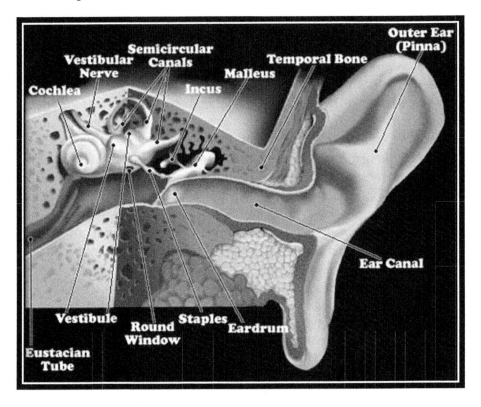

1. **Otitis externa** is inflammation of the canal between the eardrum and the external opening of the ear. It usually occurs after swimming in contaminated water or during hot, humid weather. It can also occur after trauma to the ear canal that permits detrimental microorganisms to gain entrance. This often occurs after attempts at cleaning the ear with a cotton swab, or other utensil.

2. **Otitis interna** is an inflammation of the inner ear, typically accompanied by dizziness, nausea, and loss of the sense of balance.

3. **Otitis media** is an inflammation, usually due to infection by detrimental bacteria or viruses of the middle ear (i.e. of the chamber lying behind the eardrum and containing three bony ossicles that conduct sound to the inner ear).

SYMPTOMS:

Ear pain, fever, irritability, dizziness, swelling around the ear and jaw area, nausea, vertigo.

CONVENTIONAL TREATMENTS:

Over-the-counter ear drops are gentle and effective, as long as the eardrum has not ruptured. Over-the-counter pain relievers, such as acetaminophen or ibuprofen, can provide relief for children and adults with an earache. Warning: Do **NOT** give aspirin to children. Antibiotics often clear up a bacterial ear infection. Amoxicillin is an antibiotic often chosen for treating ear infections. However, antibiotics will **not** be effective if the ear infection is caused by a virus.

NATURAL TREATMENTS:

In the treatment of otitis media, if you wish to use a local natural antibiotic, **xylitol** may help to prevent or treat this condition by inhibiting the growth of streptococcus pneumoniae (one of the detrimental bacteria that causes otitis media). Specially formulated eardrops containing **grapefruit seed extract** (GSE) may alleviate earaches associated with otitis media, as GSE has been shown to kill the haemophilus influenzae bacteria (one of the detrimental bacteria that causes otitis media).

In order to help prevent the recurrence of reoccurring otitis media, an increase in **zinc** may be very helpful. Take an extra tablet of zinc or zinc syrup (for children) in order to prevent the repeated pain and stress of recurring ear infections. An interesting fact is that children prone to recurrent otitis interna may be at greater risk of Attention Deficit/Hyperactivity Disorder (ADHD) and/or Attention Deficit Disorder (ADD): 89% of children afflicted with ADD have had three or more occurrences of otitis media or otitis interna and 74% have had eleven or more occurrences of these ailments.

The above paragraph is most important for parents to understand. Children diagnosed with ADD and ADHD (as well as many children that have not been diagnosed as such) suffer greatly from **food allergies**. The vast majority of childhood otitis interna has been due to allergic reactions to dairy, soy, and/or gluten. It has already been well established that many children diagnosed with ADD or ADHD also suffer from **other allergies**. If your child starts complaining about ear pain, work with your primary caregiver to help rule out allergies as a cause.

Our recommendation would be to **eliminate all dairy, soy, and gluten** from the diet rather than sensitivity tests. Please don't worry that children will not get enough calcium if you eliminate dairy, as dairy is far from the best source of calcium (for both children and adults). Only about 31% of the calcium content of cow's milk is absorbed by the body, while the remaining 69% is excreted from the body prior to its absorption.

Our preference is almond milk; it tastes good and most children don't notice the difference. And as a bonus, it contains about 240 mg of calcium per 100 grams, which is much better than cow's milk. Almond milk is also much less likely to cause allergic responses, and overall is much healthier than cow's milk and should be considered as a safe and nutritious replacement for the whole family.

It is always preferable to eliminate dairy and soy prior to antibiotic use unless there is absolute proof that there is an infection, since antibiotics will wipe out the beneficial bacteria that our bodies require which results in having to use probiotics to restore them. Loss of these probiotics will have detrimental effects on the immune system as well as digestion.

Otitis interna is often an active irritation and not actually an infection at all. In these cases, **vitamin A** may be beneficial to restore normal function.

Lastly, earaches may actually be nothing more than an accumulation of ear wax. As ear wax starts to block the external ear canal it can cause a very painful earache and loss of a substantial portion of hearing.

This may be easily and safely treated at home. The first thing you must understand is that Q-tips should never be used to attempt to dig out the wax. It will be much more likely to push the wax more deeply into the ear and exacerbate the problem. A much safer approach is to buy an ear bulb (a bulb with a narrow end to insert into the outer ear) and irrigate the ear. In the physician's office, **warm water** is usually used to repeatedly flush the ear until the wax softens and comes out. At home, warm water may also be used, but remember it will likely take many repetitions to completely clean the ear and alleviate the pressure. Be patient and be sure not to push the ear bulb too far into the ear. Some people find better results using **hydrogen peroxide** to flush the ear, and that is also safe.

FOR YOUR DOCTOR:

See page 324 for research and studies to share with your doctor.

ESCHERICHIA COLI
(E. COLI)

DESCRIPTION:

Escherichia coli (abbreviated "*E. coli*") bacteria normally live in the intestines of healthy people and animals. Although most strains of *E. coli* are innocuous, others can make you sick. Some strains of *E. coli* cause disease by creating a toxin called Shiga toxin, thus the bacteria which produce these toxins are called "Shiga toxin-producing" *E. coli*, or "STEC" for short. STEC live in the guts of ruminant animals (including cattle, elk, deer, sheep, and goats). Infections start when you swallow STEC — in other words, when you get tiny (usually invisible) amounts of human or animal feces in your mouth. Unfortunately, this happens more often than we would like to think about.

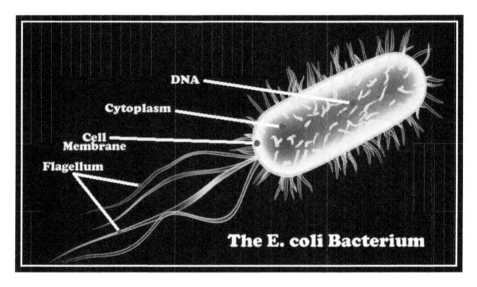

The most commonly identified STEC in the USA is *E. coli* O157:H7 (often shortened to *E. coli* O157 or even just "O157"). When you hear news reports about outbreaks of "*E. coli*" infections, they are usually talking about O157, which can cause severe abdominal cramps, bloody diarrhea, vomiting, urinary tract infections, respiratory illness, and pneumonia.

You may be exposed to 0157 from contaminated water or food (especially raw vegetables and undercooked ground beef). Healthy adults usually recover from an 0157 infection within a week, but young children and older adults can develop a life-threatening form of kidney failure called hemolytic uremic syndrome (HUS).

SYMPTOMS:

The symptoms of STEC infections vary for each person but often include severe stomach cramps, diarrhea (often bloody), slight fever, and vomiting.

CONVENTIONAL TREATMENTS:

There are no current conventional treatments that can cure E. coli, relieve symptoms, or prevent complications. For most people, the best option is to rest and drink plenty of fluids to help with dehydration and fatigue. Avoid taking an anti-diarrheal medication — this slows your digestive system down, preventing your body from getting rid of the toxins.

NATURAL TREATMENTS:

Ginger is a fabulous plant for nausea, poor appetite, and all sorts of stomach disturbances, including *E. coli*. Ginger has the ability to quell the queasiness that usually proceeds vomiting. As none of us enjoys throwing up and just about all of us feel like it at one time or another, ginger should be a must both on the spice rack and in the medicine cabinet in every home. But ginger can not only help stop vomiting, but can help promote healthy sweating, which is often helpful during illnesses.

A **good sweat** may do a lot more than simply assist detoxification. German researchers have recently found that sweat contains a potent germ-fighting agent that may help fight off infections. Investigators have isolated the gene responsible for the compound and the protein it produces, which they have named dermicidin. Dermicidin is manufactured in the body's sweat glands, secreted into the sweat, and transported to the skin's surface where it provides protection against invading microorganisms, including bacteria such as *E. coli*.

There have been about 600 scientific studies of **honey** as an infection-fighter reported in the medical literature. Honey is known to calm an upset stomach, lessen cold symptoms, and strengthen the immune system. As one of nature's natural antibiotics, honey also heals wounds while minimizing scarring. The important thing to know from the research is that raw honey can kill a wide range of infection-causing bacteria (including *E. coli)* when they are in direct contact with the disease-causing microorganisms, and that diluted honey actually works better than "straight" honey.

A product called "Ginger Wonder Syrup" is a combination of ginger and raw honey. I (Dr. Farley) have used it extensively on food poisoning cases on numerous occasions and it has never failed me. You can easily make your own at home if you wish. Simply mix the ginger from ginger capsules with raw honey, stir well, and take a teaspoon full every 30 minutes or until the symptoms stop.

Remember that your body kills foodborne infections with stomach acid, so do **NOT** take antacids before or after eating salads or rare meat. Eat bitter greens in a salad at the beginning of a meal to stimulate the production of stomach acid to kill bacteria and eliminate acid reflux by opening the pyloric valve.

FOR YOUR DOCTOR:

See page 328 for research and studies to share with your doctor.

FIBROMYALGIA

DESCRIPTION:

Fibromyalgia, in layman's terms, means "muscle pain" and is a common syndrome in which a person has long-term, body-wide pain and tenderness in the joints, muscles, tendons, and other soft tissues.

SYMPTOMS:

Widespread pain, tender spots, decreased pain threshold, sleep disturbance, fatigue, decrease in strength, depression, psychological distress.

CONVENTIONAL TREATMENTS:

There is no cure, per se, so the goal of treatment is to help relieve pain and other symptoms. Physical therapy and massage are common treatments. Also, medicines such as Duloxetine (Cymbalta), Pregabalin (Lyrica), and Milnacipran (Savella) are prescribed to treat fibromyalgia. Other common drugs prescribed for this ailment are antidepressants, pain relievers, sleeping aids, muscle relaxers, and anti-seizure medications.

NATURAL TREATMENTS:

First, make sure your problem isn't related to a chronic case of **constipation** or **diarrhea**. Either can flood the body with toxins and create achiness and soreness throughout the body. Between the small and large intestine near the appendix is a structure called the ileocecal valve. If it sticks open, you'll experience diarrhea, and toxins from the large intestine will make their way back into the small intestine where they will be absorbed into the body. If the valve sticks shut, food that should be exiting the body putrefies and causes toxic buildup. Along with these toxins comes muscle soreness, achiness, fatigue and many of the symptoms associated with fibromyalgia.

In almost every case of fibromyalgia type symptoms, the patient will have **abnormal hormone profiles** (abnormal testosterone, estradiol and progesterone have been related to fibromyalgia). This is becoming a much more common problem due to pesticides on our food, hormones being fed to livestock consumed by humans, as well as pseudoestrogens found in plastics, etc.

One common thread in fibromyalgia patients is **adrenal insufficiency**. In adrenal insufficiency, the adrenal gland is unable to produce enough cortisol to reduce chronic inflammation. In this day and age we are running under a great deal of stress in our everyday life. As we age, the adrenal glands begin to take over hormone production usually done by the ovaries and testes. If they are over worked and unable to keep up their normal pulsatile excretions, hormone levels may be low. This is especially true of cortisol, a natural anti-inflammatory. Please see the section of this book on "Adrenal Insufficiency" for more information.

In many cases, fibromyalgia is misdiagnosed and the problem is actually **osteomalacia**, a bone ailment that affects adults which involves a softening of the bones due to the loss of minerals. Osteomalacia is the adult equivalent of rickets but occurs following the cessation of bone growth. Osteomalacia (unlike rickets) does not affect the growth plates. The amounts of calcium and phosphorus in the body can be measured with a blood test to rule out osteomalacia and should also be done with your primary caregiver's support, if it has not been done already.

Before going into the herbs that may be of some benefit, we recommend that you and your physician discuss the following tests:

- ❖ A **complete hormone profile**, which must include:
  - ✓ DHEA
  - ✓ Androstenedione
  - ✓ Free Testosterone
  - ✓ Free Estradiol
  - ✓ DHT
  - ✓ SHBG
- ❖ A 24 hour **cortisol test** that includes at least a wake up level, a noon level, and an evening level.
- ❖ Since hypothyroidism has also been linked to fibromyalgia in several studies, it would be wise to have a **complete thyroid panel** to rule that out as a possibility.

A few natural supplements and herbs that may help with fibromyalgia are **coenzyme Q10, magnesium, iodine, St. John's wort, ginkgo**

biloba, aloe vera, and **chlorella.** Research on these supplements is contained in the "For Your Doctor" section.

The most important thing you can do is to find a physician that is willing to work with you to eliminate the cause of your "fibromyalgia". As you can see, the tests that are needed to determine cause or causes requires a doctor that wants to work with you for a final solution, not just attempts at treating the symptoms. Remember our personal opinion is that "fibromyalgia" is actually a symptom, not a diagnosis. **Look for the cause.**

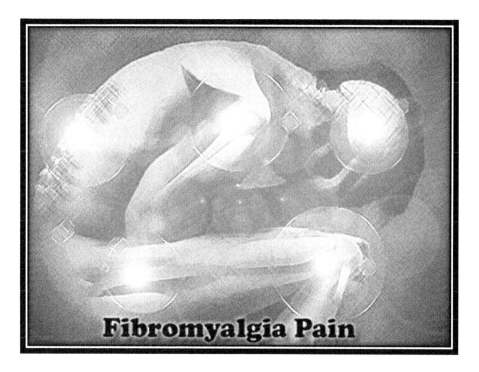

FOR YOUR DOCTOR:

See page 330 for research and studies to share with your doctor.

135

GOUT

DESCRIPTION:

Over 8 million people in the United States suffer from gout, which is one of the most frequently recorded medical illnesses throughout history. It is often related to an inherited abnormality in the body's ability to process **uric acid**, thus the body becomes overloaded with uric acid. This overload of uric acid may lead to the formation of tiny crystals of urate that deposit in tissues of the body, especially the joints. When crystals form in the joints, it causes recurring attacks of joint inflammation (arthritis).

Gouty arthritis is typically an extremely painful attack with a rapid onset of joint inflammation, which is precipitated by deposits of uric acid crystals in the joint fluid (synovial fluid) and joint lining (synovial lining). Intense joint inflammation occurs as the immune system reacts, causing white blood cells to engulf the uric acid 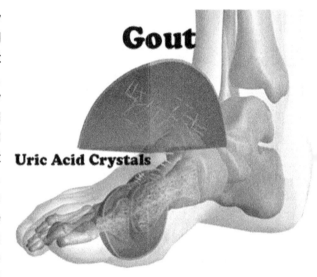 crystals and chemical messengers of inflammation to be released, leading to pain, heat, and redness of the joint tissues. As gout progresses, the attacks of gouty arthritis typically occur more frequently and often in additional joints. Chronic gout can also lead to deposits of hard lumps of uric acid in the tissues, particularly in and around the joints and may cause joint destruction, decreased kidney function, and kidney stones (nephrolithiasis).

SYMPTOMS:

Joint pain (typically big toe, knee, or ankles), red and tender skin, fever, tophi (lumps below the skin around the joints).

CONVENTIONAL TREATMENTS:

Gout is typically treated with nonsteroidal anti-inflammatory drugs (NSAIDs) such as ibuprofen or naproxen. Physicians may also prescribe strong painkillers such as oxycodone, hydrocodone, and codeine. Injecting the inflamed joint with corticosteroids can also be very effective at temporarily relieving pain. It should be noted however, that repeated cortisol injection will actually cause joint distruction. Chronic gout may be treated with daily use of allopurinol (Zyloprim) or probenecid, which both decrease uric acid levels in the blood.

NATURAL TREATMENTS:

There are several herbs that have been clinically proven to be effective without the side effects of pharmaceutical drugs.

Chrysin is a naturally occurring compound extracted from the blue passion flower. Honeycomb also contains small amounts of chrysin, as does bee propolis (the resinous "glue" bees use for hive construction) and skullcap. Chrysin has the ability to act as an anti-inflammatory compound, thus it may be effective on gout by reducing the inflammation. Chrysin also inhibits the "aromatase" enzymes (conversion compounds) in the body. This is beneficial to us because it has been shown to prevent or block the conversion of androstenedione to estrone (a basic estrogen). Other studies have shown chrysin's ability to prevent testosterone's ability to convert into estradiol (another estrogen form). Chrysin can also help lower and control the output of cortisol (the stress hormone). Chrysin has the ability to activate benzodiazapine receptors and thereby reduce cortisol output.

You should limit intake of meats, as they are rich sources of uric acid. Organ meats, sardines, and anchovies are particularly high in uric acid. Also eliminate coffee and all other caffeine sources from the diet. Drink plenty of water daily to flush uric acid from the system and prevent urate crystal deposition. Minimize alcohol consumption, since alcohol promotes dehydration and irritates the urinary tract.   Gout and hyperuricemia are aggravated by obesity, weight gain, alcohol intake, high blood pressure, high fructose corn syrup, and certain medications.

Eat **tart cherries** in all forms - fresh, or as cherry juice, or in the form of tart cherry extract. Laboratory findings at Michigan State University suggest that ingesting the equivalent of 20 tart cherries inhibits enzymes called cyclooxygenase-1 and -2, which are the targets of anti-inflammatory drugs.

FOR YOUR DOCTOR:

See page 338 for research and studies to share with your doctor.

HEADACHES

DESCRIPTION:

A headache is pain or discomfort in the head, scalp, or neck. The most common type of headaches are likely caused by tight muscles in your shoulders, neck, scalp, and jaw. These are called **tension headaches**. **Migraine headaches** are severe headaches that usually occur with other symptoms such as vision changes or nausea. **Cluster headaches** (which are rare) are sharp, very painful headaches that tend to occur several times a day for months and then go away for a similar period of time, whereas **sinus headaches** cause pain in the front of your head and face. Headaches that continually come back are sometimes referred to as **rebound headaches**.

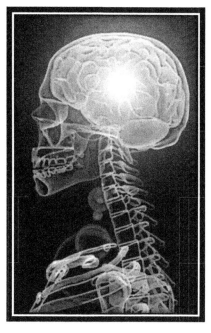

Serious causes of headaches are very rare. However, occasionally, a headache may be a sign of a brain tumor or infection, aneurysm, stroke, or high blood pressure.

SYMPTOMS:

Head pain, irritability, dizziness, nausea, vertigo, vision impairment.

CONVENTIONAL TREATMENTS:

Most tension headaches are treated with over-the-counter (OTC) medications, including **aspirin**, **ibuprofen** (Advil, Motrin, etc.), and/or **acetaminophen** (Tylenol, etc). Migraine headaches are typically treated with OTC medications, prescription drugs, rest, and cold compresses to the head and neck. OTC medications are typically not effective for treating cluster and migrain headaches, so physicians frequently resort to injectable medications, such as sumatriptan (Imitrex, Sumavel Dosepro, others), or prescription triptan nasal sprays, such as zolmitriptan (Zomig) or sumatriptan (Imitrex). Sinus headaches are typically treated with OTC medications or decongestants.

NATURAL TREATMENTS:

The treatment for cluster headaches is rather simple and requires only one herb: **cayenne pepper** (which contains capsaicin). Cayenne can be inhaled through the nose in a very small amount and has been found through research, as well as hundreds of years of use, to be extremely effective. Make no mistake; it will burn when it is inhaled through the nose for a few minutes. However,on the other hand, it is nothing compared to the pain of the headaches and will only need to be done occasionally. After the first few times it becomes easier to deal with the temporary sinus burning and while uncomfortable for a short time, it does work very quickly in most cases and the relief lasts for a very long time.

Cayenne pepper may also be used in the treatment of migraine headaches. When mixed with aloe vera gel and rubbed into the temples and other areas of pain, it has been found to be successful in many cases.

Feverfew is an herb commonly used by migraine headache sufferers. It acts by limiting the production of prostaglandins (the brain chemicals responsible for contracting blood vessels). The contraction and expansion of the blood vessels are thought to cause the "pounding" that typifies many migrain headaches, and feverfew seems to reduce it. **Ginger** has been shown to help combat nausea, so we recommend the combination of these two herbs which will create a synergistic effect. Add 20 drops of these herbs in tincture form to a cup of warm water and drink it while still warm. Add a small amount of honey to create a pleasant tasting tea. Feverfew and ginger have been combined in a sublingual tablet called LipiGesic. A recent study found that 63% of migraine sufferers using LipiGesic found some relief compared to 39% of those taking a placebo.

FOR YOUR DOCTOR:

See page 341 for research and studies to share with your doctor.

HEMORRHOIDS

DESCRIPTION:

Hemorrhoids are painful, swollen veins in the lower portion of the rectum or anus which typically result from increased pressure in the veins which causes the veins to swell. They can be either internal or external.

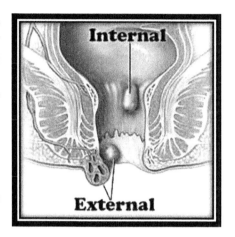

SYMPTOMS:

Anal itching and pain, anal bleeding, pain during bowel movements, lumps near the anus.

CONVENTIONAL TREATMENTS:

Typical treatments for hemorrhoids include corticosteroid creams to help reduce pain and swelling, lidocaine creams to reduce pain, and stool softeners to help reduce straining during bowel movements.

For patients with severe pain and bleeding, rubber band ligation surgery may be performed or the hemorrhoids may be surgically removed.

NATURAL TREATMENTS:

Psyllium may alleviate the pain and bleeding associated with hemorrhoids, as psyllium softens the stool, causing the passing of stools to be less painful.

Witch hazel (applied with cotton swabs) can reduce itching, swelling, and pain. Witch hazel is thought to decrease the bleeding of hemorrhoids by acting as an astringent.

Butcher's broom gets its name because it was once used by butchers in Europe to clean their chopping blocks. Butcher's broom has a long history of traditional use for hemorrhoids and varicose veins. It is often used when there is underlying poor circulation in the veins. Butcher's broom extract contains anti-inflammatory properties that are believed to improve the tone and integrity of veins and shrink the swollen tissue. The active compound is called "ruscogen." Butcher's broom is usually recommended in capsule or tea form. The tea has a slightly bitter taste, so a bit of stevia or honey can be used to sweeten it. Butcher's broom has also been shown to be effective when applied topically as an ointment or compress. **Warning:** Butcher's broom should not be used by people with high blood pressure, benign prostatic hyperplasia, by pregnant or nursing women, or by people taking alpha blocker or MAO inhibitor drugs unless otherwise recommended by their doctor.

Horse chestnut is often recommended when there is poor circulation in the veins, or chronic venous insufficiency. The active compound is believed to be aescin. Horse chestnut can be taken as a tea or in capsule form. It can also be applied externally as a compress. **Warning:** People with an allergy to the horse chestnut family, bleeding disorders, or people taking blood thinners should not take horse chestnut. Only products made from the seeds or bark of the young branches should be used. Other parts of the plant are poisonous.

Grape seed extract (150 - 300 mg per day) alleviates/prevents hemorrhoids by inhibiting the collagenase enzyme that damages the blood vessels of the walls of the anus that occurs in hemorrhoids.

Sitz baths (sitting in warm water for 10-20 minutes) promote healing and ease discomfort by encouraging blood flow to the rectal area and also relaxing the anal sphincter.

If your hemorrhoids do not get better with home treatments, you may need a type of heat treatment to shrink the hemorrhoids. This is called **infrared coagulation** and may help avoid surgery.

FOR YOUR DOCTOR:

See page 346 for research and studies to share with your doctor.

INFLUENZA ("THE FLU")

DESCRIPTION:

Sometimes people confuse colds and flu. Although they do share some of the same symptoms, most people get several colds each year, whereas they only get the flu once every few years. While a common cold (including chest cold and head cold) can be caused by more than 200 viruses, seasonal flu is caused by either influenza A or B viruses.

Most people catch the flu when they breathe in tiny droplets from coughs or sneezes of someone who has the flu. You can also catch the flu if you touch something with the virus on it, and then touch your eyes, nose, or mouth. The flu generally causes symptoms in the nose, throat, and lungs, since it is a viral infection in the respiratory tract.

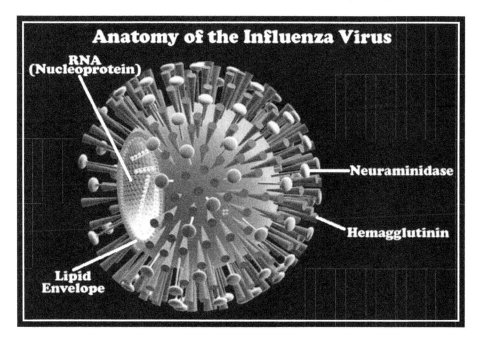

SYMPTOMS:

Fever, malaise, chilliness, headache, muscle aches and pains, sore throat, sneezing, nasal congestion, cough, watery eyes, sinus pain, nausea, and vomiting.

CONVENTIONAL TREATMENTS:

Conventional wisdom is prophylactic and is a **flu shot**. If that is your preference, by all means do so. We would suggest reading the whole section first however, and remember that the flu shot, even if it is effective, will only work against the strain expected to be the most likely for that year. Once you have acquired the flu, an antiviral (such as Tamiflu and Relenza) may be prescribed, however they have not proven to be very effective in the past, and do have side effects. Typical treatments also include **acetaminophen** (Tylenol) and **ibuprofen** (Advil, Motrin) which help lower fever. Sometimes doctors suggest you use both types of medicine. Do **NOT** use aspirin.

Also be aware that your body is running a fever for a reason. As long as it is below 102° F (or lower), if possible, let it continue. Be sure to stay well hydrated and take in extra electrolytes, because you will be losing a lot of fluid. Don't wait until you are thirsty because by then you will most likely be dehydrated. Drink small amounts all day and just before bed. The body raises its temperature in order to kill the virus causing the infection. This is one reason Native American sweat lodges were used so successfully in so many cases, and why far infrared saunas are also used effectively. Viruses, for the most part, have a very narrow range of temperature variance tolerance where they can survive. These temperature increases are frequently effective at killing the viruses.

I (Dr. Farley) remember, during my training days, coming in with a severe case of the flu. Sympathy from my Korean instructor was not high on his list. He told us what to do and we did it, or suffered the consequences. The first thing he said when he saw me was "*go for a 6 mile run, and then see me.*" I felt like I could hardly move, much less run, but I did what I was instructed to do. By the second mile I was breathing better and not feeling nearly as achy. By the end of the run, I actually felt pretty good. I went back into his office as requested and was told to take a few supplements, drink a lot of water and run again early the next day. By the next day, I had no flu symptoms at all and the run felt normal. He had me run to raise my core temperature and kill the flu viruses. It worked very well. Please do not take this as the suggested method for the treatment of the flu. I was in my twenties and worked with a special team that regularly covered 40-60 miles a day in mountainous country. We were in excellent shape and had no other health issues. I just wanted to prove the point that reducing temperature may make you feel temporarily better, but it also may prolong the symptoms.

In truth, no one really knows how many human flu viruses there are. Because flu strains are constantly mutating, and every time they mutate they act in different ways, and each mutation is given another name if it is recognized as a different stain, thus there is really no way to know how many flu types there are. Another major problem is in the discovery of different strains. In conventional medicine, the primary concern is what strains will probably be most prevalent for the next flu season and which ones pose the greatest threat to humans. At that point, an educated guess is made on what strain will be most prevalent the next season, and vaccines against that strain are produced. If you don't happen to get the flu, then it is said the vaccine worked. If you get the flu anyway, it is blamed on vaccination against the wrong strain, too late in getting the vaccination, or the theory that your immune system was compromised and you contracted the flu anyway. It must be also noted that if you contract the flu shortly after being vaccinated, you are told you should have received the vaccination earlier, and never that the vaccine actually induced the flu or other illness. Before taking the flu vaccine, we suggest reading the very well referenced work of Dr. Alan Cantwell Jr., M.D., printed below with his permission.

ARE VACCINES CAUSING MORE DISEASE THAN THEY ARE CURING?

By Alan Cantwell Jr., M.D.

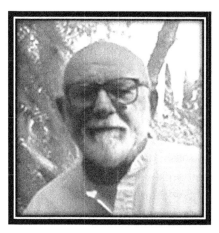

Vaccines help keep us safe from infectious diseases. Smallpox and polio epidemics have been wiped out by mass vaccine programs. People rush to get flu shots every autumn, and kids are bombarded with a barrage of 22 required vaccinations before the age of six. Even pets need their shots. The manufacture of vaccines is a giant industry and what you pay for – inoculations and doctor visits – is big business for pediatricians, family practitioners and veterinarians. So why are more and more people worried about vaccines, especially the ones for kids?

Vaccine-induced Illness

Barbara Loe Fisher, president of the National Vaccine Information Centre, a consumer's group based in Virginia, USA, claims vaccines are responsible for the increasing numbers of children and adults who suffer from immune system and neurologic disorders, hyperactivity, learning disabilities, asthma, chronic fatigue syndrome, lupus, rheumatoid arthritis, multiple sclerosis, and seizure disorders. She calls for studies to monitor the long-term effects of mass vaccination and Fisher wants physicians to be absolutely sure these vaccines are safe and not harming people.

No one can deny the dangers of vaccines. The measles, mumps, rubella (German measles) and polio vaccines, all contain live but weakened viruses. Although health officials tell you that polio has been wiped out in the US since 1979, they often fail to mention that all recorded cases of polio since that time are actually caused by the polio vaccine. Vaccine investigator Neil Z. Miller questions whether we still need the polio vaccine when it causes every new case of polio in the USA. Before mass vaccinations programs began fifty years ago, Miller insists we didn't have cancer in epidemic numbers that autoimmune ailments were barely known, and childhood autism did not exist.

Vaccine Contamination

There is also the problem of contamination that has always plagued vaccine makers. During World War II a yellow fever vaccine manufactured with human blood serum was unknowingly contaminated with hepatitis virus and given to the military. As a result, more than 50,000 cases of serum hepatitis broke out among American troops injected with the vaccine.

In the 1960s it was discovered that polio vaccines manufactured in monkey kidney tissue between 1955 and 1963 were contaminated with a monkey virus (Simian Virus, number 40). Although this virus causes cancer in experimental animals, health authorities insist it does not cause problems in humans. But evidence of SV40 genetic material has been popping up in human cancers and normal tissue. Researchers are now connecting SV40-contaminated polio vaccines to an increasing number of rare cancers of the lung (mesothelioma) and bone marrow (multiple myeloma). In a 1999 report, SV40 DNA was detected in tissue samples from four children born after 1982. Three were kidney transplant patients, and a fourth had a kidney tumour. Could SV40 be passed on from parents to their children? No one knows for sure.

Covert Vaccine Experiments

Using kids as guinea pigs in potentially harmful vaccine experiments is every parents' worst nightmare. This actually happened in 1989-1991 when Kaiser Permanente of Southern California and the US Center for Disease Control (CDC) jointly conducted a measles vaccine experiment. Without proper parental disclosure, the Yugoslavian-made "high titre" Edmonston-Zagreb measles vaccine was tested on 1,500 poor, primarily black and Latino, inner city children in Los Angeles. Highly recommended by the World Health Organization (WHO), the high-potency experimental vaccine was previously injected into infants in Mexico, Haiti, and Africa. It was discontinued in these countries when it was discovered that the children were dying in large numbers.

Unbelievably, the measles vaccine caused long-term suppression of the children's immune system for six months up to three years. As a result, the immunodepressed children died from other diseases in greater numbers than children who had never received the vaccine. Tragically, African girl babies in the experiment were given twice the dose of boys, and therefore suffered a higher death rate. The WHO pulled the vaccine off the market in 1992.

Ironically, the E-Z measles vaccine tested by Kaiser on minority babies was supposed to increase immunity in younger infants. Instead, the vaccine produced the opposite effect. A Los Angeles Times editorial (June 20, 1996) assured readers that "none of the 1,500 was injured by the unlicensed vaccine" and called upon the CDC to ensure that experiments like the E-Z measles vaccine could never occur again.

One wonders how many secret vaccine experiments are conducted by health authorities that never come to the attention of the public. During the two-year measles experiment I was employed by Kaiser and I never knew anything about it until I read the report in The Times five years later, in 1996.

In the poor inner cities across the United States the number of asthma cases is exploding and health officials don't know why. According to the CDC, 5000 asthma deaths occur annually; and it is estimated that 17.3 million people (4.8 million are children) suffer from the disease, up from 6.7 million in 1980. Asthma usually begins before age 6, and blacks are two to three times more likely to die from asthma than whites. In the Bronx and Harlem sections of New York City, the hospitalization rate for asthma is 21 times higher than in the more affluent areas of the city.

Could the sharp rise in asthma in poor children be connected with immunosuppression caused by a barrage of vaccines, as well as a lack of quality medical care and insurance, poor diet, and environmental factors? The possible connection of immunosuppressive vaccines to diseases like asthma has never been raised by health officials. With vaccine experiments frequently performed in Africa and now on black Americans, no wonder one out of every four African-Americans believes AIDS was developed as a genocide program by the US government to exterminate the black population.

But vaccine experiments in the 1990s have not been limited to blacks. Millions of female Mexicans, Nicaraguans and Filipinos have been duped into taking tetanus vaccines, some of which contained a female hormone that could cause miscarriage and sterilization. In 1995, a Catholic human rights organization called Human Life International accused the WHO of promoting a Canadian-made tetanus vaccine laced with a pregnancy hormone called human choriogonadotropic hormone (HCG). Suspicions were aroused when the tetanus vaccine was prescribed in the unusual dose of five multiple injections over a three month period, and recommended only to women of reproductive age. When an unusual number of women experienced vaginal bleeding and miscarriages after the shots, a hormone additive was uncovered as the cause.

Apparently the WHO has been developing and testing anti-fertility vaccines for over two decades. Women receiving the laced tetanus shot not only developed antibodies to tetanus, but they also developed dangerous antibodies to the pregnancy hormone as well. Without this HCG hormone the growth of the fetus is impaired. Consequently, the laced vaccine served as a covert contraceptive device. Commissioned to analyze the vaccine, the Philippines Medical Association found that

148

20 percent of the WHO tetanus vaccines were contaminated with the hormone. Not surprisingly, the WHO has denied all accusations as "completely false and without basis," and the major media have never reported on the controversy. For further details on this issue, consult the Human Life International website (www.hli.org).

Newly approved vaccines may also pose serious risks. In October 1999 a vaccine against "rotavirus" infection (which causes most cases of childhood diarrhea) was pulled off the market. One year after the RotaShield vaccine was inoculated into over a million infants, it was found to increase the risk of bowel obstruction. Almost 100 cases of bowel obstruction were reported to the government, and twenty infants developed bowel obstructions within one or two weeks after receiving the vaccine.

Vaccine Manufacture and Associated Dangers

Although the public has heard about side effects of vaccines, most people are clueless about the manufacture of vaccines. Few people know that viruses used in vaccine production need to be grown on animal parts like monkey kidneys, or in chicken embryos, or in human and fetal "cell lines." Harvesting viruses in human cell-lines can be perilous because some human cell lines are derived from cancer cells.

In *AIDS & The Doctors of Death,* I wrote about the development of the first human "HeLa" cell line - an "immortal" cell line used extensively in cancer and vaccine research for decades. Henrietta Lacks was a young black woman from Baltimore who died from a highly malignant cervical cancer in 1951. Small pieces of her tumour were donated to a laboratory specializing in tissue cell culture. In those days most attempts to grow human cells outside the body failed. But for some unknown reason Henrietta's cancer cells grew vigorously and became known as the first successful human tissue cell line in history - the now famous HeLa cell line commemorating the legendary **HE**nrietta **LA**cks.

Henrietta's cells were kept alive by feeding them a witches' brew of beef embryo extract (the ground-up remains of a three-week-old, unborn cattle embryo); fresh chicken plasma obtained from the blood of a live chicken heart; and blood from human placentas (the placenta is the sac that nurtures the developing fetus and contains powerful hormones).

It is now suspected that a sexually-transmitted papilloma virus is the cause of cervical cancer. And it is anybody's guess how many other chicken, cattle, and human viruses are incorporated into the HeLa cell line, but none of this possible viral contamination seems to bother scientists who have extensively used the cells in cancer research. What laboratory scientists did eventually discover was that HeLa cells proved so hardy that they frequently contaminated other tissue cell lines used in cancer and cancer virus research.

In the late 1960s when widespread HeLa cell contamination problems were uncovered, scientists were shocked and embarrassed to learn that millions of dollars' worth of published cancer experiments were ruined. "Liver cells" and "monkey cells" that were used in cancer experiments turned out to be Henrietta's cancer cells in disguise. Benign cells that supposedly "spontaneously transformed" into malignant cells were found to be cells contaminated with cancerous HeLa cells.

The serious problem of HeLa cell contamination in cancer and vaccine research is revealed in Michael Gold's *A Conspiracy of Cells: One Woman's Immortal Legacy and the Medical Scandal It Caused*. Even Jonas Salk, who developed the legendary Salk polio vaccine, was fooled when HeLa cells contaminated his animal cell lines. He admitted this years later in 1978 before a stunned audience of cell biologists and vaccine makers. In experiments performed in the late 1950s on dying cancer patients, Salk tried injecting them with a cell line of monkey heart tissue - the same cell line he used to harvest polio virus for his famous vaccine. He hoped the monkey cell injections would stimulate the immune system to fight cancer. However, when abscesses developed at the site of injections, Salk began to suspect that he might be injecting HeLa cells rather than monkey cells, and he stopped the experiment.

Mark Nelson-Rees, a HeLa cell expert and one of the 1978 conference attendees, offered to test Salk's line if it was still available. Salk graciously agreed and the monkey cells indeed proved to be HeLa cells which had invaded and taken over the monkey cell line. According to author Gold, Salk thought there were adequate ways to separate viruses from the tissue cell lines they were harvested in, so that it really didn't matter what kind of cells were used. Even if vaccines weren't filtered, and even if whole cancer cells were injected directly into a human, Salk believed they would be rejected by the body and cause no harm. In those days doctors didn't much believe in cancer-causing viruses. Nowadays, no researcher would dare try injecting cancer cells into a human being. But in the 1950s Salk had done it accidentally. He had injected HeLa cells into a few dozen patients and it hadn't bothered him a bit.

Is There a Vaccine Contamination Connection to AIDS?

Most people assume vaccines are "sterile" and germ free. But sterilizing a vaccine can destroy the necessary immunizing protein that makes it work. Thus, contaminating viruses or viral "particles" can sometime survive the vaccine process.

Animal viruses are also contained in fetal calf serum, a blood product commonly used as a laboratory nutrient to feed various tissue cell cultures. Vaccine contamination by fetal calf serum and its possible relationship to HIV was the subject of a letter by J. Grote, published in the Journal of the Royal (London) Society of Medicine in October 1988. Bovine visna virus (which looks similar to HIV) is a known contaminant of fetal calf serum used in vaccine production and virus-like particles have been detected in vaccines certified for clinical use. Grote warns that "*It seems absolutely vital that all vaccines are screened for HIV prior to use, and that bovine visna virus is further investigated as to its relationship to HIV and its possible role in progression towards AIDS.*"

Could virus-contaminated vaccines lie at the root of AIDS? A few researchers, including myself, believe HIV was "introduced" into gays during the experimental hepatitis B vaccine trials when thousands of homosexuals were injected in Los Angeles, San Francisco, and New York, during the years 1978-1981. The AIDS epidemic first erupted in gays living in those cities in 1981. In 1980, one year before, already 20% of the gays inoculated in Manhattan with the experimental vaccine were already HIV-positive. This was several years before definite AIDS cases were diagnosed in Africa. In the early 1970s the hepatitis B vaccine was developed in chimpanzees, now wildly accepted as the animal from which HIV supposedly evolved.

Hepatitis B vaccine was developed to protect people from the sexual spread of the hepatitis B virus. Now the government recommends that all newborn babies be given the vaccine [this is also the case in Australia]. Such recommendations do not make sense to many parents. And people are still fearful of the hepatitis B vaccine because of its original connection to gay men and AIDS. The original experimental vaccine was made from the pooled blood serum of hepatitis-infected homosexuals and, as mentioned, serum-based vaccines cannot be sterilised.

Another theory of AIDS is that HIV originated from polio vaccines contaminated with chimp and monkey viruses, and administered to Africans in the late 1950s. In *The River: A Journey to the Source of HIV and AIDS*, published in 1999, Edward Hooper details how polio vaccine was made using monkey (and possibly chimp) kidneys and how the ancestor virus of HIV could have jumped species (via the vaccine) to produce the outbreak of AIDS in Africa. Hooper's well-researched book greatly expands the polio vaccine theory of AIDS first reported by Tom Curtis in Rolling Stone magazine in 1992, and The River is a must-read for anyone interested in the possible man-made origin of AIDS.

Other researchers think it more likely that the various WHO-sponsored vaccine programs (particularly the smallpox program) in Africa in the 1970s are responsible for unleashing AIDS in Africa in the 1980s. Hooper, who has worked as a United Nations official, has discounted the research pointing to AIDS as a man-made disease, as proposed by Dr. Leonard Horowitz in *Emerging Viruses*, and in my two books *AIDS & The Doctors of Death: An Inquiry into the Origin of the AIDS Epidemic* and *Queer Blood - The Secret AIDS Genocide Plot*.

Horowitz and I both suspect contaminated smallpox vaccines as the source of HIV in Africa. Certainly the smallpox (vaccinia-cowpox) virus is an excellent virus to use for the genetic engineering of new, multipurpose vaccines. By splicing into the DNA genes of the vaccinia virus, scientists can add on parts of disease-producing viruses like influenza, hepatitis, and other viruses. The safety of this technique has not been fully evaluated, prompting one vaccine maker at a Vaccinia Virus Workshop in 1984 to ask if this could lead to another form of AIDS.

Vaccine Connection to Gulf War Illness and Huntsville Mystery Illness

The cause of Gulf War Illness (GWI) is unknown. For years this debilitating illness (which now affects one-half of the Gulf War vets) has been ignored by Pentagon officials who claim the disease does not exist and that vets are simply reacting to stress. GWI is also thought to be contagious. Vets insist their disease has been passed on to spouses, other family members, and even pets.

Some people suspect multiple vaccines, particularly the experimental anthrax vaccine, are implicated in the disease. Currently, soldiers who refuse to take the mandatory anthrax vaccine are being court-martialled and dismissed from the service.

Researchers Dr. Garth Nicolson and his wife Nancy have found a tiny bacterial microbe (a "mycoplasma") in the blood of nearly half the ill vets with GWI. Amazingly, this infectious agent has a piece of HIV (the AIDS virus) attached to it. This microbe could never have occurred naturally. On the contrary, the composition of the microbe suggests a man-made and genetically-engineered biological warfare agent.

Garth Nicolson's scientific credentials are impeccable. For 16 years he was a professor of medicine at the University of Texas M.D. Anderson Cancer Center in Houston, as well as professor of pathology and laboratory medicine at the University of Texas Medical School, also in Houston. Nancy Nicolson, a molecular biophysicist, was on the faculty at Baylor College of Medicine.

Six months after returning home from the Gulf War, the Nicolson's daughter contracted GWI. Her mother Nancy had contracted a similar illness in 1987 when she was working with Mycoplasma incognitus in infectious disease research. Finally suspecting that this research had biowarfare implications, Nancy Nicolson became a whistle-blower and angered officials. As a result, she believes she was deliberately infected with the mycoplasma. After partial paralysis and a long illness, she finally regained her health with the antibiotic Doxycycline.

The Nicolson's discovery of a similar mycoplasma (but without the attachment of HIV) in a mysterious illness that erupted in the Huntsville, Texas area among prison guards and their families has all the drama of a 'Movie of the Week'. Although the Huntsville disease broke out in the late 1980s (shortly before the Gulf War), it has many of the same signs and symptoms of GWI. Many locals are convinced the sometimes deadly disease originally spread from prisoners incarcerated in several large prisons around Huntsville.

In experiments conducted during the 1970s and 80s, the prisoners were inoculated with flu vaccines containing genetically engineered viruses and mycoplasma. It is suspected that vaccines were being covertly developed and deployed as biological warfare weapons. Nobel prize winner James Watson, world famous for his discovery of the molecular structure of DNA and a leading researcher of the still ongoing Human Genome Project, was involved in these prison experiments. The guards are convinced the Huntsville mystery illness is intimately connected to these experiments, jointly conducted by the Medical School and the military. Like GWI, health officials deny the disease exists.

The Nicolsons continue to developed antibiotic treatments, which have helped some vets. But they have paid a heavy price for their controversial research and unprecedented discoveries. Garth Nicolson was forced to resign from M.D. Anderson in 1996. His career and reputation destroyed, the Nicolsons have since moved to California and head The Institute for Molecular Medicine in Huntington Beach.

Dangerous Animal and Human Cell Lines in Vaccine Manufacture

In an effort to quell concerns about the safety of vaccines, scientists are finally taking another look at the "non-infectious" particles of bird-cancer viruses (avian leukosis virus) in the mumps/measles/rubella vaccines routinely given to kids. Could this be the reason the US Food and Drug Administration held a meeting in September, 1999, to reconsider using human tumour cell lines (like HeLa) rather than monkey kidneys and chicken embryos which are no longer guaranteed 100% safe?

Writing in *Science*, Gretchen Vogel admits public trust in vaccines is a bit shaky. In Wales anti-vaccine parents are holding "measles parties" to infect their children with the disease rather than vaccinate them. She cites the danger of using immortal cell lines for live vaccine production because cancer genes or other hazardous factors might be transferred to people receiving vaccines. But manufacturers also realise vaccine critics are becoming more wary of vaccines made in animal and bird tissue. And vaccine makers want to use immortal cell lines to grow their viruses because obviously viruses can't grow on their own.

The big question everyone seems to avoid is: Can vaccines cause cancer? There is certainly evidence connecting contaminated vaccines

154

to AIDS. And HIV is a cancer-causing virus. Robert Gallo, the co-discoverer of HIV in 1984, has clearly stated AIDS is an epidemic of cancer. Animal and avian viruses can contaminate vaccines and have all been studied as cancer-causing agents. And cancer and vaccine research would be much more difficult without the use of cell lines, some of which are derived from cancer.

Vaccines and Public Paranoia

Is the fear of vaccines justified? It is clear that vaccines can be dangerous. The contamination of vaccines is a reality, and vaccine experiments can be hazardous to one's health. AIDS, unknown two decades ago, is now an increasing worldwide epidemic with millions of death predicted for the next decade. Could vaccines contaminated with cancer-causing and immunosuppressive viruses unleash new plagues in the New Millennium? If so, the new plagues may be far worse than the diseases we eradicated by vaccine programs in the twentieth century.

References

"Anti-diarrheal vaccine for babies recalled," Los Angeles Times, October 16, 1999.

Butel JS, Arrington AS, Wong C, et al.: Molecular evidence of simian virus 40 infections in children. J Infect Dis 180:884-887, 1999.
Cantwell A: AIDS & the Doctors of Death. Aries Rising Press, Los Angeles, 1988.

Cantwell A: Queer Blood. Aries Rising Press, Los Angeles, 1993.

Gold M: A Conspiracy of Cells. State University of New York Press, Albany, 1986.

Hooper E: The River: A Journey to the Source of HIV and AIDS. Little, Brown and Company, Boston, 1999.

Horowitz L: Emerging Viruses- AIDS & Ebola. Tetrahedron, Inc, Rockport, MA, 1996.

Jaroff Leon: "Vaccine Jitters," TIME, September 13, 1999.

Likoudis P: "Gulf war illness probe to advance with new study," The Wanderer, January 21, 1999.

"Measles, government and trust " (Editorial), Los Angeles Times, June 20, 1996.

Miller NZ: Immunization: Theory vs Reality. New Atlantean Press, Santa Fe, 1996.

Miller NZ: Immunizations: The People Speak! New Atlantean Press, Santa Fe, 1996.

Quinnan GV: Vaccinia Viruses as Vectors for Vaccine Antigens. Elsevier, New York, 1985.

Stolberg SG: "Poor fight baffling surge in asthma," New York Times, October 18, 1999.

Alan Cantwell is a physician and AIDS researcher. His book on the man-made epidemic of AIDS entitled *AIDS & The Doctors of Death: An Inquiry into the Origin of the AIDS Epidemic*, is available on the internet through Amazon and Barnes and Noble, and in Australia through Infinity Bookshop in Sydney, Tel: (02) 92122225. Comprehensive information on the dangers of vaccines is available at the following website: http://209.1.224.11/HotSprings/1158/Vaccines.htm.

The above article appeared in New Dawn No. 63 (Nov-Dec 2000). Reprinted from: www.newdawnmagazine.com/Articles/Vaccine_Genocide.html

NATURAL TREATMENTS:

Multiple studies show that **elderberry extract** is extremely effective at curing up to 10 strains of the flu virus. In one study published in the Journal of International Medical Research, 90% of Norwegian influenza patients who took elderberry extract were back to normal within three days, compared to six days for the control group, which took placebos. Nearly all of the scientific studies conducted on elderberry have used a commercial product called Sambucol, which is available as a liquid supplement from a number of different companies.

Though **licorice root** has shown itself to be a very well documented antiviral, it needs to be taken with the knowledge that it has other effects which may be detrimental if they are not understood. As far as its ability to kill a broad spectrum of influenza viruses, it compares to black elderberry. When used in conjunction with black elderberry, its ability to kill a broad spectrum of influenza-causing viruses will be dramatically increased. However, it must be used with another supplement to be safe.

Licorice root causes the body to excrete potassium at an accelerated rate, thus supplemental potassium should be taken while you are on licorice root. The reason for this is that the active constituent, glycyrrhizin, mimics the actions of aldosterone, which is a steroid hormone produced by the adrenal cortex in the adrenal gland. It acts on the kidneys and causes the conservation of sodium, secretion of potassium, increased water retention, and increased blood pressure. Therefore, if you have high blood pressure, licorice root should be used only with the supervision of your healthcare provider. Also, due to its ability to mimic aldosterone, people with kidney problems should not use licorice root.

Licorice root also stimulates the aromatase enzyme, which will lower serum testosterone levels by increasing the conversion of testosterone to estradiol. Licorice has also been known to very rarely cause (ventricular) tachycardia. Though licorice root comes with some cautions, it has also been found to be effective against the hepatitis C virus as well as the herpes virus. Due to its well documented effects on a wide spectrum of viruses, we feel it should be a part of one's antiviral arsenal, if it is not contraindicated with other conditions.

Green tea is an excellent choice as a beverage due to its many health benefits. It is not only effective in treating the influenza virus, but it is capable of preventing the viral infection as well. It is much better to prevent a disease then treat one. The primary actives in green tea are the catechins which are able to inhibit the replication of the influenza virus. It is a safe and very effective way to both prevent and treat the influenza virus.

FOR YOUR DOCTOR:

See page 349 for research and studies to share with your doctor.

LUPUS

DESCRIPTION:

Systemic lupus erythematosus (commonly referred to as lupus) is an autoimmune disorder that occurs when the body engages in "friendly fire" against its own tissues and organs (including the skin, joints, kidneys, brain, heart, lungs, and blood). It affects close to 1.5 million Americans and eventually leads to chronic inflammation.

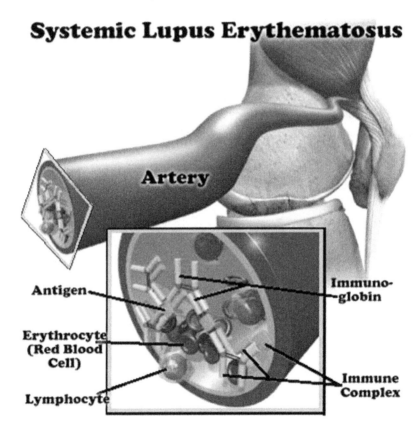

Systemic Lupus Erythematosus

Artery

Antigen

Immuno-globin

Erythrocyte (Red Blood Cell)

Immune Complex

Lymphocyte

SYMPTOMS:

Each person with lupus has different symptoms. However, some of the most common symptoms include painful or swollen joints, fatigue, unexplained fever, red skin rash ("butterfly" rash), sensitivity to sunlight (photosensitivity), cold hands, kidney problems, and malaise.

CONVENTIONAL TREATMENTS:

According to conventional medical wisdom, there is no cure for lupus. The goal is to control symptoms. Common treatments include **nonsteroidal anti-inflammatory medications** (NSAIDs), **cortico-steroid creams** (like prednisone, prednisolone, medrol, and deltasone) to treat skin rashes and decrease the immune response, and **hydroxychloroquine** (an antimalaria drug) for skin and arthritis symptoms. In most cases, symptomatic relief is less than optimal and has various side effects.

NATURAL TREATMENTS:

Our own findings (in the many identified "autoimmune" diseases) run contrary to current methodologies. After treating many of these cases, we have found that understanding the immune system and providing methods to actually normalize its reactions enables us to achieve a superior outcome than is achieved by trying to suppress it or inhibit it. When the immune system is working properly, it does not attack its own tissues and systems.

We feel it is also important to note that many lupus patients are **adrenally insufficient**. If your adrenals are not able to deliver the normal pulsatile secretions of both sex hormones and cortisol, inflammation will result. We have found that insufficiencies of cortisol secretions are best controlled with physiological doses of hydrocortisone to increase cortisol to normal levels. Since we know the adrenals normally secrete between 20-30 mg/day, simply restoring them to normal levels with bio-identical cortisol (like hydrocortisone) will result in reduced symptoms and have virtually no side effects, especially when compared to large dose (and very long lasting) pharmaceuticals such as prednisolone.

Another symptom of adrenal insufficiency is imbalances of sex hormones, due to the fact that the adrenals have a large part to play in sex hormone production. Most lupus patients (including men and women) have a low testosterone/estradiol ratio. Testosterone deficiencies can cause a decrease in pain tolerance, loss of muscle mass, increased inflammation, decreased flexibility, and poor recovery from work. This being so, the most sucessful treatments include

testosterone, pregnenolone, and **DHEA** along with a few herbs that have proven beneficial.

LifeOne is specially formulated and scientifically proven to repair a malfunctioning immune system, such as the case with Lupus. You can purchase LifeOne at this website: www.healthpro.com.dm/lifeone.html. Dietary supplementation with **omega-3 fish oils** improves lupus symptoms. In a 2007 study of 60 people with lupus, participants who took 3 grams of omega-3 fish oil supplements daily for six months showed improvements in their symptoms. **Cordyceps**, one of the better-known traditional Chinese medicines, has a broad range of pharmacological and biological actions on the liver, kidneys, heart, and immune system. It has been successfully used to treat lupus.

Remember that complete hormone profiles should be done for all lupus patients, since most patients have never had this done and have no idea where they stand, and correcting any hormonal deficiencies is essential. These must be done with the help of your primary caregiver. We also suggest a 24 hour cortisol saliva test, since it is much more reliable than a challenge test.

FOR YOUR DOCTOR:

See page 359 for research and studies to share with your doctor.

LYME DISEASE

DESCRIPTION:

Lyme disease ("Lyme Borreliosis") is an inflammatory disease caused by Borrelia burgdorferi which is a species of detrimental bacteria that is transmitted by a specific type of tick ("Ixodes dammini"), which is caried by deer, mice, and other mammals. Borrelia burgdorferi is able to burrow into tendons, muscle cells, ligaments, and directly into organs. Borrelia burgdorferi is capable of transforming into three distinct bacterial forms: spirochete, cell-wall-deficient, and cyst. It has also been suggested that Lyme disease can also be transmitted by other insects including fleas, mosquitos and mites.

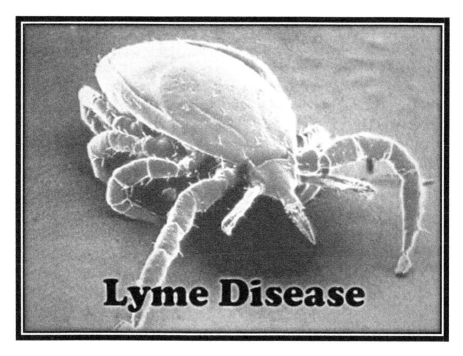

The incidence of Lyme disease is increasing. Part of this may be due to more common knowledge of the disease by physicians and more testing as well as an increase in its prevalence. It has moved from America into Canada at an alarming rate. Lyme disease is most prevalent in the Northern Hemisphere, particularly in the USA, Europe, Russia, Japan, and China.

Symptoms:

Lyme disease progresses through three distinct stages which offer different symptoms. The symptoms of **stage I** ("early localized" Lyme disease), where the infection is not yet widespread in the body, usually manifest within two to three weeks of infection. Symptoms include: fever, fatigue, swelling of the lymph nodes ("lymphadenopathy"), and arthralgia (muscle pain). Headaches are also common at this stage as well as a skin rash, known as erythema migrans. This skin rash is usually red circular lesion that looks like a bull's-eye and is larger than 5 cm in diameter. The rash, which occurs in 60%-80% of serologically confirmed cases, is usually not painful, but may increase in size up to 50 cm in size.

The symptoms of **stage II** ("early disseminated" Lyme disease), where the bacteria have begun to spread throughout the body, are too non-specific to be of much use. You may experience an increase in joint and muscle pain, especially in the knees. The symptoms of **stage III** ("late disseminated" or "chronic" Lyme disease), where the bacteria have spread throughout the body, may occur in months or even years after the tick bite. Symptoms include: an erosive arthritis of large joints (especially found in the knees), backache, muscle weakness, a stiff neck, nausea, vomiting, chills, insomnia, sudden hearing loss, sore throat ("pharyngitis").

Interestingly, the symptoms of Lyme disease can mimic Amyotrophic Lateral Sclerosis (ALS), also known as "Lou Gehrig's Disease," as well as Parkinson's disease, Multiple Sclerosis (MS), Bell's Palsy, reflex sympathetic dystrophy, neuritis, psychiatric illnesses (schizophrenia), autism, lupus, and many other conditions.

Conventional Treatments:

Conventional therapy includes pharmaceutical drugs (including **Amoxicillin** and **Doxycycline**) if the disease has not progressed past stage I. Broad-spectrum **cephalosporins** are used to treat Lyme disease if it has reached stage II or stage III. However, if the disease has reached stage III, treatment is less successful.

Another point which needs to be addressed is that Lyme disease affects the normal flora of the gut and tends to destroy the beneficial bacteria. The drugs used to treat the disease also destroy beneficial bacteria. Therefore, it is vital to supplement with probiotics and digestive enzymes in order to both preserve and replace the beneficial flora.

NATURAL TREATMENTS:

Before starting any therapy, it is imperative that there has been a serological test to verify the accuracy of the diagnosis. Quite often, a patient is diagnosed with ALS (or other disease) when Lyme disease is the true culprit.

The following natural treatments have shown to be effective during the spore stage as well as the early stage. If desired by your physician, both therapies may be used to increase the odds of a quick and complete recovery.

Colloidal silver (CS) has been shown to alleviate symptoms of Lyme disease. There are hundreds of websites and dozens of books about the groundbreaking and remarkable antibiotic capabilities of CS, which possesses a broad-spectrum, extremely powerful action against many microbes. However, the quality of available CS varies greatly. Remember that good CS is a powerful antibiotic, whereas poorly made CS is virtually worthless.

Cat's claw comes from a woody vine with claw-shaped thorns native to the Amazon highlands of Peru and other areas of South and Central America. This wonder herb is considered to be one of the main herbs that can help lower, or even eliminate, lyme spirochete loads in the body and support the innate immune function to help respond to the borrelia infection. It also helps alleviate central nervous system confusion, skin problems, and arthritic inflammation. Cat's claw is specifically good for helping treat stage III Lyme disease and that which does not respond to antibiotics.

Grapefruit seed extract is a powerful natural antibiotic that has produced herxheimer ("herx") reactions in Lyme disease sufferers. Herx reactions are a temporary worsening of symptoms which occurs because the Bb bacteria, under attack from the antibiotics (pharmaceutical or natural), start to break up and die, releasing toxins and other harmful debris as they do so. This, in turn, causes the body's immune system to temporarily go into overdrive in order to cope with the abrupt deluge of toxins and debris. This by no means indicates you should not use grapefruit seed extract. It means that it is very effective and should be started at a low dose, then worked up.

Berberine, as well as **N-acetylcysteine** (NAC), **olive leaf, cat's claw** and **grapefruit seed extract**, when combined, have been found to be very effective. They act synergistically and seem to act very quickly on killing the offending organism, regardless of stage.

Please note that our natural Lyme disease protocol includes taking CS, cat's claw, and GSE **together** with the addition of **probiotics** twice daily and **digestive enzymes** at every meal. Regardless of the therapy you and your primary caregiver choose, it is very important to take serological tests to be sure you are clear of all infection. Due to the difficulty in eliminating Lyme disease, it is recommended that serological testing be repeated every 30 days for a period of three months after the first clean serological report. This will assure you that the disease has been completely irradicated.

FOR YOUR DOCTOR:

See page 365 for research and studies to share with your doctor.

MARFAN SYNDROME

DESCRIPTION:

Marfan syndrome is a genetically passed disorder of connective tissue (tissue that strengthens the body's structures) which affects the skeletal system, cardiovascular system, eyes, and skin. It is believed to be carried by a gene called FBN1 which encodes a connective protein called "fibrillin-1." All people have a pair of FBN1 genes, and because Marfan syndrome is dominant, people who have inherited one affected FBN1 gene (from either parent) will have Marfan syndrome, which accounts for approximately 70% of Marfan syndrome cases. However, approximately 30% of cases have no family history. People with Marfan syndrome are at risk of aortic enlargement. Without proper management, the aorta (the large blood vessel that carries blood away from the heart) is prone to enlarge and could dissect (tear) or rupture. An aortic rupture is usually fatal.

SYMPTOMS:

Marfan syndrome has a range of expressions that range from mild to very severe. People with Marfan syndrome are usually tall with long, thin arms and legs and spider-like fingers (a condition called "arachnodactyly"). Other symptoms include defects of the heart valves and aorta, lungs, eyes, spinal cord, and skeleton, as well as a chest that sinks in or sticks out, flat feet, crowded teeth, and a thin, narrow face.

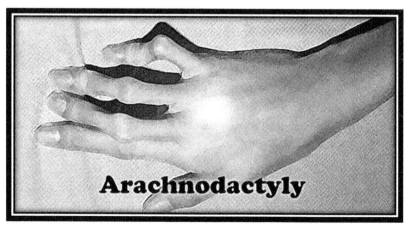

Arachnodactyly

CONVENTIONAL TREATMENTS:

There is no conventional cure for Marfan syndrome. However, a range of treatment options can minimize and sometimes prevent complications. Conventional therapy includes beta-blockers like Atenolol, which lowers blood pressure by blocking adrenaline receptor sites in the muscles. Also, annual echocardiograms to monitor the size and function of the heart and careful monitoring of the skeletal system by an orthopedist are common methods to monitor the disease.

NATURAL TREATMENTS:

Copper is an essential trace mineral of which humans need from 2 to 3 mg per day. Almost all Marfan syndrome patients are copper deficient. Desmosine is an amino acid specific to elastin, and the content of desmosine in urine is used to measure degradation of elastin content in the body. Copper is one of the factors known to influence elastin, and studies consistently show that Marfan syndrome patients have low desmosine content in their urine, providing another clue that perhaps copper deficiency may play an important role in the syndrome.

Another well-known problem with Marfan is abnormally high homocysteine levels. Homocysteine is an amino acid that inflicts damage to the inner arterial lining (endothelium) and other cells of the body. Elevated homocysteine levels have been found to be more relevant to heart failure than cholesterol. Research studies have documented that the nutraceutical, **N-acetylcysteine (NAC)**, can lower plasma homocysteine levels and improve endothelial function.

Many studies show that most people (60 - 85%, depending on the study) with mitral valve prolapse are low in **magnesium**. Not surprisingly, magnesium supplementation has been shown to alleviate the symptoms of mitral valve prolapse. Heart valves with mitral valve prolapse show abnormalities of hyaluronic acid. People with connective tissue disorders (like Marfan syndrome) commonly have mitral valve prolapse, and studies show they always have hyaluronic acid abnormalities. Here's the connection: hyaluronic acid depends upon magnesium for its synthesis.

A review of the studies on Medline shows that hyaluronic acid is linked to mitral valve prolapse, mitral valve prolapse is linked to a wide variety of disorders, especially connective tissue disorders like Marfan syndrome, and most connective tissue disorders are linked to anomalies of hyaluronic acid. One proven causative factor in mitral valve prolapse is low magnesium levels.

FOR YOUR DOCTOR:

See page 365 for research and studies to share with your doctor.

MULTIPLE SCLEROSIS (MS)

DESCRIPTION:

Multiple Sclerosis (MS) is a chronic neuromuscular ailment in which the myelin sheaths surrounding the nerves in the brain and spinal cord are damaged. The term "multiple sclerosis" is derived from the multiple lesions which occur on the myelin sheath during the progression of MS. This damage inhibits their ability to transmit signals throughout the central nervous system. There are several theories on the cause of MS. One theory is that it is a disorder of the immune system in which the myelin is attacked by immune system cells as if it were a foreign invader. Some scientists believe this may be started by a foreign agent such as a virus, which turns on the immune system and causes it to be unable to distinguish the myelin sheath from a foreign invader. Some scientists believe that varying environmental toxins and other environmental factors play a major role in MS.

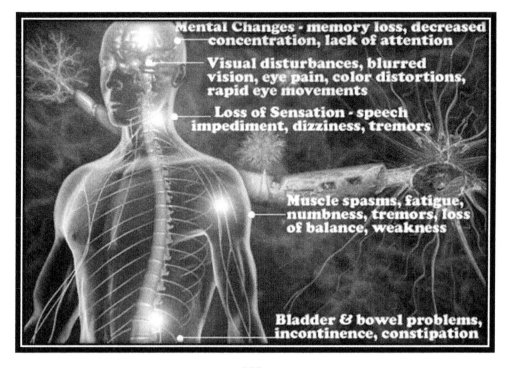

Mental Changes - memory loss, decreased concentration, lack of attention

Visual disturbances, blurred vision, eye pain, color distortions, rapid eye movements

Loss of Sensation - speech impediment, dizziness, tremors

Muscle spasms, fatigue, numbness, tremors, loss of balance, weakness

Bladder & bowel problems, incontinence, constipation

Simply put, there is really no proven positive cause for the development of MS. Once the nerves have been stripped of their myelin sheaths, scar tissue develops at the site of the lesion. The scars, called plaques, are unable to transmit signals. You will find the same type of plaques forming in the brains of Alzheimer's patients, with the same result of faulty nerve transmission.

One of the primary problems with MS is that it occurs during the impairment of the blood-brain barrier, a process which increases until the activated and inactivated cells of the immune system enter the brain through the blood-brain barrier. These cells then start an autoimmune process that begins to destroy the myelin sheaths of the axons of the neurons. The extent to which the symptoms increase directly correlates to the myelin sheath loss.

Demographically, MS occurs mainly in the Caucasian populations of westernized nations, with the highest incidence in the USA, Canada, Western Europe, Australia and New Zealand. In these countries the incidence of MS currently runs between 50-100 cases per 100,000 of the population. Another interesting finding is that in the higher latitudes with the more temperate climates there is a higher incidence of MS. It should also be noted that MS is more prevalent in women than in men. It is also noteworthy to understand that MS usually begins at an early age, most often beginning in the early adult years. There is also some scientific data which suggests a childhood infection may trigger an autoimmune response later in life.

Our personal belief is that there are probably numerous causes for this disease and that demyelization can be induced by multiple factors. Once this demyelization occurs, regardless of the causative factors, it will be diagnosed as MS. As an example, it has been presented and proven that heavy metal poisoning can cause sclerotic lesions to the myelin sheath as well various carbon based poisons which may induce lesions as well as many pesticides. It has been shown in numerous studies that the damage done from environmental contamination can do great damage to the myelin sheath and the rest of the nervous system as well as the cardiovascular system. At times, this contamination may actually be induced by Western medicine, as well as the combination of diet and pollution.

SYMPTOMS:

MS symptoms vary. Episodes can last for days, weeks, or months. Fever, hot baths, sun exposure, and stress can trigger or worsen attacks. **Muscle symptoms** include tremors and weakness in the arms and legs, problems walking, muscle spasms, loss of balance, and numbness. **Eye symptoms** include double vision, vision loss, and uncontrollable rapid eye movements. **Bowel and bladder symptoms** include incontinence, constipation, difficulting urinating, and frequent urination. **Other symptoms** include facial pain, decreased attention span, dizziness, hearing loss, slurred speech, difficulty chewing, and depression. Chronic fatigue is also a common MS symptom.

There are several clinical expressions of MS. During an acute attack, sudden deterioration in normal physical abilities (ranging from mild to severe) will occur. This is referred to as an exacerbation of MS, which will typically last for more than 24 hours and often will last for a few weeks, though usually not more than four weeks.

Approximately 65%-80% of patients begin with what is called relapsing-remitting (RR) MS, which is the most common type of the disease. During RR MS, the patient will suffer a series of attacks followed by either complete or partial disappearance of the symptoms. This remission will last anywhere from weeks to decades before another attack occurs, and the patient will feel normal during remission.

About 10-20% of patients suffer from what is called primary-progressive, (PP) MS. In PP MS there is a continuing decline in a person's physical strength and abilities without periods of remission.

The third type of recognized MS is called secondary-progressive. These patients start with RR MS, but over time their disabilities worsen. It is thought that about 50% of RR MS patients will become secondary-progressive MS patients, resulting in increased severity of attacks as well as a steady decline in abilities. It should also be known that in rare cases there is a rapid progression of the disease symptoms which is sometimes fatal. This variant is called "malignant" or "fulminant" MS, but is very rare.

Conventional Treatments:

There is no conventional cure for MS. However, a range of treatment options can minimize and sometimes prevent complications and slow the progression of the disease.

Common medications include:

- ❖ Intravenous immunoglobulin (IVIg)
- ❖ Interferons (Avonex, Betaseron, or Rebif) for the immune system
- ❖ Natalizumab (Tysabri)
- ❖ Glatiramer acetate (Copaxone)
- ❖ Mitoxantrone (Novantrone)
- ❖ Fingolimod (Gilenya)
- ❖ Azathioprine (Imuran)
- ❖ Methotrexate
- ❖ Cyclophosphamide (Cytoxan)
- ❖ Lioresal (Baclofen) or tizanidine (Zanaflex) to control spasms
- ❖ Antidepressants
- ❖ Amantadine (Symmetrel) for fatigue
- ❖ Acyclovir (due to its ability to inhibit the Human Herpes Virus Type 6)
- ❖ Alemtuzumab
- ❖ Aspirin
- ❖ Antibiotics (Doxycycline and Minocycline)
- ❖ Low-dose Naltrexone
- ❖ Olmesartan
- ❖ Prednisone

Natural Treatments:

It is generally accepted that MS is neither preventable nor curable, although many patients have gone into remission for many years and various therapies have been demonstrated to alleviate the symptoms of MS.

An interesting study was done in France which correlated **sunlight exposure** to MS as well as the difference between a male and female response to sunlight exposure. Their research showed a direct link between the time exposed to UVB radiation and the incidence of MS.

This comes at the same time that the importance of **vitamin D3** is becoming understood as it relates to preventing some types of cancer as well as its many other functions. Since vitamin D comes from both sunlight exposure and diet, avoidance of UVB radiation may be important for the health of some MS patients, but making sure that low exposure to sunlight is coupled with proper vitamin D3 supplementation is imperative.

Many have become overzealous in the use of sunscreens in the hope of stopping the harmful effects of sunburn and other future problems. The one caution we would recommend is to read the ingredients of any sunscreen product you choose very carefully. There is reliable research that has shown many of the chemicals used in widely used sunscreens actually may induce cancer as well as increase the possibility of other medical problems.

Our own personal opinion is that we require sunlight and it is an important part of everything from setting our internal clocks for normal pulsatile hormone release as well as for the natural production of vitamin D. Low vitamin D levels are dangerous, and lack of sunlight has also been linked to depression. Our recommendation is to take natural antioxidants to prevent free radical damage from the sunlight and limit your exposure time so that you never burn.

There are numerous naturally occurring plant chemicals that have been proven to not only protect us from the harmful effects to our skin, but also help repair DNA damage that sunlight may cause. Among them are the polyphenols found in **green tea** as well as silymarin which is a constituent of **milk thistle**.

In the year 2010, many experts using vitamin D found that it worked best if dosed at a rate based on body weight. The optimal dose is now considered to be 77 IU per kg of body weight per day in divided doses. Some studies have actually shown a decline in MS cases in people consuming high levels of vitamin D. The idea of preventing this debilitating disease is very appealing, so consumption of adequate vitamin D should be a staple for both those with currently diagnosed MS as well as young people concerned with developing MS or with a family history of the disease.

It should also be noted that there is such a thing as "pediatric onset" MS. Vitamin D has been shown to not only dramatically reduce the number of these cases, but be very beneficial in the treatment of this form of the disease. The normal recommended dosage ranges from 200 to 600 IU's per day.

Before going into what may be helpful in the management of MS, we would like to address two foods that have been repeatedly shown to make the condition worse. Both **animal fats** and **dairy products** should be avoided completely. The numerous studies that support this statement go back to work done on MS in the 1970s. The advertisement that states *"milk does a body good"* is not accurate when referring to cow's milk. Other animal fats, such as found on beef, pork, and butter have all been found to detrimental to MS patients.

Though the title of the book mentions curing various conditions, we cannot offer a "cure" for MS to either you or your primary caregiver. There are however, proven supplements that have been shown to be effective at both limiting the symptoms and their duration as well as the prevalence of acute attacks, and in some cases, even stopping the progression of the disease.

Acetyl-L-carnitine (ALC) has been found useful in MS patients due to its ability to suppress neuronal degradation as well as attenuate oxidative damage. The dosage usually recommended is 2000 mg/day in divided doses. It is considered a safe supplement with very few if any side effects.

N-acetylcysteine (NAC), which is a derivative of the amino acid L-cysteine, has also been shown to offer protections against continuing neuronal injury as well as possessing antioxidant properties. Be cautious when using NAC, since a few studies found that at very high doses it can place stress on the heart and respiratory system. It needs to be emphasized that the doses used in these experiments far exceeded what a healthcare practitioner would recommend, plus these exceedingly high doses are not required for NAC to have beneficial effects. At a dosage of 600 mg twice daily, all of the desired benefits are attainable. It has been found to be safe at 10,000 mg per day, so you will be well within the very safe range.

L-carnitine fumarate is a combination of L-carnitine and fumaric acid. This addition of fumaric acid to the L-carnitine has been shown to be beneficial in numerous ways and is supported in numerous studies. It acts by reducing the inflammatory response and, perhaps more importantly, by facilitating production of cells which protect dendritic cells from further damage. One caution is that L-carnitine may increase seizure activity if you have a seizure disorder, so be sure to discuss this with your primary caregiver. The normal dosage range is from 100 to 300 mg daily, divided into three doses. If you are taking L-carnitine fumarate, additional L-carnitine is not needed.

Calcium AEP is 10% calcium bound to 90% Amino Ethanol Phosphate (AEP). It is the AEP portion of the complex that gives this product its most beneficial characteristics, since AEP is directly attracted to cell membranes. It was first discovered by a biochemist, Erwin Chargaff, in 1941. It was Chargaff who found AEP to be extremely protective to cell membranes, but it was a German physician, Dr. Hans Nieper, that made the first great strides in its uses in the 1960s. Protecting the cell membranes has made calcium AEP one of the most used and most highly regarded of dietary supplements for MS patients. The normal recommended dosage runs from 1000 to 2000 mg per day in two divided doses.

After evaluating the treatment of over three thousand MS patients over many years, Dr. Nieper found not only that calcium AEP reduced recurrence of MS remarkably, but also that almost none of the patients had developed cancer. Also, in a 6-year study of 8 patients with repeated surgery for colon cancer, there were no further recurrences with calcium AEP therapy.

In 1971, Monninghoff in Munster, Germany, published electron microscopic findings that showed conslusively that the sealing of these cell membranes was able to prevent penetration of peroxidase granules. It is penetration of peroxidase granules which induce the state called "lipid peroxidation" which (by definition) causes great oxidative stress within the cells.

There seems to be general agreement that the addition of **calcium orotate** with the calcium AEP may prove to be even more beneficial, but not enough studies have been done to state this as fact. Our opinion is that some trials have shown it to be helpful and no trials have shown it not to be helpful, so we tend to recommend its use in conjunction with the calcium AEP. It is a very safe supplement and can be used very effectively at a recommended dosage of 300 mg twice daily.

As a word of caution, calcium orotate may decrease the absorption of other drugs such as bisphosphonates (alendronate), tetracycline antibiotics (doxycycline, minocycline), estramustine, levothyroxine, and quinolone antibiotics (ciprofloxacin, levofloxacin). Due to this fact, you would be wise to work with your primary caregiver to help work out a schedule that separates the doses of these medications as far as possible from the calcium orotate to make sure you are able to get the maximum benefit from all medications. The dosages range from 250 to 1200 mg per day in two divided doses. Dosage is dependent on age, sex, and pregnancy status. Speak with your caregiver for advice on required dosage for your case.

Many MS patients exhibit low levels of **vitamin B12** (methylcobalamin). Supplemental vitamin B12 (in the methylcobalamin form only) has been shown to counteract the degeneration of the myelin sheaths of the central nervous system that occurs during the progression of MS. Though very large doses of B12 taken orally have shown the ability to improve visual and brain stem nerve potentials, the dose is 60 mg and it does not improve motor function. However, when given by small needle injection, or in a sublingual tablet, it has been shown to be extremely effective. Though there are other forms of B12, methylcobalamin is the only form that shows maximum effect. The normal dosage ranges from 500 to 4000 micrograms daily. To obtain the maximum benefit, be sure to discuss with your primary caregiver to determine your current levels and raise it to the high normal levels.

Vitamin B3 (the niacinamide form) may be useful for the treatment of MS, while another form of vitamin B3 (niacin) has also been shown to have beneficial effects but may need to be administered through I.V. injection. Though it has been found to be very safe, "niacin flush" may be noticed until the patient becomes used to it. Both forms of vitamin B3 are presently being used to prevent autoimmune-mediated demyelization of nerve tissue. Due to its extreme safety and its proven ability to protect the nerves from demyelization, vitamin B3 seems to be a worthwhile supplement. Though most physicians use injectable forms, oral forms are available at a very reasonable price. The normal dosage range for niacinamide capsules is from 100 to 500 mg. Be aware that when first taking this supplement, many people feel a hot flush for a short time. This is normal and will pass as your body becomes used to it and your serum levels increase.

Magnesium has been found to have several beneficial effects in the comprehensive treatment of MS. It has been found to decrease the relapse rate of MS, decrease the inflammatory response, decrease muscle spasticity, as well as reduce the dysfunction of the nerve cells. It has also been shown to concentrate in the white matter of the brain and offer neurological protection of these cells. The most used dosages run from 200 to 500 mg per day in two divided doses.

Proteolytic enzymes are defined as a group of enzymes that increase the rate that proteins are decomposed or destroyed. It is the destruction of these foreign proteins that eliminates their ability to produce autoimmune actions. The enzymes **bromelain** and **trypsin** have been combined into a product called Phlogenzym. This product has gone through several small studies in several countries, but no large scale studies. Personally, we find the consistency of the results more important than large numbers of patients with inconsistent results. Do to the consistency of Phlogenzyme against T-cell mediated autoimmune disease (and specifically MS), we are comfortable in recommending its use in conjunction with the other well researched supplements. Whether you choose this product or purchase the two enzymes separately, due to their mechanisms of action, we suggest giving these enzymes several months to have full effect. Normal recommended dosage for Phlogenzyme is 3 tablets twice daily or 2 tablets three times daily.

Naturally occurring antioxidants are found in numerous plants and many have undergone substantial research, specifically targeting MS due to the oxidative damage that occurs to the myelin sheath. It has been determined that by reducing this oxidative stress, less neuronal damage is likely to follow. By keeping oxidative stress to a minimum, MS patients are more capable of maintaining intact myelin sheaths and neuronal conductivity, thus limiting damage that would otherwise occur. These naturally occurring plant antioxidants are also capable of functioning as free radical scavengers, which are capable of inactivating any compound that reacts with free radicals and reducing free radical damage. Three vitamins that have reliable research behind them in preventing this free radical damage are the **vitamins A, C,** and **E.**

The normal recommended doses for these vitamins are:

- ❖ Vitamin A – 400 to 1,600 IU per day.
- ❖ Vitamin C – 2000 to 10,000 mg per day in divided doses. Much larger doses are sometimes used as therapeutic.
- ❖ Vitamin E – 400 to 1,600 IU per day with the higher dose being used therapeutically (in the form of mixed tocopherols).

Some of the most important natural antioxidants for MS patients have been found to be **quercetin, resveratrol, daidzein, genistein,** and **catechins** such as those found in green tea polyphenols. These should also be considered for supplementation. Dosages for all of these will depend on the product you choose. Use the advised dosage as a guideline to discuss with your provider.

It is important to remember that supplementation of at least all of the vitamins as well as a few of the natural antioxidants (such as quercetin, resveratrol, and green tea polyphenols) should be combined, thus creating a synergistic effect and enhancing the overall response. If these are combined with the other well documented natural aids (such as vitamin D), dietary changes, and proper hormone regulation (which we will cover next), we believe that it will be possible to see a drastic reduction of acute attacks, much longer remissions, and a drop in the severity of the acute episodes.

The term "estrogen" is a word that includes not a single hormone but a substantial family of hormones, consisting primarily of estrone (E1), estradiol (E2), and estriol (E3). Along with these three principal estrogens, we know that there are at least two dozen other identified estrogens produced in the body.

Though steroids are often used to alleviate the chronic fatigue suffered by many MS patients, we believe that long term use of corticosteroids causes more long term harm than good. An option that is supported by very favorable research findings is the use of **estriol**. It is one of the safest of estrogens, while estradiol has been found to be detrimental in many instances. Estriol supplementation will, in all probability, cause a drop in estradiol levels due to the fact that the endocrine system works through negative feedback. This means that if there is an adequate supply of estriol, estradiol production will be inhibited.

Estriol has been found to be more effective with less side effects than corticosteroids, so a complete hormone panel should be done on all MS patients. If estradiol levels are high (in relation to DHEA, testosterone, or other hormones) or if estriol levels are in the low to low normal range, then estriol should definitely be considered for supplementation. The dosage of hormones will be directly decided by the results of your personal hormone profile in conjunction with your primary caregiver.

Other hormones (such as testosterone, DHEA, hGH, melatonin, progesterone, pregnenolone, and IGF-1) have been shown to be helpful in some MS patients. A complete hormone panel, if read by a knowledgeable primary caregiver, will give a very good indication of what needs to be supplemented. Since all of these hormones have been shown to be helpful in MS patients, they should all be considered. However, in this book, we will deal with only one of these hormones, due to the data that substantiates its use. That hormone is **testosterone**.

Unfortunately, many primary caregivers seem to forget that testosterone is as important to women as it is to men. Not only does it increase libido, muscular strength, and fight estradiol dominance when used with an aromatase inhibitor (like DeAromatase), but it also has been shown to have a neuroprotective effect. Our feeling is that with proper management, testosterone levels should be kept at the upper limits of normal. The reason we believe it should be kept in the upper levels (with aromatase control) is that human testosterone levels have been falling dramatically over the last decade. This skews the normal range so that what now falls in the "normal" range at the low end is actually very low and would have been considered very low on the scale of normal ranges 10 years ago. The dosage of hormones will be directly decided by the results of your personal hormone profile in conjunction with your primary caregiver.

MS patients are also often particularly deficient in **docosahexaenoic acid** (DHA), a non-essential omega-3 fatty acid which can be synthesized within the body or obtained via the diet. However, its categorization as "non-essential" is far from true, as the mere fact that the body produces DHA proves that it is essential for numerous mechanisms. Among these mechanisms is DHA's ability to reduce inflammation of neurons, modulate immune cell production, and increase cell survival. Most MS patients are deficient in DHA, therefore supplementation should be considered. The normal dosage range is between 600 to 2000 mg per day.

MS patients are also often found to have low **copper** and **zinc** levels. These minerals play an important part in controlling proper brain function (on several levels) and supplementation is warranted. It is interesting to note that although low levels may be present in the brain, the levels may appear normal in cerebral spinal fluid and other parts of the body. Since there is evidence of malabsorption, it may be wise to work with your primary caregiver to determine (through a comprehensive stool analysis) if the proper good flora is present to facilitate this absorption or if pathogenic bacteria are present that may inhibit their absorption. The normal dosage range for zinc is between 30 and 60 mg per day. The normal range for copper is 1 to 3 mg per day, but it should not be taken at the same time as vitamin C or zinc.

In some trials, **gingko biloba** has shown only modest benefits and in some it has been disappointing with only minor or transitory effects. If you choose to try it, the recommended dosage would vary dramatically, depending on the form you use. Start at the recommended dosage on the bottle for a start and see if it is helpful. The dosage may be slowly increased if you find it beneficial in your case. Speak with your caregiver about dosage adjustment.

Though there are many other herbs that have shown beneficial effects on MS, few have passed enough peer reviewed research to positively say that they will be effective on most patients. That is not to say they are not worthy of consideration, however they will need to be evaluated on an individual basis. These would include: aloe vera (orally), olive leaf, andrographis, and milk thistle. All of these should be started at the recommended dose and should be added one at a time to determine which are most helpful.

The most commonly used pharmaceutical drugs for symptomatic relief of MS **that will not interfere with a more comprehensive approach** as outlined above are as follows:

- ❖ Alemtuzumab (which is used to reduce the number of attacks experienced by people with RR MS)
- ❖ Aspirin (1,300 mg per day) has been shown to reduce fatigue associated with MS.

❖ Prednisone at relatively high doses of 60 mg per day for 5 to 7 days may facilitate recovery of acute attacks of MS, but due to its numerous toxic side effects, should be used sparingly. It is primarily masking the problem by temporarily decreasing the inflammation associated with MS.

❖ Baclofen is used to temporarily reduce muscle spasms associated with MS.

❖ Doxycycline at a normal dosage of 100 mg per day for 21 days is sometimes used when it is determined that the infection of chlamydia pneumoniae may be the cause of MS.

❖ Low-dose Naltrexone is sometimes used in the treatment of Multiple Sclerosis, though research is scant.

❖ Natalizumab, which is administered via intravenous injection, is sometimes used to prevent recurrences and worsening of the symptoms of MS.

❖ Olmesartan at the normal dosage of 160 mg per day taken as one 40 mg dose each six hours has been found to be useful for some cases of MS.

FOR YOUR DOCTOR:

See page 374 for research and studies to share with your doctor.

PARKINSON'S DISEASE

DESCRIPTION:

Parkinson's disease (aka idiopathic parkinsonism, primary parkinsonism, PD, or paralysis agitans) is named after the English doctor James Parkinson, who published the first detailed description in *An Essay on the Shaking Palsy* in 1817.

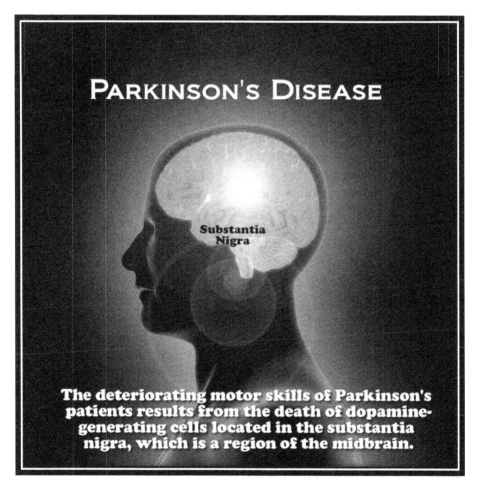

PD is a chronic disease of the central nervous system that is characterized by slowness and uncoordinated movement, rigid muscles and shaking, as well as difficulty with walking in the earlier stages. The deteriorating motor skills of PD result from the death of dopamine-generating cells located in the substantia nigra, which is a region of the midbrain. There are many theories as to the cause of this cell death, and the truth is that there are likely multiple causes, including aluminum toxicity, heavy metals, pesticides, and pathogenic organisms.

Currently, PD is known as an idiopathic disease, meaning *"a disease of unknown cause,"* and usually occurs after the age of 40. Several specialists and researchers (including the authors of this book) have come to conclude that environmental toxins and contaminated well water are primarily to blame for PD, but it also may have genetic links. It is universally agreed, however, that PD results from the degeneration or destruction of nerve cells that produce dopamine.

Despite the fact that PD is known as an idiopathic disease, we know of several factors that increase the likelihood of developing it. For instance, there is an increase in PD in workers that are around certain pesticides and various heavy metals. Also, smokers are actually less likely to develop PD due to the fact that nicotine has been shown to be an effective treatment. This is not an endorsement of smoking on any level, but facts are facts, and there are other deliveries of nicotine that are far safer and that have controlled dosages.

PD is characterized by an accumulation of a protein called "alpha-synuclein" into Lewy bodies within the neurons. It also affects the formation and activity of dopamine which is produced by particular neurons within parts of the midbrain. It is actually the pathology of the Lewy bodies that lead the distinguishing factors of PD, since the distribution of these Lewy bodies varies from individual to individual. In most PD cases, diagnosis is made through the observation of symptoms, such as uncontrollable shaking of the hands, but is normally verified through neuroimaging.

Although both AD and MS are frequently believed to be painless diseases, that is almost never the case. Neuropathy is almost always accompanied by painful spasms and neuropathic pain. It is interesting to note that schizophrenia and the psychotic features of bipolar disorder are directly associated with imbalances of both dopamine and serotonin in the brain.

SYMPTOMS:

Parkinson's symptoms may be mild in the beginning of the disease. For instance, you may have a mild tremor or a slight feeling that one leg or foot is stiff and dragging. As the disease progresses, other symptoms include drooling, difficulty swallowing, constipation, slow blinking, difficulty balancing, difficulty with facial expressions, difficulty moving, tremors, slowed or slurred speech, low blood pressure, memory loss, hallucinations, depression, confusion, and anxiety, amongst others. Cognitive and behavioral problems (associated with dementia) occur in the late stages of the disease. Emotional problems as well as sleep disorders may also present as part of the disease process.

CONVENTIONAL TREATMENTS:

Although there is no conventional cure for PD, there are a number of medicines that can help to improve symptoms, chiefly by increasing the levels of dopamine in the brain.

Currently the pharmaceutical drug of choice in the early stages of PD is Levodopa, or L-Dopa. Levodopa is converted into dopamine in the body, thereby elevating the dopamine levels inhibited by the disease. Dopamine is a very important monoamine neurotransmitter formed in the brain which is usually formed from the amino acid, tyrosine, but PD interferes with its production. Dopamine is essential for the normal function of the central nervous system and has multiple functions including regulating emotions, perception, and movement.

Although L-Dopa may provide substantial relief of the symptoms of PD, it does not actually retard the progress of the disease. In the normal PD patient, the effectiveness of L-Dopa usually begins to decline after 5 to 7 years. Although L-Dopa increases dopamine levels, it does not repair the damage to the dopamine receptors nor does it regenerate the damaged dopaminergic neurons (neurons whose primary neurotransmitter is dopamine). It must also be noted that L-Dopa's oxidative byproducts may actually increase the destruction of dopaminergic neurons. In recent studies it has actually been shown that the use of L-dopa has shortened the expected lifespan of patients taking it.

The primary results of elevating dopamine levels in early stage PD are reduction of stiffness, reduction of tremors, spasms and increased muscle control. There are numerous other pharmaceuticals that cannot be taken with L-Dopa (such as nardil, parnate, marplan, and isocarboxazid). There are also several possible side effects, so L-Dopa should not be taken if you suffer from any type of heart or cardiovascular disease, or have narrow-angle glaucoma, malignant melanoma, kidney or liver disease, respiratory disease (such as COPD or asthma), endocrine disorder, depression, wide-angle glaucoma, or any psychiatric disorder. As PD progresses, more dopaminergic neurons are destroyed and the use of L-Dopa is no longer effective. It is at this time that a common complication called dyskinesia (which involves involuntary writhing movements) begins. Later in this chapter, we will discuss safer methods of raising dopamine levels that do not have the harmful effects of L-Dopa.

There are also pharmaceuticals that are used to aid in sleep disturbances, as well as emotional problems that often accompany PD. Another popular drug in use for PD is called rasagiline. Rasagiline is a monoamine oxidase-B (MAO-B) inhibitor which is used to treat the symptoms of PD and is often used in conjunction with L-Dopa. Certain medicines should not be taken together with rasagiline; therefore it is imperative to work closely with your primary caregiver when using this drug.

At their official site is the following warning:

"Before you take this medication, tell your doctor about all other medications you are using, especially muscle relaxers, narcotic pain medicine, over-the-counter cough medicine, or St. John's wort. Do not use rasagiline if you have taken another MAO inhibitor such as furazolidone (Furoxone), isocarboxazid (Marplan), phenelzine (Nardil), selegiline (Eldepryl, Emsam), or tranylcypromine (Parnate) in the last 14 days. Serious, life threatening side effects can occur if you use rasagiline before the other MAO inhibitor has cleared from your body. Before you take rasagiline, tell your doctor if you have liver disease … Side effects include but are not limited to; changes in vision, chest pain, confusion, hallucination, high blood pressure, fast, irregular heartbeat, feeling faint or lightheaded, falls, fever, memory loss, muscle or neck stiffness or spasm, numbness or pain in the arms or legs, especially on one side only, problems with balance, talking, or walking, seizures, sudden severe headache, suicidal thoughts or other mood changes, unexpected weight loss, unexplained nausea or vomiting, unusual sweating, bruising, diarrhea or consti-

pation, dry mouth, loss of appetite, muscle pain or cramps, stomach upset or heartburn."

Did you notice that a large number of possible side effects **are exactly the same** as the known symptoms of PD? You and your healthcare provider will have to determine if this is a medication you will want to use. There is a much safer alternative (deprenyl) which actually has advantages over this drug which we will discuss later in this chapter.

NATURAL TREATMENTS:

Comprehensive treatment for PD will rely heavily on honesty and cooperation with your primary caregiver. Sometimes the patient is unaware of deterioration, so their spouse or close friend may be very helpful in aiding the doctor understand the progression and symptoms more thoroughly.

Research at Harvard School of Public Health has found that caffeine may have a protective affect against the development of PD. The research was performed on over 120,000 people, which is a very large sample size. The evidence supported the theory that moderate **caffeine** intake may be protective against developing PD. In our opinion, it should definitely be considered as a treatment. **Green tea** may offer additional protection due to its content of polyphenols. Research has actually shown that tea drinkers also have a lower incidence of PD, but the researchers typically do not understand why. Apparently they are unaware that tea also contains caffeine.

Acetyl-L-carnitine (ALC) has been researched extensively and it offers some protection against oxidative damage as well as relief from neuronal originating pain. It has also been shown to act as a mitochondrial energy transporter, which means it is able to transport energy to the mitochondria of the cell. Mitochondria are specialized compartments present in every cell of the body (with the exception of red blood cells) and are responsible for creating more than 90% of the energy needed by the body to sustain life. In AD, the mitochondria do begin to fail, and as the number of failed mitochondria increases, there is less and less energy generated within the cell, which eventually results in cell injury and cell death.

Two additional attributes of ALC are its ability to aid in the release of dopamine and its ability to protect these dopamine releasing cells from certain toxins. It is very safe and there has been no toxicity found even in very high doses. The usual recommended dose is 500 to 2,000 mg per day, with many people obtaining benefits using the lower dosage of 500 mg per day.

Creatine monohydrate (α-methyl-guanidinoacetic acid) is a naturally occurring nitrogenous organic acid which is produced within the body. Dietary meat provides about half of the typical person's creatine intake. Whatever creatine is not taken in as food is synthesized in the liver and pancreas from glycine, methionine, and arginine (with the aid of two enzymes). Because these two enzymes are not concentrated in the liver and pancreas, synthesis begins in the kidneys and is completed through a process called "methylation" in the liver. The largest concentration of creatine is found in skeletal muscle followed by cardiac muscle, but neither skeletal muscle nor cardiac muscle are able to produce creatine.

Creatine is capable of effecting multiple cellular tasks, including increasing muscle strength, decreasing oxidative damage to neuronal cells, and (perhaps most importantly) reducing mitochondrial damage to cells, thus increasing cellular function. It has yet to be researched for its long-term effects on AD patients, but there is hope that it may at least diminish the effects of AD and perhaps inhibit the disease progression.

Methionine sulfoxide reductase A (MsrA) is an extremely important antioxidant repair enzyme; its primary function is reducing oxidized methionine to methionine. Since oxidation of methionine in proteins impairs their function, an absence of MsrA leads to abnormalities in the human brain. Any substance that is able to effectively reduce this oxidative process in neurodegenerative disease will be able, at the very least, to slow its progression in a worst case scenario, and perhaps even reduce the incidence and severity of recurrent acute attacks.

N-acetylcysteine (NAC) comes from the amino acid L-cysteine. All amino acids are building blocks of proteins. One of the common uses of NAC is to counteract acetaminophen (Tylenol) and carbon monoxide poisoning. It has many other uses, including treatment for unstable angina and spasms of the heart muscle, and is used for several neurodegenerative diseases such as ALS (Lou Gehrig's disease), Alzheimer's disease, and PD.

In neurodegenerative diseases its actions are numerous. NAC has been shown to preserve dopamine receptors and prevent oxidative stress on both dopamine receptors and dopamine production cells. It also offers some cellular protection from several of the neurotoxins which cause PD. Neuroprotective affects can be achieved with 500 mg twice daily. The toxic dosage is considered to be 10,000 mg per day. It can be taken effectively orally and should definitely be discussed with your primary caregiver.

There are several other amino acids that are sometimes recommended for PD patients. All of them have claims, but few have enough consistent positive research for us to recommend them. Some recommended supplements that have showed promise are SAMe, taurine, tyrosine, theanine, and glutamic acid. Yet in later research these same products have been shown to be potentially counterproductive. For this reason we have left them out. Hopefully further research will be done to validate more amino acids for the future.

The biggest problem is that pharmaceutical companies cannot patent naturally occurring molecules, so there is little motivation for them to fund research. Without well done consistent research findings, we feel it is irresponsible to recommend them. Also, please make sure that any claims being made by any doctor for any new "miracle drug" are backed by unbiased and credible research and that the doctor is not just stepping into a sales position for profit. This happens all too often in the pharmaceutical industry where doctors are given trips, gifts, or other rewards for selling a pharmaceutical drug.

Astaxanthin is considered to be a "xanthophyll dihydroxycarotenoid"; it does not convert to vitamin A within the body. Astaxanthin contains two additional oxygenated groups on each ring structure (compared with other carotenoids), which results in it having more powerful antioxidant activities than most other antioxidants. Another of astaxanthin's important attributes is the ability to protect neuronal cells from toxin induced cell death. In addition to these vital properties, it has also been shown to protect the mitochondria of the cells.

Maximum levels of astaxanthin are reached about 6½ hours after it is orally taken. One important thing to remember is to either find an astaxanthin supplement that contains some type of dietary fat or take it in conjunction with a dietary fat (such as fish oil). This will dramatically increase its absorption and enable it to readily pass through the blood-brain barrier, which is required for it to have its neuroprotective and antioxidative effects.

Astaxanthin appears to be a very safe compound and in animal studies; it has shown a complete lack of toxicity. The normal therapeutic dose ranges from 2 to 8 mg (2,000 mcg to 8,000 mcg) per day. It may be taken in divided doses or in a single dose. Because its half-life is less than 24 hours, and it reaches its peak in just over 6 hours, we recommend taking it in divided doses about 12 hours apart.

Coenzyme Q10 (CoQ10) is a fat-soluble coenzyme Q ("quinone") which is considered the single most important Q coenzyme for humans. It is interesting to note that its structure is very similar to other molecular structures that offer some of the same benefits, such as idebenone, vitamin E, and vitamin K. There has been an enormous amount of research on CoQ10 which has found it to be a valuable tool in anti-aging, cardiovascular disease, kidney disease, eye disease, pancreatic and gastrointestinal disease, allergies, viral and bacterial infections, and cancer. The reason it affects so many systems is that it is contained in almost every cell in the body.

CoQ10 has been shown to directly reduce the oxidative stress of PD on the mitochondria of the cell. It has also been shown to reduce disease progression up to 40% in some research, but that is at a high dosage. An interesting study showed there was a significant reduction in CoQ10 concentrations in the cortex region of the brain, which is the region of the brain most affected by PD.

So to simplify the findings, it can be said that research has shown that CoQ10 offers neuroprotection in PD via its positive affects on mitochondrial function, cellular bioenergetics, and oxidation. We also know that there is a lack of CoQ10 in the regions of the brain that directly affect PD, and since it is harmless to take, it seems that supplementation would be wise. Unfortunately, CoQ10 is a relatively expensive supplement and the best results have been found in studies using 1200 mg per day in divided doses. It is also strongly suggested it be taken with vitamin E to insure its transport across the blood-brain barrier.

Based on recent research, we believe that CoQ10 acts synergistically with creatine and vitamin E. This synergy allows us to reduce the amount of each substance and increase the efficacy of what is taken. In Europe, physicians regularly use 600 mg of CoQ10 daily without ill effects and with good results. Our advice is to take 200 mg three times daily with vitamin E and creatine.

NADH stands for "nicotinamide adenine dinucleotide (NAD) + hydrogen (H)." This chemical occurs naturally in the human body and is responsible for a major role in the chemical process that generates energy. NADH is often used for improving mental acuity, concentration, alertness, and memory; it is also used in the treatment of AD. NAD is used by athletes to increase their energy and endurance, and it is also used in the treatment of chronic fatigue syndrome (CFS).

NADH is also used in the treatment of PD since it both protects and increases the energy of the cell. It is easily taken sublingually at a dosage from 2.5mg to 10mg. Alzheimer's patients often take up to 20mg. It should not be taken orally due to the fact that stomach acids destroy it, so physicians often administer via injection for the treatments of PD and depression. However, this may make regular use difficult for most patients, so our suggestion is to use the sublingual NADH.

Melatonin is a neurohormone which is produced from the amino acid tryptophan by the pineal gland when the eyes detect no light (in darkness or blindness, or during sleep). The lymphocytes, mast cells, the retina of the eye, and cells in the gastrointestinal tract also produce melatonin, but to a much lesser extent. Through a series of enzyme-catalyzed reactions, tryptophan is partially converted to 5-hydroxytryptophan (5-HTP), which is partially converted to serotonin, which is partially converted to melatonin. Many suggest taking melatonin with NADH, as melatonin has a very well researched role in protection of nerve cells from free radical damage. Another advantage is that research has shown that melatonin replaces the hydrogen atom on NADH when it is used, thus stabilizing active levels of NADH.

The timing of taking melatonin supplements is very important. It is best to take melatonin on a nightly basis approximately 2 to 3 hours before normal sleep time. If possible, it is best taken at the same time each night since the body has its own circadian rhythm of sleep and skipping a dose can have the effect of disrupting the normal sleep patterns. If you have an unusually late night out, it is best to skip that night's dosage and begin again the following night.

Melatonin will require a bit of experimentation due to the variability of dosage required from one person to the next. Actual therapeutic doses for neuropathic diseases can vary by a factor of as much as 2,000. Some patients will require as little as .1 mg per night and others may require from 1 to 10 mg per night; it is best to start low and slowly work your way up. Smaller doses of .1 mg or less have been found to be more effective for promoting sleep in some research, but in neurodegenerative diseases, the goal is much more than just a sleep aid. Find the dose that best helps you to sleep and makes you feel better, with higher daytime energy levels. Melatonin is very safe and some clinical trials have used as much as 300 mg per night, so working within the range of 1 to 10 mg per night is exceedingly safe.

Deprenyl (aka Selegiline) is considered a "smart drug", or a drug that increases memory and cognitive ability. Many smart drugs are used in anti-aging medicines and some are available by mail order from other countries. All of the smart drugs have been found to be safe when used as labeled and many have proven helpful in various neurological and cerebral dysfunctions. Deprenyl was discovered approximately 40 years ago in Hungary by Dr. Joseph Knoll and colleagues as they were attempting to develop an effective anti-depressant drug. Deprenyl is chemically related to phenetylamine (PEA), a substance found in chocolate and are produced in higher-than-normal amounts in the brains of people who are "in love."

After conducting a 2-year lifespan study on rats using the drug, they found that deprenyl had anti-aging properties as well. Since then, many other lifespan studies on deprenyl have been conducted in other countries, the majority of which have confirmed Dr. Knoll's initial findings. Available in Europe under the trade names Eldepryl and Jumex, deprenyl's primary function in PD is the inhibition of an enzyme found in the brain called monoamine oxidase-B (MAO-B). Like most enzymes, MAO-B has only one function, which, in this case is to break down dopamine and other compounds known as neurotransmitters. By inhibiting this breakdown of dopamine and neurotransmitters, it is possible to radically slow the progression of PD. Another additional benefit of deprenyl is that some studies have shown that it actually increases the lifespan of PD patients.

Although **vitamin D** is commonly called a vitamin, it is not actually classified as an essential dietary vitamin due to the fact it can be synthesized in adequate amounts by all mammals from an interaction between sunlight and cholesterol. It actually acts more like a hormone within the body than an essential vitamin. The majority of PD patients are deficient in vitamin D, which plays innumerable roles in the body, and even today, several new ones are still being investigated. It is needed for prevention of rickets, several forms of cancer, bone remodeling and fracture repair, as well as neuronal health and function.

Vitamin D is actually a group of fat-soluble secosteroids (molecules similar to steroids but with "broken" rings in their molecular structures). In humans, vitamin D is unique due to the fact that it can be ingested as cholecalciferol (vitamin D3) or ergocalciferol (vitamin D2) and because the body can also synthesize it from cholesterol with the help of direct sun exposure. Unfortunately in Western society, sunlight exposure has become either "frightening" due to skin cancer fear or unavailable due to working inside an office all day long. In the liver, vitamin D is converted to calcidiol (also known as calcifediol INN, 25-hydroxycholecalciferol, or 25-hydroxyvitamin D), which is the specific vitamin D metabolite that is measured in serum to determine a person's vitamin D status. Part of the calcidiol is converted by the kidneys to calcitriol, which is the biologically active form of vitamin D. Calcitriol circulates as a hormone in the blood, regulating the ratios of calcium and phosphate in the bloodstream and facilitating the healthy growth and remodeling of bone. Calcidiol is also converted to calcitriol outside of the kidneys for other purposes, such as the proliferation, differentiation, and apoptosis of cells. Calcitriol also affects neuromuscular function, repair, and inflammation.

It is very important for PD patients to obtain **complete hormone profiles** in order to see if they are low in progesterone and to make sure they are not estradiol dominant. This is true for all neurodegenerative disease patients, thus complete hormone profiles need to become a much more prominent part of comprehensive medical care for several other diseases as well. Unfortunately, they are rarely done, and if they are done, they are almost always incomplete.

Monitoring of the free unbound levels of estradiol and testosterone as well as DHEA, progesterone, estriol and pregnenolone is vital in the comprehensive management of PD.

Both **vitamin C** and **vitamin E** are well known and have been mentioned in much of the research in this book. Of particular import to PD patients are their free radical scavenging abilities and antioxidative properties. In addition to being an antioxidant, vitamin C also helps the production of L-dopa from tyrosine. There are innumerable herbs that have a few studies that show some efficacy in the treatment of PD. We have read them all, from ashwagandha to yerbamate, and almost everything in between. The problem is that almost all of them would be "inference" studies in this book, and we prefer to stick to correctly performed and published peer reviewed studies. By inference studies, we mean studies that show an herb's mehanisms of action are desirable, thus the reader would infer that it would be helpful. However, we prefer to include only studies that use the actives of herbs on the specific disease we are discussing. In other words, we have a sort of "*show us the beef*" attitude when it comes to patient welfare.

Ginkgo biloba has been thoroughly studied and published. The vast majority of studies have shown it to have little to no effect on neurological disorders, hypertension in the elderly, or significant help in retaining cognitive function. There are a few positive articles published, but we question the sources of the publication. Also in most of the positive research, changes were small enough to be questioned.

In numerous studies, **iron** has been found in much higher than normal levels in the brains of PD patients. Though our bodies require iron and cannot live without it, excessively high levels within the brain cause extreme oxidative damage. There are now several agents which chelate iron that are being used to reduce these high levels found in the brain. Though we believe it may be helpful in some cases, and certainly is worth trying in many cases, we would like to offer a word of caution. Chelating agents remove not only heavy metals from the blood but they also remove many needed minerals as well. Make certain that you primary healthcare provider is experienced in chelation therapy and knows proper protocols for removal of heavy metals.

In proper chelation therapy, zinc, copper, magnesium, calcium, potassium and several other substances will need to be replaced.

When you are receiving chelation therapy, there is an easy rule to remember: metals are removed in the same order they appear on the periodic table. Be sure to keep track of your iron levels and never remove too much. If you do not keep track of all of these factors, a very promising therapy may end up being harmful to you. Many oral chelating agents are on the market as well as I.V. chelation. Whatever your health care provider recommends, chelation should never be done more than three days out of every seven, with replacement of needed minerals every day. It is also important to have an idea of your renal and liver function before you begin, as it is through these organs that the toxins will be removed, and they need to be healthy to accomplish this task.

In order to make the best progress, it is best to start with the appropriate dietary changes for several months, since these changes don't typically work very quickly with neurodegenerative diseases. Try to be patient. You may want to keep a journal of your feelings, as this will enable you to look back over months and see patterns as well as determine which supplements resulted in improvement and how long it took for you to feel improvement. Increase supplements one at a time. Each person is different and what is effective for one may be ineffective for another. Give each new supplement time to work; look at the results after several weeks and not after a few days. All of them will require time for noticeable change to occur, with the possible exception of CoQ10 which often gives additional energy fairly quickly. If you find that a supplement has been helpful, continue taking it while you add another single supplement. This technique will allow you to develop the best personal supplemental regime.

New research is being done all over the world on neurodegenerative diseases. The more we understand the more treatment options that will come to light, whether they are herbs, vitamins, mineral or medicines. The new knowledge of how the brain cleans its waste offers new hope that with the correct treatment we may be able to much more effectively and thoroughly break down, clean and remove the harmful plaques and chemicals that are responsible for causing Alzheimer's, Parkinson's and other cerebral neurodegenerative diseases.

FOR YOUR DOCTOR:

See page 405 for research and studies to share with your doctor.

PLAGUE

DESCRIPTION:

The plague is a severe and potentially deadly bacterial infection. It is caused by the bacterium **Yersinia pestis**. Rodents, rabbits, squirrels, and prairie dogs carry the disease; it is spread by their fleas. People can get the plague when they are bitten by a flea that carries the plague bacteria from an infected rodent, or if they are bitten by the infected animal itself. Once established, Yersinia pestis can rapidly spread to the lymph nodes and multiply. Complications include

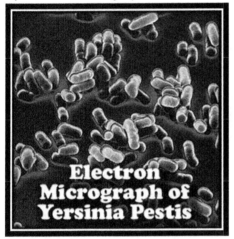

Electron Micrograph of Yersinia Pestis

septicemia (blood poisoning) and when it spreads to the lungs, it becomes pneumonic plague. If a victim isn't treated quickly, the bacteria will flood the body with toxins leading to internal bleeding, organ failure and death. Pneumonic plague can spread from human to human when an infected person coughs and spreads the bacteria in the air for someone else to breathe.

In the Middle Ages in Europe, massive plague epidemics killed almost 100 million people. The plague has caused more fear and terror than perhaps any other infectious disease in history. In total, the plague has killed nearly 200 million people and has produced monumental changes, such as marking the end of the Dark Ages and causing the advancement of clinical research in medicine.

The three most common forms of plague are:

1. **Bubonic plague** -- an infection of the lymph nodes
2. **Pneumonic plague** -- an infection of the lungs
3. **Septicemic plague** -- an infection of the blood

The time between being infected and developing symptoms is typically 2 to 7 days, but may be as short as 1 day for pneumonic plague.

SYMPTOMS:

Fever, chills, headache, seizures, muscle pain, swelling of the lymph glands (groin, armpits, and/or neck), profuse sweating, coughing, subcutaneous hemmorhaging in the skin, fever, spitting up blood, chest pain, difficulty breathing, abdominal pain, bleeding, nausea, fever, vomiting, diarrhea.

CONVENTIONAL TREATMENTS:

People with the plague need immediate treatment. If treatment is not received within 24 hours of when the first symptoms occur, death may occur.

Antibiotics such as **streptomycin, gentamicin, chloramphenicol, tetracyclene, doxycycline,** or **ciprofloxacin** are used to treat plague. Oxygen, intravenous fluids, and respiratory support usually are also needed.

NATURAL TREATMENTS:

"Coptis chinensis Franch" (Ranunculaceae) is a natural herb widely used in China for prevention and treatment of infectious diseases, including the plague. **Berberine** is the major constituent of Coptis chinensis Franch extract. The herbs with the highest amounts of berberine are **Oregon grape root, goldenseal**, and **barberry**. We recommend 150 mg of berberine, twice daily.

Angelica sinensis, commonly called dong quai, is native to China and has been used there as a medicine for thousands of years. At least six chemicals related to coumarin have been identified in dong quai. These include bergapten, imperatorin, oxypeucedanin, osthole, and psoralen. Due to its natural antibiotic properties and blood building attributes, we recommend 1 gram of angelica sinensis, twice daily.

LifeOne is specially formulated and scientifically proven to boost the body's natural immune system. The immune system performs two types of key functions: humoral activity, which results in the production of antibodies, essentially defending the body from viruses; and cellular immunity, which involves the interaction of cell mediated actions, which defend the body against bacteria. A healthy immune system allows cells to differentiate and attack invading harmful organisms, such as

Yersinia pestis. You can purchase LifeOne at this website: www.healthpro.com.dm/lifeone.html.

Garlic has been used as a medicinal substance by many cultures around the world for thousands of years. In the 1700s, gravediggers drank garlic crushed in wine or ate fresh garlic in an effort to ward off plague. Garlic is a potent natural antibiotic whose properties may be able to protect against the plague and destroy the bacteria. Garlic is also high in antioxidants that destroy free radicals, helping the body's immune system become stronger. The active ingredient in garlic, allicin, contains antibacterial, antifungal and antiviral properties known to kill a variety of disease-causing bacteria.

FOR YOUR DOCTOR:

See page 443 for research and studies to share with your doctor.

RHEUMATOID ARTHRITIS

DESCRIPTION:

Rheumatoid arthritis (RA) is a long-term disease that leads to inflammation of the joints and surrounding tissues. It can also affect other organs. The cause of RA is unknown. It is an autoimmune disease, which means the body's immune system mistakenly attacks healthy tissue.

SYMPTOMS:

RA usually affects joints on both sides of the body equally. Wrists, fingers, knees, feet, and ankles are the most commonly affected. The disease often begins slowly, usually with only minor joint pain, stiffness, and fatigue.

Joint symptoms may include:

- ❖ Morning stiffness
- ❖ Joint pain
- ❖ Over time, joints may lose their range of motion and may become deformed.

Other symptoms include:

- ❖ Difficulty sleeping
- ❖ Burning, itching eyes
- ❖ Chest pain when taking a breath (pleurisy)
- ❖ Dry eyes and mouth (Sjogren syndrome)
- ❖ Numbness, tingling, or burning in the hands and feet

CONVENTIONAL TREATMENTS:

RA usually requires lifelong treatment. Disease modifying antirheumatic drugs (DMARDs) are the first drugs usually tried in patients with RA. They are prescribed in addition to anti-inflammatory drugs. Methotrexate (Rheumatrex) is the most commonly used DMARD for RA, while leflunomide (Arava) and chloroquine may also be used. Hydroxychloroquine (Plaquenil) is an antimalarial medication that is usually used along with methotrexate.

Anti-inflammatory medications (such as aspirin) and nonsteroidal anti-inflammatory drugs (NSAIDs – such as ibuprofen and naproxen) are frequently used for RA patients. However, NSAIDs can cause ulcers, bleeding, and heart problems if used for a long period of time. Celecoxib (Celebrex) is another anti-inflammatory drug, but it is labeled with strong warnings about heart disease and stroke. Be sure to talk to your primary caregiver about whether COX-2 inhibitors (like Celebrex) are right for you.

NATURAL TREATMENTS:

The first step we would recommend is to ask your physician to run a **full hormone profile**. We are aware that we have repeatedly suggested hormone profiles, but understand that the pollutants, pesticides and other medications have been causing increases in estradiol dominance and testosterone deficiencies. This fact may be verified in innumerable studies. It is hardly a coincedence that this fact accompanies more frequent diagnosis of these disease processes.

RA has been linked in a large volume of studies to low testosterone levels. Make sure you ask the doctor to include a free testosterone and free estradiol level in the panel. Totals are useless because ounce they are bound to sex hormone-binding globulin (SHBG) they can no longer be used by the body.

If your levels are low and he is willing to supplement you with **testosterone**, please read and request politely he read about **De Aromatase**, which is a supplement that should be taken with testosterone. It is a natural and effective supplement that raises bioavailable testosterone levels and lowers estrogen. The website is www.healthpro.com.dm/dearomatase.html

Research has shown that RA may be helped with supplementation of **ginger**, **green tea**, and **fish oil**. Also, eat **tart cherries** in all forms - fresh, or as cherry juice, or in the form of tart cherry extract. Laboratory findings at Michigan State University suggest that ingesting the equivalent of 20 tart cherries inhibits enzymes called cyclooxygenase-1 and -2, which are the targets of anti-inflammatory drugs.

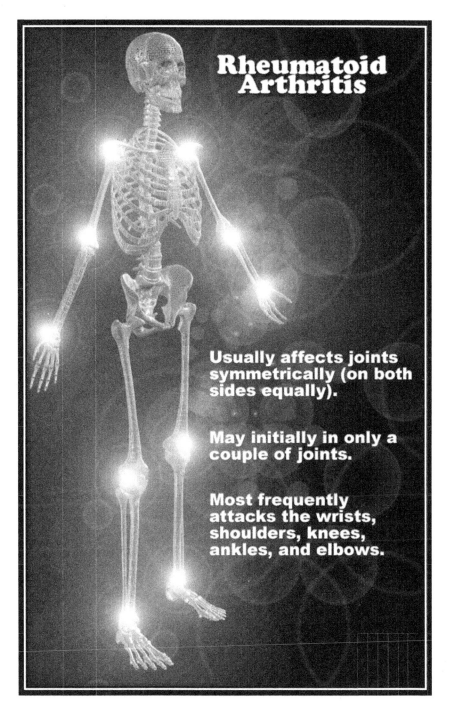

FOR YOUR DOCTOR:

See page 445 for research and studies to share with your doctor.

TUBERCULOSIS (TB)

DESCRIPTION:

Tuberculosis (TB) may present as either an acute or chronic infectious disease caused by inhalation of infected droplets of the detrimental bacteria – *Mycobacterium tuberculosis*. In most instances, TB remains localized and asymptomatic (without symptoms) in the lungs but can progress to its active form, even after years of latency. This is called chronic pulmonary TB, due to the fact that it primarily affects the lungs.

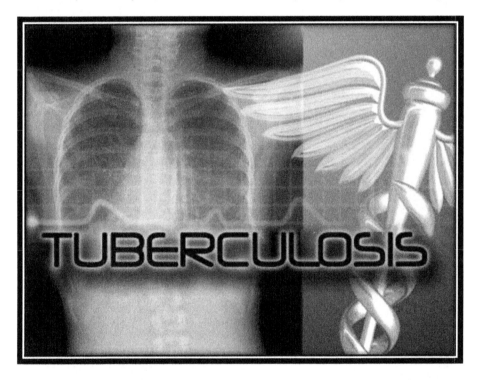

The World Health Organization (WHO) has currently estimated that 33% of the world's population is latently infected with TB at this time. It is transmitted from person to person via droplets from the throat and lungs of an infected person, when they cough. These droplets can then be either ingested in contaminated food (handled by an infected person that may be coughing) or simply breathing the same air from someone that is coughing near you.

In healthy people, infection with *Mycobacterium tuberculosis* oftentimes causes no visible symptoms, since the person's immune system acts to "wall off" and protect the person from the bacteria. This is what takes place if the immune system is intact. If the immune system is compromised, the disease may go into its active form. One of the seldom talked about problems with illegal immigration is that they are not screened for TB and may be unknown carriers that very often end up working either harvesting food or preparing it.

SYMPTOMS:

The most common symptoms of active pulmonary TB are coughing (sometimes with bloody sputum), wheezing, difficulty breathing, chest pains, night sweats, fever, weakness, and weight loss.

CONVENTIONAL TREATMENTS:

TB is typically treated with a 6-month course of **antibiotics** which fight the *Mycobacterium tuberculosis* bacterium. Treatment of active pulmonary TB will always involve a combination of many drugs (usually four drugs). The most common combination is **Pyrazinamide, Rifampin, Isoniazid,** and **Ethambutol.** Other drugs such as **Streptomycin** and **Moxifloxacin** are sometimes used as well.

When people do not take their TB medications as recommended, the infection may become much more difficult to treat. The TB bacteria may become resistant to treatment, and sometimes, the drugs no longer help treat the infection.

NATURAL TREATMENTS:

Do to the number of cases worldwide and the multiple antibiotic resistances that are occurring, supplemental treatment is often advised by experienced practitioners. The following have been found to be very effective in ridding the body of *Mycobacterium tuberculosis*.

One of the aloes (**Aloe secundiflora**) has a reputation as the "Aloe vera" of Kenya, and its roots are frequently stewed to inhibit the growth of TB and diarrhea-causing bacteria. Avocados have also been identified as a good source of **beta-sitosterol**, which has been studied for the treatment of TB in combination with antituberculosis medications.

Several studies have shown that **green tea** may be used as adjuvant therapy for the existing TB therapies. This is because green tea contains polyphenol compounds that can inhibit the proliferation of mycobacteria, namely epigallocatechin gallate (EGCG). Each gram contains 30 to 50 milligrams of green tea EGCG, which acts as an immunomodulator. This mechanism is not found in TB drugs in use today.

Data from a study published in the January 2007 *Journal of International Medicine and Research* found that **astragalus** destroyed Mycobacterium tuberculosis. We recomend taking 250 mg to 500 mg of a standardized extract of astragalus three or four times daily to treat TB.

Vitamin C, **vitamin A**, **vitamin D**, as well as supplemental **zinc** have been shown to be beneficial to aiding in recovery from TB when used in conjunction with antibiotic therapy, and would be well worth the discussion with your doctor, even if you are already using antibiotic therapy. Research shows that **vitamin D** has several health benefits, including enhancing the immune response to tuberculosis infection. In 2011, researchers at UCLA showed how the immune system depends on vitamin D to mount a response against the causative bacterium, *Mycobacterium tuberculosis*. A study published January 6, 2011 in *The Lancet* indicate that vitamin D can also speed up antibiotic treatment of TB. **Vitamin A** deficiency has been commonly observed in patients with TB, so supplementing with this vitamin is recommended. Also, repeated studies have shown that **vitamin C** helps against TB.

FOR YOUR DOCTOR:

See page 458 for research and studies to share with your doctor.

ULCERATIVE COLITIS

DESCRIPTION:

Ulcerative colitis (UC) is a type of inflammatory bowel disease that affects the lining of the large intestine (colon) and rectum.

SYMPTOMS:

Symptoms vary, depending upon the severity of the UC attacks. However, common symptoms include fever, bloody stool, diarrhea, abdominal pain, gurgling abdominal sounds, nausea, vomiting, rectal bleeding, and gastrointestinal bleeding.

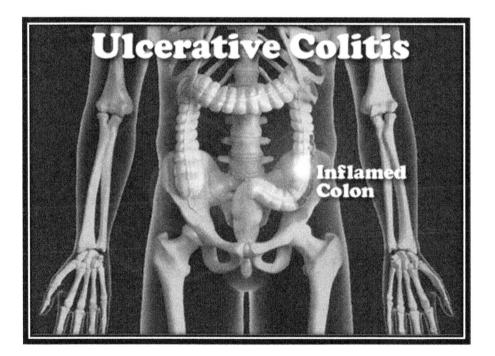

CONVENTIONAL TREATMENTS:

The goals of treatment are to control the attacks and help heal the colon.

Medications that may be used to decrease the number of attacks include:

- ❖ **5-aminosalicylates** (such as mesalamine or sulfazine)
- ❖ **Corticosteroids** (prednisone and methylprednisolone) to reduce inflammation
- ❖ **Immunomodulators** (such as azathioprine)

Sometimes, surgery to remove the colon is recommended for patients who have not responded to pharmaceuticals.

NATURAL TREATMENTS:

A Japanese study evaluated the role of **dietary factors** on inflammatory bowel disease. Included in the study were 111 people with UC who were given food questionnaires. The survey found a higher consumption of sweets was positively associated with risk of developing UC.

Other dietary suggestions include eating small amounts of food throughout the day, drinking plenty of water, avoiding high-fiber foods (bran, beans, nuts, seeds, and popcorn), and avoiding fatty, greasy, and/or fried foods.

Aloe vera has been found in studies to have an anti-inflammatory effect. A double-blind, randomized trial examined the effectiveness and safety of aloe vera gel for the treatment of UC. Researchers gave 30 patients 100 milliliters of oral aloe vera gel and 14 patients 100 milliliters of a placebo twice daily for four weeks. Clinical remission, improvement, and response occurred in nine (30%), 11 (37%) and 14 (47%) respectively, of aloe vera patients compared with one (7%), one (7%) and two (14%), respectively of patients taking the placebo.

Probiotics ("friendly" bacteria that reside in the gut) have been found to be effective in managing UC, as they help control the number of potentially harmful bacteria, reduce inflammation, and improve the protective mucus lining of the gut. In an Italian study, researchers gave 25 UC patients a supplement containing 250 milligrams of Saccharomyces boulardii three times a day for four weeks during maintenance treatment with the drug mesalazine. Of the 24 patients who completed the study, 17 had clinical remission, which was confirmed by endoscopic exam.

Boswellia (aka "frankincense") is an herb that comes from a tree native to India. The active ingredient is the resin from the tree bark, which has been found to block chemical reactions involved in inflammation. Unlike anti-inflammatory medication, boswellia does not seem to cause gut irritation that can occur with many conventional pain relievers.

Studies have shown that **American ginseng** and **ginkgo biloba** can prevent and treat UC and colon cancer, which sometimes results. The Chinese and Native Americans have used American ginseng to treat digestive disorders for hundreds of years. Scientists believe that ginkgo biloba may be effective in the treatment of UC due to its scavenging effect on oxygen-derived free radicals.

FOR YOUR DOCTOR:

See page 467 for research and studies to share with your doctor.

URINARY TRACT INFECTION (UTI)

DESCRIPTION:

A urinary tract infection (UTI) is almost exclusively caused by bacteria that travel to the bladder through the urethra. The bacteria clings to the urethra's opening and multiplies. The most common culprit is Escherichia coli (*E. coli*). UTIs are 10 times more common among women than men.

SYMPTOMS:

UTIs may cause different symptoms in some people even if caused by the same infection. Symptoms include abdominal pains, foul smelling urine, chills, fever, bloody urine, nausea, malaise, pain during urination, night sweats, and frequent urination.

CONVENTIONAL TREATMENTS:

Antibiotics are usually recommended because there is a risk that the infection can spread to the kidneys.

Commonly used antibiotics include:

- ❖ **Trimethoprim-sulfamethoxazole**
- ❖ **Amoxicillin**
- ❖ **Doxycycline**
- ❖ **Augmentin**

Your doctor may also recommend drugs to relieve the burning pain and the urgent need to urinate. **Phenazopyridine hydrochloride** (Pyridium) is the most common of this type of drug.

NATURAL TREATMENTS:

Mustard oils (derived from **horseradish** and **nasturtium**) can be used as treatment for UTI, according to a 2006 study published in the Arzneimittel-Forschung journal. The study found that a combination of these extracts demonstrated antimicrobial properties, thus their combination is a rational treatments for UTI. In another 2006 study published in the *Arzneimittel-Forschung* journal, participants took either antibiotics or an herbal drug combining horseradish and

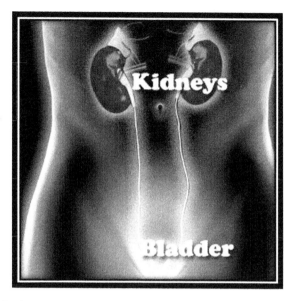

nasturtium. The group who took the antibiotics experienced a 87.9% decrease in symptoms versus 81.2% in patients who took the herbal drug. However, researchers found that the herbs had a clear advantage because those patients needed fewer supportive procedures and less supportive medications.

Used by both Native Americans and the Chinese for centuries for UTIs, the effects of **uva ursi** (aka **bearberry**) are well-established. Bearberry leaves contain arbutin, which exhibits an antibacterial effect in alkaline urine, where arbutin breaks down into glucose (sugar) and hydroquinone (an antiseptic agent). However, bearberry is **not** a daily supplement to be used for prevention. Rather, it is a reactive herbal treatment which should only be employed once a problem appears. Bearberry is an herb that teeters on the boundary between stiff cure and potent poison, so it should not be taken by children, pregnant women, or anyone with existing liver problems. The normal therapeutic dosage of Bearberry capsules (standardized to contain 20% Arbutin) varies from 750 - 1,500 mg per day for 7-10 days.

Scientists report that within eight hours of drinking **cranberry juice**, the juice could help prevent bacteria from developing into an infection in the urinary tract. Previous studies have suggested that the active compounds in cranberry juice are not destroyed by the digestive system after people drink them, but instead work to fight against bacteria, including *E. coli*. This latest study, presented at the national meeting of the American Chemical Society in Boston, affirms that and provides evidence of the medicinal value of cranberries. The research suggests that the beneficial substances in cranberry juice could reach the urinary tract and prevent bacterial adhesion within eight hours. **Grapeseed extract** may also be an effective treatment for UTI and other infections. Grapeseed extract is antibacterial, antifungal, and antiviral. **Goldenseal** can stop bacteria from adhering to the bladder walls and reduce the likelihood of an infection.

FOR YOUR DOCTOR:

See page 471 for research and studies to share with your doctor.

WHOOPING COUGH (AKA PERTUSSIS)

DESCRIPTION:

Whooping cough (aka pertussis) is an acute and extremely contagious bacterial disease resulting from an infection in the mucous membranes that line the entire respiratory system. The responsible pathogenic bacterium, *bordetella pertussis*, which characteristically reside in the mucous membranes of the respiratory tract. The infection typically causes uncontrollable, spasmodic, violent coughing, and a deep "whooping" sound is often heard when the patient tries to take a breath and is more prominent in children than in adults.

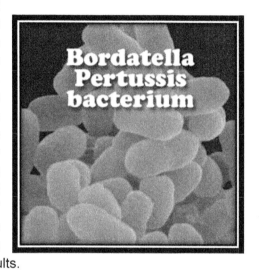

In the pre-vaccination era, pertussis was one of the leading causes of infant death. The number of cases reported had decreased by more than 99% from the 1930s to the 1980s. Whether this drastic decrease in pertussis resulted from vaccinations, improved sanitary conditions, other factors, or a combination thereof is beyond the scope and purpose of this book. Interestingly, due to many local outbreaks, the number of cases reported in the USA increased by more than 2300% between 1976 and 2005, when the recent peak of 25,616 cases were reported. The disease is still a significant cause of morbidity and mortality in infants younger than 2 years, despite the fact that vaccinations that are now mandated in most states.

Truth be told, pertussis is **not** what has been responsible for the vast majority of deaths in juvenile cases. It is the development of pneumonia and other opportunistic infections that has caused most pertussis related deaths. In the vast majority of adult cases, the symptoms are much less severe and are often simply shrugged off as a cold. The problem is that the bacteria causing pertussis is very virulent and spreads very easily. It is often a working parent that may bring it home from an infected co-worker, or a child interacting with material at the store that has been touched by a carrier, or an in school interaction with another infected child that causes such a rapid spread of the disease. It is most dangerous to young children, and it is young children with the highest mortality rate.

It is interesting to note that pertussis vaccinations (like all vaccinations) are implied to give lifelong protection. That is not at all the case. Most vaccines are only effective for a maximum of 7 years, with the majority being effective for a much shorter period of time. Despite the fact that pertussis vaccinations and booster vaccinations are recommended, many children that have followed this vaccination regime have still developed pertussis.

As in the measles outbreak during the Reagan Presidency, in which almost all of the infected mothers had been vaccinated against measles, the pertussis outbreaks once again force us to reconsider the efficacy of mass vaccinations, their true value, and their true cost. The primary caregivers are being asked to re-vaccinate children and in many cases the elderly in the hopes of preventing pertussis, but unfortunately this does not seem to be having much of a beneficial effect.

SYMPTOMS:

Symptoms typically last 6 to 10 weeks, but may last longer, and usually occur in 3 stages.

Stage 1: Stage 1 symptoms include common cold symptoms, such as sneezing, runny nose, mild coughing, watery eyes, and sometimes a mild fever. This stage lasts several days to 2 weeks. It is at this stage that the infected person is most contagious.

Stage 2: During stage 2, cold-like symptoms typically diminish, but the cough worsens, changing from a dry, hacking cough to bursts of uncontrollable and often violent coughing. During a coughing episode, it is sometimes temporarily impossible to take a breath because of the intensity and close repetition of coughs. When the victim is able to breathe, the individual may take in a sudden gasp of air through airways that have been narrowed by inflammation, and this sometimes causes a "whooping" noise. It is common for vomiting and extreme exhaustion to often follow a coughing spell, but then the infected person may actually appear normal. This is considered the most dangerous stage of whooping cough and usually lasts between 2 and 4 weeks.

Stage 3: During stage 3, the patient may improve and feel stronger, but at the same time, the cough may become louder and sound worse. Coughing spells will oftentimes occur irregularly for weeks to months and may become worse if a cold or other upper respiratory problem develops.

CONVENTIONAL TREATMENTS:

Pertussis should always be included in the possible diagnosis of any prolonged cough in infants as well as young children exhibiting cyanosis (lack of oxygen) or vomiting, persistent rhinorrhea (runny nose), as well as marked lymphocytosis (an abnormal increase in the number of lymphocytes in the blood). The diagnosis of lymphocytosis must be done through blood work.

The normal diagnostic procedure should include a throat culture and sensitivity, a nasopharyngeal culture and sensitivity, as well as a complete history and physical exam. The reason we are suggesting sensitivity (along with the cultures) is that when there is an outbreak and there are numerous cases, bacteria tend to mutate, thus one antibiotic may be much less effective than what is typically prescribed. As a matter of fact, the most commonly used antibiotics used in the treatment of pertussis have shown themselves to be ineffective and are now used to prevent the patient from infecting others rather than heal the patient. Before allowing antibiotics to be used, please understand that research has shown that antibiotics do **not** alter the course of the disease whatsoever.

In fact, antibiotics can often make the problem worse due to the fact that they kill the good flora in the digestive tract, which account for approximately 70% of the immune system. In children, this can result in diarrhea (which can accelerate dehydration and further complicate the disease) as well as nausea and vomiting in some cases, as a result of antibiotic reactions. If you or a loved one develops pertussis and decides to take antibiotics, please be aware that they will kill the beneficial bacteria which will need to be replaced with the use of a probiotic. Probiotics are harmless and can at least partially restore normal gut flora which the body requires.

In Western medicine, the most commonly prescribed antibiotic is **erythromycin**. Also, other macrolide antibiotics such as **azithromycin** and **clarithromycin** are sometimes used. In some cases an albuterol inhaler may be given to assist in breathing, and corticosteroids are frequently prescribed as well. These treatments do not provide a cure for the patient, and they also destroy the beneficial bacteria in the gut.

Because a child's immune system is immature and not fully functional and the elderly frequently have compromised immune systems, and in light of the fact that antibiotic therapy has shown no real, consistent studies of its efficacy in treating the disease, perhaps the wisdom of medical care of the 1930s and 1940s should be revisited. We will address this in the next section.

The following is a quote from the Cochrane Library:

> *"Antibiotics are effective in eliminating B. pertussis from patients with the disease, rendering them non-infectious, **but do not alter the subsequent clinical course of the illness**. Effective regimens include: three days of azithromycin, seven days of clarithromycin, seven or 14 days of erythromycin estolate, and 14 days of erythromycin ethylsuccinate. Considering microbiological clearance and side effects, three days of azithromycin or seven days of clarithromycin are the best regimens. Seven days of trimethoprim/sulfamethoxazole also appeared to be effective for the eradication of B. pertussis from the nasopharynx and may serve as an alternative antibiotic treatment for patients who cannot tolerate a macrolide. **There is insufficient evidence to determine the benefit of prophylactic treatment of pertussis contacts."***
> ~ Cochrane Database Syst Rev. 2005 Jan 25;(1):CD004404.

Even according to this primary database, it is made clear that, at best, an antibiotic will render the patient less contagious to others and clear pertussis from the nasal passages, but it does not alter the clinical course of the disease. In other words, antibiotic therapy has **not** been show to cure pertussis and actually may make the patient worse, though less infective to others. Antibiotics have shown themselves to be ineffective in preventing the disease from occurring in a disease populated area, so prophylactic use of antibiotics should be seriously discussed. As we have already mentioned, there is a real concern over risk vs. benefit in antibiotic treatment to prevent infection.

NATURAL TREATMENTS:

Vitamin C (ascorbic acid) has been very well researched as a treatment modality for many years; it has been shown to be safe and effective when other modalities have failed. It is certainly one of the safest treatments and may be used in conjunction with almost any other treatment being utilized. Most research is from the 1930s, but should not be discounted, since medicine was actually much more open and progressive then and research was much less influenced by pharmaceutical companies. Please note that recent research has been done in Canada which backs up the effectiveness of vitamin C use for pertussis.

My own opinion (Dr. Farley) concerning pertussis comes entirely from research and discussion with physicians in their late 70s that had seen several cases during their careers. Fortunately, in my own practice of over 30 years, I have never had a pertussis case. One of my closest friends was a physician that practiced until his death at 78. He had treated numerous cases of pertussis in his career, and he verified to me that the only effective therapy he had found was vitamin C. He suggested oral vitamin C taken every four hours, with the dosage determined by weight in infants and by tolerance in juveniles and adults. By tolerance, he meant that you take increasing doses of vitamin C until your stools become loose. At that point, you decrease it by 500 mg per day until your stools are normal. This is also called the "saturation dosage" and is the dosage you will maintain until all symptoms have been gone for a period of 5 days.

Vitamin C is very safe and toxicity is very rare because the body cannot store and it is excreted within about 4 hours after ingestion. It is considered to be one of safest of all nutrients. Due to the fact that it is water soluble, any excess is rapidly removed from the body through the kidneys and is excreted in the urine. The only people that should moderate its use are those with iron overload (vitamin C increases iron absorption) or kidney disease.

There has been some concern that pregnant women should not take high doses of vitamin C. Progesterone, necessary for the maintenance of a pregnancy, has been shown in some studies to be inhibited by doses of vitamin C above 1000 mg per day. However, this must be taken with a grain of salt. In a 1943 study of 79 women with threatened, previous spontaneous or habitual abortion, Javert and Stander had 91% success with 33 patients (who received vitamin C together with bioflavonoids and vitamin K), with only 3 abortions, whereas all of the 46 patients who did not receive the vitamins aborted.

Most LD50 (the dose that will kill 50% of a population) was taken from rats. Translated to humans it would equate to about 1.2% of your body weight taken at one time. For a 150 pound human, that would equate to 1.85 pounds taken orally. As you can see, overdosing on vitamin C would be very difficult.

If you and your primary healthcare provider choose to use vitamin C as the primary therapy, make sure they are confident in the appropriate dosage and make sure they follow the case closely and are able to tell you when the therapy may be discontinued.

Perhaps the article by Dr. Suzanne Humphries, MD puts treatment with vitamin C in the best light:

Why is nobody studying vitamin C in whooping cough? ~ Conventional medicine's hypocrisy

by Suzanne Humphries, MD

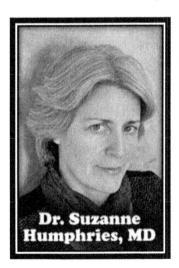

Dr. Suzanne Humphries, MD

"Just as ignorance of the law is no sound defense to legal charges brought against you, ignorance of medical fact is ultimately no sound defense for a doctor withholding valid treatment, especially when that information can be easily accessed." ~ Thomas Levy, MD, JD, author

Last year I wrote a document entitled 'The Vitamin C treatment of Whooping Cough' in order to meet the needs of parents who seek treatment that is safe

214

and effective. I have first hand experience of its effectiveness and there is old literature to suggest that even low doses of Vitamin C help reduce the severity and duration of the cough.

Currently, the conventional approach to whooping cough (pertussis) is to vaccinate infants, and to give older children booster injections. Adults have recently been encouraged to get vaccinated to curb the spread as well. It is my opinion, based on conventional information that this approach is unlikely to make much difference in the presence of pertussis. Because both vaccinated and unvaccinated people get pertussis, we need a safe and effective treatment when the cough occurs.

The Pertussis vaccine has failed us miserably. Here is a very good BLOG regarding the failure of whooping cough vaccine that I wholeheartedly agree with. To me, it makes no sense that more vaccines are tossed to the world as a solution to the problem, simply because doctors and health officials have nothing else to offer. As noted in the BLOG, 'The medical system believes its own self-fulfilling prophecy that whooping cough is a disease that has limited treatments. That is after all, why they have vastly expanded the age range of people recommended to receive the very vaccine which doesn't work, and which has had a hand in creating today's problem.'

The medical establishment's own literature, as I outlined in my original document, admits that the vaccine is a failure. For this reason, research has been under way for years to develop an improved vaccine. Thus far it appears that the new vaccine will simply be added to the current vaccine schedule rather than used as a replacement.

The other approach to active pertussis infection is to give antibiotics to those infected and to close contacts. This is an intervention that carries its own risks, including alteration of bowel flora, drug reactions and possibly even worsen the cough. The reason most cited for using antibiotics in pertussis is not actually to treat the disease so much as to limit the spread, and data on that remains sketchy. The CONSENSUS is that antibiotics may limit the period of infectivity but do not alter the clinical course and are not indicated in close contacts. Most cases that come to *treatment have already been coughing and spreading the disease, and antibiotics are of limited if any use. Yet we still see antibiotics being used rampantly in all contacts, and in infected children who have had the infection long enough that they have already passed the stage where antibiotics would render them non-infectious. If a child is admitted to a hospital with pertussis, the first intervention will be an antibiotic, even though there is no proof that the clinical course will change. But there is an intervention that will limit the duration and the severity. Vitamin C.*

Critics of vitamin C bring up the fact that there are only a handful of studies suggesting that vitamin C decreases cough severity and duration, and they are not modern studies.

OTANI in 1936, should be considered a pilot study as he did document improvement more rapidly than expected in the majority of his cases, though his dosing is far lower than what I would recommend. He used 50-200 mg per injection. Had he used fifty times that, his results would have been unquestionable.

VERMILLION in 1938 published a study 'In this small series of twenty-six cases of whooping cough, cevitamic acid seemed to be strikingly effective in relieving and checking the symptoms in all but two of the cases which apparently received little if any relief. It is our opinion that it should be given further trial in all cases of whooping cough regardless of the age of the patient, or the length of time already elapsed since the original symptoms.' He also used very low doses of cevitamic acid.

ORMEROD in 1937 reported in a small study group: 'Ascorbic acid has a definite effect in shortening the period of paroxysms from a matter of weeks to a matter of days.' His doses were also very low 150 mg to 500 mg. Given that pertussis is a toxin-mediated disease, these low doses would not have reached anywhere near saturation.

Sessa (1940) and Meier (1945) also reported positively on low dose vitamin C in pertussis.

I agree with the critics that there are no randomized controlled trials (RCT) to demonstrate the effect of high-dose vitamin C on the duration and severity of pertussis. However, I have a friend who has been taking care of very young infants and children for thirty years using high dose vitamin C and they have not lost or damaged one of these children. There are thousands of happy mothers out there who know that vitamin C saved their children from suffering the feared ravages of pertussis – even in very young infants.

Now I have my own series of documented cases and testimonials where parents witnessed the rapid reduction in cough and improvement in symptoms. They now know that whooping cough does not have to be the dreaded '100 day cough.'

At this point, while I recognize that RCTs are thought to be the gold standard of proof in medical treatments, I would be reluctant to sign any child up for such a study since the half that is untreated would be knowingly deprived of a potentially life-saving intervention. If such a study was ever performed, it would have to be unblinded and open-label in order to minimize the risk to the untreated. I believe that after just a few days the placebo half would quickly reveal the detriment of withholding vitamin C.

As a nephrologist and internist, I am well aware that many decisions made by doctors every day not only have no RCT to support them, but that doctors are also using drugs off-label and attempting salvage with some hair-raising interventions, after their suppressive treatments have ended poorly.

To download an excellent special report entitled *"The Vitamin C Treatment of Whooping Cough (Pertussis)"* by Dr. Humphries, please visit the following website:

www.vaccinationcouncil.org/wp-content/uploads/2012/07/final-vit-C-and-WC.pdf

FOR YOUR DOCTOR:

See page 475 for research and studies to share with your doctor.

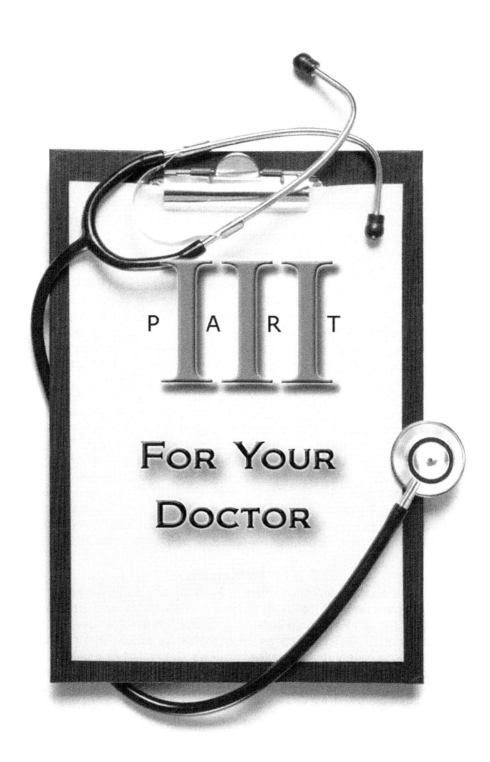

P A R T

III

FOR YOUR
DOCTOR

ACID REFLUX

Betaine Hydrochloride (Betaine HCl)

The prevalence of gastroesophageal reflux disease (GERD) is increasing. GERD is a chronic disease and its treatment is problematic. It may present with various symptoms including heartburn, regurgitation, dysphagia, coughing, hoarseness or chest pain. The aim of this study was to investigate if a dietary supplementation containing: melatonin, l-tryptophan, vitamin B6, folic acid, vitamin B12, methionine and betaine would help patients with GERD, and to compare the preparation with 20 mg omeprazole. Melatonin has known inhibitory activities on gastric acid secretion and nitric oxide biosynthesis. Nitric oxide has an important role in the transient lower esophageal sphincter relaxation (TLESR), which is a major mechanism of reflux in patients with GERD. Others biocompounds of the formula display anti-inflammatory and analgesic effects. A single blind randomized study was performed in which 176 patients underwent treatment using the supplement cited above (group A) and 175 received treatment of 20 mg omeprazole (group B). Symptoms were recorded in a diary and changes in severity of symptoms noted. All patients of the group A (100%) reported a complete regression of symptoms after 40 days of treatment. On the other hand, 115 subjects (65.7%) of the omeprazole reported regression of symptoms in the same period. There was statiscally significant difference between the groups (P < 0.05). This formulation promotes regression of GERD symptoms with no significant side effects. *Reference: Pereira R. S. Regression of gastroesophageal reflux disease symptoms using dietary supplementation with melatonin, vitamins and aminoacids: comparison with omeprazole. Journal of Pineal Research. 41(3):195-200, 2006.*

Melatonin

Gastro-Esophageal Reflux Disease (GERD) defined as a condition that develops when the reflux of stomach contents causes troublesome symptoms and/or complications. Many drugs are used for the treatment of GERD such as omeprazole (a proton pump inhibitor) which is a widely used antiulcer drug demonstrated to protect against esophageal mucosal injury. Melatonin has been found to protect the gastrointestinal mucosa from oxidative damage caused by reactive oxygen species in different experimental ulcer models. The aim of this study is to evaluate the role of exogenous melatonin in the treatment of reflux disease in humans either alone or in combination with omeprazole therapy. 36 persons were divided into 4 groups (control subjects, patients with reflux disease treated with melatonin alone, omeprazole alone and a combination of melatonin and omeprazole for

4 and 8 weeks). Each group consisted of 9 persons. Persons were subjected to thorough history taking, clinical examination, and investigations including laboratory, endoscopic, record of esophageal motility, pH-metry, basal acid output and serum gastrin. Melatonin has a role in the improvement of Gastro-esophageal reflux disease when used alone or in combination with omeprazole. Meanwhile, omeprazole alone is better used in the treatment of GERD than melatonin alone. The present study showed that oral melatonin is a promising therapeutic agent for the treatment of GERD. It is an effective line of treatment in relieving epigastric pain and heartburn. However, further studies are required to confirm the efficacy and long-term safety of melatonin before being recommended for routine clinical use. **Reference:** *Kandil, T. S., et al. The potential therapeutic effect of melatonin in gastro-esophageal reflux disease. BMC Gastroenterol. 10(1):7, 2010.*

Reflux esophagitis (RE), a major gastrointestinal disorder results from excess exposure of the esophageal mucosa to acidic gastric juice or bile-containing duodenal contents refluxed via an incompetent lower esophageal sphincter. Recent studies implicated oxygen derived free radicals in RE induced esophageal mucosal damage resulting in mucosal inflammation. Thus, control over free radical generation and modulation of inflammatory responses might offer better therapeutic effects to counteract the severity of RE. In this context the authors investigated the effect of melatonin against experimental RE in rats. Melatonin pretreatment significantly reduced the haemorrhagic lesions and decreased esophageal lipid peroxidation aggravated by RE. Moreover, the depleted levels of superoxide dismutase and glutathione observed in RE were replenished by melatonin signifying its free radical scavenging properties and antioxidant effects resulting in the improvement of esophageal defense mechanism. Further melatonin repressed the upregulated levels of expression of proinflammatory cytokines like, TNF-alpha, IL-1beta and IL-6 in RE. However, increased levels of the anti-inflammatory cytokine IL-10 remained unaltered after melatonin administration signifying its immunomodulatory effect through suppression of Th1-mediated immune responses. The involvement of receptor dependent actions of melatonin against RE were also investigated with MT2 receptor antagonist, luzindole (LUZ). LUZ failed to antagonize melatonin's protective effects against RE indicating that melatonin mediated these beneficial effects in a receptor-independent fashion. Thus, esophageal mucosal protection elicited by melatonin against experimental RE is not only dependent on its free radical scavenging activity but also mediated in part through its effect on the associated inflammatory events in a receptor-independent manner. **References:** *Lahiri, S., et al. Melatonin protects against experimental reflux esophagitis. Journal* *of Pineal Research. 2008. -- Neuropharmacology Unit, Division of Pharmacology, Central Drug Research Institute, Lucknow, UP, India.*

The prevalence of gastroesophageal reflux disease (GERD) is increasing. GERD is a chronic disease and its treatment is problematic. It may present with various symptoms including heartburn, regurgitation, dysphagia, coughing, hoarseness or chest pain. The aim of this study was to investigate if a dietary supplementation containing: melatonin, l-tryptophan, vitamin B6, folic acid, vitamin B12, methionine and betaine would help patients with GERD, and to compare the preparation with 20 mg omeprazole. Melatonin has known inhibitory activities on gastric acid secretion and nitric oxide biosynthesis. Nitric oxide has an important role in the transient lower esophageal sphincter relaxation (TLESR), which is a major mechanism of reflux in patients with GERD. Others biocompounds of the formula display anti-inflammatory and analgesic effects. A single blind randomized study was performed in which 176 patients underwent treatment using the supplement cited above (group A) and 175 received treatment of 20 mg omeprazole (group B). Symptoms were recorded in a diary and changes in severity of symptoms noted. All patients of the group A (100%) reported a complete regression of symptoms after 40 days of treatment. On the other hand, 115 subjects (65.7%) of the omeprazole reported regression of symptoms in the same period. There was statiscally significant difference between the groups ($P < 0.05$). This formulation promotes regression of GERD symptoms with no significant side effects. ***Reference:*** *Pereira R. S. Regression of gastroesophageal reflux disease symptoms using dietary supplementation with melatonin, vitamins and aminoacids: comparison with omeprazole. Journal of Pineal Research. 41(3):195-200, 2006.*

The enterochromaffin cells of the gastrointestinal (GI) tract secrete 400 times as much melatonin as the pineal gland; therefore, it is not surprising that research is finding that this indole plays an important role in GI functioning. In animal studies, it protects against GI ulcerations, and randomized clinical trials suggest its efficacy in treating functional dyspepsia and irritable bowel syndrome. Melatonin administration has been shown to protect against esophageal lesions in animals. Moreover, in a randomized, single-blind clinical trial of subjects with gastroesophageal reflux disease (GERD), the combination of melatonin with other natural supplements was found to be superior to omeprazole, a proton pump inhibitor (PPI). Its administration as a single treatment for GERD has not been previously reported. A 64-year-old Caucasian female who required treatment with a PPI for symptoms of GERD wished to substitute a natural treatment because of the risk of worsening her osteoporosis. She experienced a return of symptoms following each of three 20-day trials of a proprietary blend of D-limonene when attempts were made to discontinue the PPI. She then underwent a trial of a natural formula consisting of melatonin 6 mg, 5-hydroxytryptophan 100 mg, D,L-methionine 500 mg, betaine 100 mg, L-taurine 50 mg, riboflavin 1.7 mg, vitamin B6 0.8 mg, folic acid 400 microg, and calcium 50 mg. After 40 days, the PPI was withdrawn without a return of symptoms. Subsequently, an attempt to reduce melatonin to 3 mg resulted in symptoms, while all other ingredients were withdrawn with minimal symptoms during 10 months of follow-up. *Reference:* *Werbach, M. R. Melatonin for the treatment of gastroesophageal reflux disease.Werbach MR. Altern Ther Health Med. 14(4):54-58, 2008.*

Limonene

These studies involved subjects who had heartburn or reflux. In the first experiment, 21 people took 1,000 mg d-limonene in capsule form either every day for 10 days or every other day for 20 days. Of the 19 study participants who returned questionnaires, 89% reported substantial relief on both severity and frequency indexes. The second experiment was a double-blind, placebo-controlled study in which 15 patients took d-limonene and 10 took a placebo. After 14 days, 83% of the d-limonene group reduced their heartburn severity and frequency from 6.9 and 7.2, respectively, on a 10-point scale, to between 1 and 2. Only 30 percent in the placebo group experienced relief. Of the 20 participants from the two studies who were followed up six months later, 10 remained free of symptoms. The researchers concluded d-limonene at 1,000 mg, when taken daily or every other day "provides long-lasting relief from heartburn and GERD." *Reference:* *Willette, R. C., et al. Journal of Complementary and Alternative Medicine.*

Limonene been used to relieve heartburn, because of its potential for gastric acid neutralization and its support for healthy peristalsis. *Reference:* *Sung, J. D-Limonene: Safety and clinical applications. Alternative Medicine Review. 12(3):259-264, 2007.*

The author (a chemist) suffered painful symptoms of GERD for years and did not like the idea of taking a proton-pump inhibitor drug on a chronic basis. He experimented with d-limonene, an extract from the orange peel, as a long-term approach to controlling GERD symptoms. Based on both anecdotal and as yet unpublished clinical research studies, the intake of just one 1000-mg capsule of purified d-limonene every other day for 20 days has been shown to reduce or eliminate GERD symptoms in most people for six months or longer. *Reference:* *Willette, R. C., et al. Purified d-limonene: an effective agent for the relief of occasional symptoms of heartburn. Proprietary study. WRC Laboratories, Inc. Galveston, TX, USA.*

There is no clearly established mechanism by which d-limonene is so effective for the treatment of heartburn. Researchers have speculated that d-limonene works in several ways to eliminate GERD-related pain. Since d-limonene is lighter than water, it floats to the surface of gastric juices in the stomach. Some researchers believes that the minor burping that occurs with d-limonene causes this orange peel extract to be directly carried into the esophagus. By coating the esophagus, d-limonene may protect the esophagus against caustic contents that would have otherwise been regurgitated from the stomach. D-limonene may promote quicker movement of food and gastric juices out of the stomach so that these esophageal irritants do not promote as much reflux. D-limonene may also provide a barrier in the stomach and esophagus against bacterial infection. It is well established that stomach cancer risk is increased in those infected with the H. pylori bacteria. Finally, d-limonene may reduce the amount of gastric juices that reflux (regurgitates) back into the esophagus. **Reference:** *Martin, R. Natural relief from heartburn. Life Extension. September 2006.*

Adrenal Insufficiency
(aka Addison's Disease)

Epimedium Flavonoids

The objective of this study was to investigate the regulatory effects of epimedium flavonoids (EF) on adrenocortical regeneration in rats with inhibited hypothalamic-pituitary-adrenal (HPA) axis. Cell distribution in cell cycle and cell apoptotic rate were measured with PI stain and flow-cytometry; apoptosis cells were showed by in situ terminal-deoxynucleotidyl transferase-mediated deoxy-uridine triphosphate-fluorescene nick end labeling assay (TUNEL), and the genome-wide gene mRNA expression was detected by oligonucleotide microarrays. Compared to the normal control, adrenal cells isolated from the HPA axis inhibited model group were arrested in Go/GI phase, and showed a higher apoptotic rate ($P < 0.05$). After treated with EF, cells in G0/G1 phase decreased and those in G2/M phase increased ($P < 0.01$), and the elevated apoptotic rate reduced significantly ($P < 0.05$). TUNEL assay showed the number of apoptotic cells per section was 4.67 1.53 in the normal control group, 70.67 +/- 9.29 in the model group, and 18.67 +/- 7.64 in the EF-treated group respectively (n=3). Gene expressions in adrenal were mostly restrained in the model group, including 7 cytocycle promoting genes, including V-ras, V-jun, etc., while after treatment with EF, 6 cytocycle promoting genes, 1 anti-apoptotic gene, and genes that closely related with adrenocortical regeneration as IGF-II and FGF7 and their receptors, as well as 7 steroid biosynthesis participated genes were all up-regulated. EF can accelerate adrenocortical cell proliferation, inhibit its apoptosis, and promote steroid biosynthesis so as to enhance adrenocortical regeneration in HPA axis inhibited rats, which may contribute to the beneficial effects of EF in protecting adrenocortical function during glucocorticoid withdrawal. *Reference: Huang, J. H., et al. [Exploration on molecular mechanism of epimediun flavonoids in regulating adrenocortical regeneration in rats with inhibited hypothalamic-pituitary-adrenal axis using oligonucleotide microarrays.] Zhongguo Zhong Xi Yi Jie He Za Zhi. 26(5):423-426, 2006. -- Institute of Integrated Western and Chinese Medicine, Huashan Hospital, Fudan University, Shanghai.*

Licorice Root

Licorice root is one of the most highly regarded herbs used to treat conditions associated with diminished adrenal function. Licorice possesses adrenocorticoid-like activity. The active constituents of licorice with adrenocorticoid activity are glycyrrhizine and glycyrrhetinic acid. Both of these constituents bind to glucocorticoid and mineralocorticoid receptors, possibly displacing endogenous steroids thus contributing to an increase in availability of free cortisol within the body. They may also increase the half-life of circulating cortisol in the body by inhibiting its metabolism or breakdown. *Reference: Rouse, J. Herbal support for adrenal function. Clinical Nutrition Insights. 6(9):1-2, 1998.*

Vitamin B1 (Thiamin)

Experimental and clinical results have shown thiamin to be an effective nutrient to protect the adrenal gland from functional exhaustion secondary to surgery. *Reference: Kelly, G. S. Nutritional and botanical interventions to assist with the adaptation to stress. Alternative Medicine Review. 4(4):249-265, 1999.*

Intramuscular injections of thiamin (120 mg per day), starting several days prior to surgery and 1.5 - 2.0 hours immediately prior to surgery, reduced the cortisol reaction, both prior to the operation and at the height of the surgery. Continued administration of thiamin post-surgery prevented the usual post-surgery reduction in blood cortisol levels. *Reference: Vinogradov, V. V., et al. Thiamine prevention of the corticosteroid reaction after surgery. Probl Endokrinol. 27:11-16, 1981.*

Vitamin C

The authors recommend the use of 3,000 mg of vitamin C per day for the treatment of adrenal insufficiency. Vitamin C acts as a reducing agent for the mixed function oxidase enzyme used in the synthesis of steroid hormones in the adrenal glands. *Reference: Meletis, C. D. et al. Adrenal fatigue: enhancing quality of life for patients with a functional disorder. Alternative & Complementary Therapies. 8(5), 2002.*

ALLERGIES

Ginger

In the present study on five pure phenolic compounds (1-5) isolated from the rhizomes of Zingiber officinale (ginger) and investigated for their antiallergic potency, rat basophilic leukemia (RBL-2H3) cells were incubated with these compounds and the release of beta-hexosaminidase was measured kinetically. The data obtained suggest that ginger rhizomes harbor potent compounds capable of inhibiting allergic reactions and may be useful for the treatment and prevention of allergic diseases. *Reference: Chen, B. H., et al. Antiallergic potential on RBL-2H3 cells of some phenolic constituents of Zingiber officinale (Ginger). Journal of Natural Products. 2009.*

Ginkgo Biloba

The authors investigated the effects of BN 52021 (a specific PAF antagonist derived from Ginkgo biloba) on PAF-induced human eosinophil and neutrophil chemotaxis. In response to an optimal concentration of PAF (10(-6) mol/L), the drug was significantly more potent in inhibiting eosinophil as compared to neutrophil locomotion. These inhibitory effects were observed in a dose-dependent manner with a concentration of drug required to produce 50% inhibition of 7.0 (+/- 2.2) X 10(-6) mol/L and 2.3 (+/- 0.2) X 10(-5) mol/L for eosinophils and neutrophils, respectively. Sodium cromoglycate, nedocromil sodium, salbutamol, and dexamethasone (preincubated with cells up to 6 hours) had no effect over a wide dose range (10(-3) to 10(-9) mol/L). BN 52021 was significantly more effective in inhibiting chemotaxis when the cells were preincubated with the compound for up to one hour before commencement of the locomotion assay, whereas washing the cells completely abolished this effect. Inhibition by BN 52021 was specific for PAF in that it had no effect on chemotaxis induced by either leukotriene B4, N-formyl-methionyl-leucyl-phenylalanine, or a purified human mononuclear cell-derived neutrophil chemotactic factor. BN 52021 also inhibited the specific binding of [3H]-PAF (10(-8) mol/L) to eosinophils and neutrophils in a concentration-dependent fashion with a concentration of drug required to produce 50% inhibition of 1.5 (+/- 0.3) X 10(-6) mol/L and 9.1 (+/- 2.5) X 10(-7) mol/L, respectively. BN 52021 has potential as an anti-inflammatory agent in conditions associated with PAF-induced accumulation of neutrophils and eosinophils. *Reference: Kurihara, K., et al. Inhibition of platelet-activating factor (PAF)-induced chemotaxis and PAF binding to human eosinophils and neutrophils by the specific ginkgolide-derived PAF antagonist, BN 52021. J Allergy Clin Immunol. 83(1):83-90, 1989.*

Stinging Nettle

This double-blind, randomized study comparing the effects of a freeze-dried preparation of Urtica dioica (stinging nettles) with placebo on allergic rhinitis in 98 patients. 69 patients completed the study. Assessment was based on daily symptom diaries, and global response recorded at the follow-up visit after one week of therapy. Urtica dioica was rated higher than placebo in the global assessments. *Reference: Mittman, P. et al. Randomized, double-blind study of freeze-dried Urtica diocia in the treatment of allergic rhinitis. Planta Medica. 56(1):44-47, 1990.*

A nettle (Urtica dioica) extract shows in vitro inhibition of several key inflammatory events that cause the symptoms of seasonal allergies. These include the antagonist and negative agonist activity against the Histamine-1 (H(1)) receptor and the inhibition of mast cell tryptase preventing degranulation and release of a host of pro-inflammatory mediators that cause the symptoms of hay fevers. The nettle extract also inhibits prostaglandin formation through inhibition of Cyclooxygenase-1 (COX-1), Cyclooxygenase-2 (COX-2), and Hematopoietic Prostaglandin D(2) synthase (HPGDS), central enzymes in pro-inflammatory pathways. The IC(50) value for histamine receptor antagonist activity was 251 (+/-13) microg mL(-1) and for the histamine receptor negative agonist activity was 193 (+/-71) microg mL(-1). The IC(50) values for inhibition of mast cell tryptase was 172 (+/-28) microg mL(-1), for COX-1 was 160 (+/-47) microg mL(-1), for COX-2 was 275 (+/-9) microg mL(-1), and for HPGDS was 295 (+/-51) microg mL(-1). Through the use of DART TOF-MS, which yields exact masses and relative abundances of compounds present in complex mixtures, bioactives have been identified in nettle that contribute to the inhibition of pro-inflammatory pathways related to allergic rhinitis. These results provide for the first time, a mechanistic understanding of the role of nettle extracts in reducing allergic and other inflammatory responses in vitro. *Reference: Roschek, B., et al. Nettle extract (Urtica dioica) affects key receptors and enzymes associated with allergic rhinitis. Phytotherapy Research. 23(7):920-926, 2009], [HerbalScience Group LLC, Naples, FL, USA].*

The authors previously found that the O-methylated derivative of (-)-epigallocatechin-3-O-gallate (EGCg), (-)-epigallocatechin-3-O-(3-O-methyl)-gallate (EGCG' '3Me), has potent antiallergic activity. The high-affinity IgE receptor, FcepsilonRI, is found at high levels on basophils and mast cells and plays a key role in a series of acute and chronic human allergic reactions. To understand the mechanism of action for the antiallergic EGCG' '3Me, the effect of EGCG' '3Me on the cell surface expression of FcepsilonRI in human basophilic KU812 cells was examined. Flow cytometric analysis showed that EGCG' '3Me was able to decrease the cell surface expression of FcepsilonRI. Moreover, immunoblot analysis revealed that total cellular expression of the FcepsilonRI alpha chain decreased upon treatment with EGCG' '3Me. FcepsilonRI is a tetrameric structure comprising one alpha chain, one beta chain, and two gamma chains. The level of mRNA production of each subunit in KU812 cells was investigated. EGCG' '3Me reduced FcepsilonRI alpha and gamma mRNA levels. The cross-linkage of FcepsilonRI causes the activation of basophils, which leads to the secretion of inflammatory mediators including histamine. EGCG' '3Me treatment inhibited the FcepsilonRI cross-linking-induced histamine release. These results suggested that EGCG' '3Me can negatively regulate basophil activation through the suppression of FcepsilonRI expression. **Reference:** *Fujimura, Y., et al. Antiallergic tea catechin, (-)-epigallocatechin-3-O-(3-O-methyl)-gallate, suppresses FcepsilonRI expression in human basophilic KU812 cells. J Agric Food Chem. 50(20):5729-5734, 2002.*

ALZHEIMER'S DISEASE

Gingko Biloba

Ginkgo biloba extract is prescribed in psychic and behavioural disorders of the elderly, in peripheral vascular deficiency and in functional disorders of ischaemic origin in the E.N.T. and eye areas. Numerous controlled clinical trials justify these prescriptions and are in agreement with the pharmacological data currently available. Experimentally, Ginkgo biloba extract has proved active on the circulatory and rheological functions, on neuronal metabolism threatened by ischemia or hypoxia, on neurotransmission and on membrane lesions caused by free oxygenated radicals. In Alzheimer's disease and dementia, no firm conclusion can be drawn for the time being due to the lack of animal model. However, experimental data suggest that the product may act on a number of major elements of Alzheimer's disease and dementia. From what is already known about Ginkgo biloba extract, it appears that it fulfills the conditions laid down by the WHO concerning the development of drugs effective against cerebral aging. **Reference:** *Allard, M. Traitement des troubles du vieillissement par extrait de Ginkgo biloba. De la pharmacologie a la clinique. [Treatment of the disorders of aging with Ginkgo biloba extract. From pharmacology to clinical medicine.] Presse Medicale. 15(31):1540-1545, 1986.*

Substantial evidence suggests that the accumulation of beta-amyloid (Abeta)-derived peptides, and to a lesser extent free radicals, may contribute to the aetiology and/or progression of Alzheimer's disease (AD). Ginkgo biloba extract (EGb 761) is a well-defined plant extract containing two major groups of constituents, i.e. flavonoids and terpenoids. It is viewed as a polyvalent agent with a possible therapeutic use in the treatment of neurodegenerative diseases of multifactorial origin, e.g. AD. The authors investigated here the potential effectiveness of EGb 761 against toxicity induced by (Abeta)-derived peptides (Abeta25-35, Abeta1-40 and Abeta1-42) on hippocampal primary cultured cells, this area being severely affected in AD. A co-treatment with EGb 761 concentration-dependently (10-100 microg/mL) protected hippocampal neurons against toxicity induced by Abeta fragments, with a maximal and complete protection at the highest concentration tested. Similar, albeit less potent protective effects were seen with the flavonoid fraction of the extract (CP 205), while the terpenes were ineffective. EGb 761 (100 microg/mL) was even able to protect (up to 8 h) hippocampal cells from a pre-exposure to Abeta25-35 and Abeta1-40. EGb 761 was also able to both protect and rescue hippocampal cells from toxicity induced by H_2O_2 (50-150 microM), a major peroxide possibly involved in mediating Abeta toxicity. Moreover, EGb 761 (10-100 microg/mL), and to a lesser extent CP 205 (10-50 microg/mL), completely blocked Abeta-induced events, e.g. reactive oxygen species accumulation and apoptosis. The neuroprotective effects of EGb 761 are partly associated with its antioxidant properties and highlight its possible effectiveness in neurodegenerative diseases, e.g. AD via the inhibition of Abeta-induced toxicity and cell death. *Refereces: Bastianetto, S., et al. The Ginkgo biloba extract (EGb761) protects hippocampal neurons against cell death induced by beta-amyloid. Eur J Neurosci. 12(6):1882-1890, 2001. -- Douglas Hospital Research Centre, Department of Psychiatry, McGill University, 6875 Bld LaSalle, Verdun, Quebec, Canada.*

Bacopa monniera and Ginkgo biloba are well-known cognitive enhancers in Indian and Chinese traditional medicine systems. Standardized extracts of B. monniera and G. biloba were used to evaluate the antidementic and anticholinesterase activities in adult male Swiss mice. Antidementic activity was tested against scopolamine (3 mg/kg ip)-induced deficits in passive avoidance test. Three different extracts of B. monniera (30 mg/kg) and extract of G. biloba (15, 30 and 60 mg/kg) were administered postoperatively, daily for 7 days and 60 min after the last dose, i.e., on Day 7, first trial was conducted. In passive avoidance test, increased transfer latency time (TLT) and no transfer response (NTR) were taken as criteria for learning. TLT and NTR were significantly increased and decreased in second trial, 24 h after the first trial in control group and scopolamine-dementia group, respectively. The B. monniera- and G. biloba-treated groups produced significant increase in TLT and NTR on second trial (40-80%) after scopolamine treatment, thus, attenuating its antidementic effect. Both the extracts showed a dose (10-1000 &mgr;g)-dependent inhibitory effect on acetylcholinesterase (AChE) activity (in vitro), performed spectrophotometrically. IC(50) of G. biloba was 268.33 &mgr;g, whereas none of the extracts of B. monniera showed more than 50% inhibition. At a dose concentration of 30 and 60 mg/kg, extracts of G. biloba showed a cognitive enhancing property and, at the same time, a significant decrease in AChE-specific activity in both per se and scopolamine-dementia groups. These extracts possess a significant anticholinesterase and antidementic properties, which may be useful in the treatment of dementia. *References: Das, A., et al. A comparative study in rodents of standardized extracts of Bacopa monniera and Ginkgo biloba. Anticholinesterase and cognitive enhancing activities. Pharmacol Biochem Behav. 73(4):893, 2002. -- Division of Pharmacology, Central Drug Research Institute, Lucknow, India.*

Researchers assessed 40 Alzheimer's disease patients with a

comprehensive battery of tests which included the SKT (which tests cognitive function, memory and attention span), the Sandoz Clinical Assessment Geriatric Scale, reaction time, saccadic eye movements, and EEG. Significant improvements were observed in all parameters after thirty days of daily treatment with 240 mg of Ginkgo biloba and continued steady improvement continued throughout the three month study. The authors concluded that Ginkgo biloba extract is an effective treatment for Alzheimer's disease. *Reference: Hofferberth, B. The efficacy of EGb 761 in patients with senile dementia of the Alzheimer type, a double-blind, placebo-controlled study on different levels of investigation. Human Psychopharmacol. 9:215-22, 1994.*

The efficacy of the ginkgo biloba special extract EGb 761 in outpatients with presenile and senile primary degenerative dementia of the Alzheimer type (DAT) and multi-infarct dementia (MID) according to DSM-III-R was investigated in a prospective, randomized, double-blind, placebo-controlled, multi-center study. After a 4-week run-in period, 216 patients were included in the randomized 24-week treatment period. These received either a daily oral dose of 240 mg EGb 761 or placebo. In accordance with the recommended multi-dimensional evaluation approach, three primary variables were chosen: the Clinical Global Impressions (CGI Item 2) for psychopathological assessment, the Syndrom- Kurztest (SKT) for the assessment of the patient's attention and memory, and the Nurnberger Alters-Beobachtungsskala (NAB) for behavioral assessment of activities of daily life. Clinical efficacy was assessed by means of a responder analysis, with therapy response being defined as response in at least two of the three primary variables. The data from the 156 patients who completed the study in accordance with the study protocol were taken into account in the confirmatory analysis of valid cases. The frequency of therapy responders in the two treatment groups differed significantly in favor of EGb 761. The intent-to-treat analysis of 205 patients led to similar efficacy results. The clinical efficacy of the ginkgo biloba special extract EGb 761 in dementia of the Alzheimer type and multi-infarct dementia was confirmed. *Reference: Kanowski, S., et al. Proof of efficacy of the ginkgo biloba special extract EGb 761 in outpatients suffering from mild to moderate primary degenerative dementia of the Alzheimer type of mlti-infarct dementia. Pharmacopsychiaatry. 29(2): 47-56, 1996.*

In 1996, Kanowski et al. reported about the beneficial effects of ginkgo biloba special extract EGb 761(R) (240 mg/day) in outpatients with pre-senile and senile primary degenerative dementia of the Alzheimer type (DAT) and multi-infarct dementia (MID) of mild to moderate severity. The comparison of the results of this double-blind, placebo-controlled, randomized, multi-center study with other dementia studies is hampered by the fact that only the responder analysis of the per-protocol (PP) population, which was pre-specified in the protocol as confirmatory analysis, has been published in detail so far. Moreover, cognitive functioning was measured using the Syndrom-Kurztest (SKT), whereas results of other studies are based on the Alzheimer's Disease Assessment Scale-Cognitive Subscale (ADAS-cog). Therefore, the conventional intention-to-treat (ITT) analysis of this study is provided with an estimation of ADAS-cog scores based on measured SKT scores. After 24 weeks of treatment, the ITT analysis of the SKT and estimated ADAS-cog scores revealed a mean decrease in the total score by -2.1 (95 % CI: -2.7; -1.5) points and -2.7 (95 % CI: -3.5; -1.9) points, respectively, for the EGb 761(R) group, which indicates an improvement in cognitive function. On the contrary, the placebo group exhibited only a minimal change of -1.0 (95 % CI: -1.6; -0.3) and -1.3 (95 % CI: -2.0; -0.4) points, respectively. The changes from baseline differed significantly between treatment groups by 1.1 (SKT) and 1.4 (estimated ADAS-cog) points, respectively (P = 0.01). The Clinical Global Impression of Change (CGI, Item 2) favored the EGb 761 group with a mean difference of 0.4 points (P = 0.007). Changes in the rating related to activities of daily living (Nurnberger-Alters-Beobachtungs-Skala, NAB) showed a favorable trend for EGb 761. A subgroup analysis regarding patients with DAT yielded comparable results. Using a decrease of at least 4 points on the estimated ADAS-cog scores as cutoff criterion for treatment response, 35 % of EGb 761-treated patients were considered responders versus only 19 % for the placebo group (P = 0.01). The results of this ITT analysis substantiate the outcomes previously obtained with a responder analysis of the per-protocol population and confirm that EGb 761 improves cognitive function in a clinically relevant manner in patients suffering from dementia. *Reference: Kanowski, S., et al. Ginkgo biloba Extract EGb 761(R) in Dementia: Intent-to-treat Analyses of a 24-week, multi-center, double-blind, placebo-controlled, randomized trial. Pharmacopsychiatry. 36(6): 297-303, 2003.*

This double-blind, placebo-controlled human study determined that 3 months of Ginkgo biloba supplementation in Alzheimer's disease patients resulted in significant improvement in attention span and memory. Improvements were also noted in psycopathology, psychomotor performance, functional dynamics and neurophysiology. The initial benefits of Ginkgo biloba begin to occur after one month of Ginkgo biloba use. *Reference: LeBars, P., et al. A placebo-controlled, double-blind randomized trial of an extract of ginkgo biloba for dementia. Journal of the American Medical Association. 278(16):1327-1332, 1997.*

Alzheimer's disease (AD) is affecting larger and larger proportions of our population as lifespan increases. Thus, the means to prevent or reduce the rate of this disorder is a high priority for medical research. A standardized extract of Ginkgo biloba leaves EGb 761 is a popular dietary supplement taken by the general public to enhance mental focus and by the elderly to delay onset of age-related loss of cognitive function. EGb 761 has been used for treatment of certain cerebral dysfunctions and dementias associated with aging and AD. Substantial evidence indicates that EGb 761 has neuroprotective effects. But, mechanisms of action of the components of the extract are, unfortunately, poorly understood. Research in the author's laboratory focuses on understanding mechanisms of action of the components of the herbal extract EGb 761 in protection against Alzheimer's disease. The author has demonstrated that EGb 761 inhibited amyloid beta aggregation in vitro and attenuates reactive oxidative species (ROS) in a model organism - the round worm Caenorhabditis elegans. Furthermore, EGb 761 eased its toxicity in the transgenic C. elegans. Only a certain size of the amyloid beta aggregates is toxic to the worms. These findings suggest that EGb 761 has a clear therapeutic potential for prevention and/or treatment of AD. A better understanding of the mechanisms of neuroprotection by EGb 761 will be important for designing therapeutic strategies, for basic understanding of the underlying neurodegenerative processes, and for a better understanding of the effectiveness and complexity of this herbal medicine. **Reference:** *Luo, Y. Alzheimer's disease, the nematode Caenorhabditis elegans, and Ginkgo biloba leaf extract. Life Sciences. 2006.*

Dementia of Alzheimer's type (DAT), together with vascular dementia, is the most important indication for Ginkgo biloba extract (EGb). The therapeutic efficacy of this extract is founded on neuroprotective, metabolic and rheological effects. In addition to these mechanisms - which also form the basis of the activity of the older synthetic nootropics--the hypothesis that DAT is due to a "cholinergic deficit" at central synapses has led, over the last decade, to the development of a new group of drugs for this indication, the cholinesterase (ChE) inhibitors. Thus nowadays, EGb is competing, on the synthetic side, with the ChE inhibitors tacrine, donepezil, rivastigmine and galantamine. No direct comparative trials have been undertaken, but long-term studies lasting 24-56 weeks to demonstrate efficacy have been carried out with both groups of substances in accordance with current EU guidelines. To date, only one psychometric scale has gained general acceptance as the primary criterion of efficacy, namely the cognitive subscale of the Alzheimer's Disease Assessment Scale (ADAS-Cog), whose scores range from 0 to 70 (the lower the better). The initial scores of patients in the trials were between 20 and 30; the improvements after 6 months treatment (less those seen with placebo) were about 2 points under Ginkgo extract and 2 to 4 points with the ChE inhibitors. However, the relatively small differences are called into question by the occurrence of drug-specific side effects with the ChE inhibitors. Unlike the treatment with EGb, up to 90% of the patients given the ChE inhibitors developed nausea and vomiting, so there is a suspicion that methodological reasons in the sense of an "unblinding" of the treatment groups caused the apparent superiority in the intensity of the effect. In addition, the benefits of treatment were rapidly reversed after ending administration of ChE inhibitors, which did not occur to the same extent with EGb. Adverse drug reactions are more than 10 times more common with the ChE inhibitors and the treatment costs about five times higher than with EGb. Given the limited therapeutic options for DAT, treatment with EGb still appears to be the method of choice compared to the ChE inhibitors. *Reference: Schultz, V. Ginkgo extract or cholinesterase inhibitors in patients with dementia: what clinical trials and guidelines fail to consider. Phytomedicine. 10(Supplement 4):74-79, 2003.*

The role of amyloid beta-peptide (Abeta) in the free-radical oxidative-stress model of neurotoxicity in Alzheimer's disease (AD) has received much attention recently. The authors employed both in vitro and in vivo models displaying endogenous Abeta production to study the effects of Abeta on intracellular free radical levels. They employed a neuroblastoma cell line stably expressing an AD-associated double mutation, which exhibits both increased secretion and intracellular accumulation of Abeta when stimulated, as well as transgenic Caenorhabditis elegans constitutively expressing human Abeta. A rise in levels of hydrogen peroxide (H2O2) was observed in both in vitro and in vivo AD-associated transgenic models expressing the Abeta peptide compared with the wild type controls. Treatment of the cells or C. elegans with Ginkgo biloba extract EGb 761 significantly attenuated the basal as well as the induced levels of H2O2-related reactive oxygen species (ROS). Among individual EGb 761 components tested, kaempferol and quercetin provided maximum attenuation in both models. Furthermore, an age-dependent increase in H2O2-related ROS was observed in wild type C. elegans, which is accelerated in the AD-associated C. elegans mutant. These results support the hypothesis of the involvement of Abeta and ROS in association with AD. *References: Smith, J. V., et al. Elevation of oxidative free radicals in Alzheimer's disease models can be attenuated by Ginkgo biloba extract EGb 761. J Alzheimers Dis. 5(4):287-300, 2003. -- Laboratory of Cellular and Molecular Neuroscience, Department of Biological Sciences, The University of Southern Mississippi, Hattiesburg, MS, USA.*

Alzheimer's disease (AD) is characterized by cognitive decline and deposition of beta-amyloid (Abeta) plaques in cortex and hippocampus. A transgenic mouse AD model (Tg2576) that overexpresses a mutant form of human Abeta precursor protein exhibits age-related cognitive deficits, Abeta plaque deposition, and oxidative damage in the brain. The authors tested the ability of Ginkgo biloba, a flavonoid-rich antioxidant, to antagonize the age-related behavioral impairment and neuropathology exhibited by Tg2576 mice. At 8 months of age, 16 female Tg2576 and 15 female wild-type (wt) littermate mice were given ad lib access to tap water or Ginkgo biloba (70 mg/kg/day in water). After 6 months of treatment, all mice received Morris water maze training (4 trials/day for 10 days) to assess hippocampal dependent spatial learning. All mice received a 60-s probe test of spatial memory retention 24 h after the 40th trial. Untreated Tg2576 mice exhibited a spatial learning impairment, relative to wt mice, while Ginkgo biloba-treated Tg2576 mice exhibited spatial memory retention comparable to wt during the probe test. Spatial learning was not different between Ginkgo biloba-treated and untreated wt mice. There were no group differences in learning to swim to a visible platform. Soluble Abeta and hippocampal Abeta plaque burden did not differ between the Tg2576 groups. Brain levels of protein carbonyls were paradoxically elevated in Ginkgo biloba-treated mice. These data indicate that chronic Ginkgo biloba treatment can block an age-dependent decline in spatial cognition without altering Abeta levels and without suppressing protein oxidation in a transgenic mouse model of AD. **References:** *Stackman, R.W., et al. Prevention of age-related spatial memory deficits in a transgenic mouse model of Alzheimer's disease by chronic Ginkgo biloba treatment. Exp Neurol. 184(1):510-520, 2003. -- Department of Behavioral Neuroscience, Oregon Health & Science University, Portland, OR, USA.*

The efficacy of four cholinesterase inhibitors (tacrine, donepezil, rivastigmine, metrifonate) and Ginkgo special extract EGb 761 in Alzheimer's disease were compared. The differences in the effects of the active substance and placebo on cognition were measured on the ADAS-Cog scale, taking into account the different degrees of dementia in the various studies and the dropout rate due to adverse drug reactions. Efficacy, expressed as the delay in symptom progression or the difference in response rate between active substance and placebo, showed no major differences between the four cholinesterase inhibitors and the Ginkgo special extract. Only tacrine exhibited a high dropout rate due to adverse drug reactions. In view of this, the subject of new prescriptions should be critically reviewed. Second-generation cholinesterase inhibitors (donepezil, rivastigmine, metrifonate) and Ginkgo special extract EGb 761 should be considered equally effective in the treatment of mild to moderate Alzheimer's dementia.

References: Warburton, D. M., [Clinical psychopharmacology of Ginkgo biloba extract.] La Presse Medicale. 15(31):1595-604, 1986. -- Wettstein, A., et al. Cholinesterase inhibitors and Gingko extracts-- are they comparable in the treatment of dementia? Comparison of published placebo-controlled efficacy studies of at least six months' duration. Phytomedicine. 6(6):393-401, 2000.

Standardized Ginkgo biloba extract EGb 761 exhibits beneficial effects to patients with Alzheimer's disease (AD). It was previously demonstrated that EGb 761 inhibits amyloid beta (Abeta) oligomerization in vitro, protects neuronal cells against Abeta toxicity, and improves cognitive defects in a mouse model of AD (Tg 2576). In this study, the neurogenic potential of EGb 761 and its effect on cAMP response element binding protein (CREB) were examined in a double transgenic mouse model (TgAPP/PS1). EGb 761 significantly increases cell proliferation in the hippocampus of both young (6 months) and old (22 months) TgAPP/PS1 mice, and the total number of neuronal precursor cells in vitro in a dose-dependent manner. Furthermore, Abeta oligomers inhibit phosphorylation of CREB and cell proliferation in the hippocampus of TgAPP/PS1 mice. Administration of EGb 761 reduces Abeta oligomers and restores CREB phosphorylation in the hippocampus of these mice. The present findings suggest that 1) enhanced neurogenesis by EGb 761 may be mediated by activation of CREB, 2) stimulation of neurogenesis by EGb 761 may contribute to its beneficial effects in AD patients and improved cognitive functions in the mouse model of AD, and 3) EGb 761 has therapeutic potential for the prevention and improved treatment of AD. *References: Tchantchou, F., et al. EGb 761 enhances adult hippocampal neurogenesis and phosphorylation of CREB in transgenic mouse model of Alzheimer's disease. FASEB J. 2007. -- Department of Pharmaceutical Sciences, School of Pharmacy, Center for Integrative Medicine, School of Medicine, University of Maryland, Baltimore, Maryland, USA.*

This randomized, double-blind study included 410 outpatients who received either a once-daily dose of 240 mg of the patented Ginkgo biloba extract EGb 761 or a corresponding placebo for 24 weeks. The primary outcome measure in the cognitive domain was the change in the total score of the SKT test battery, an internationally and cross-culturally validated measure to test cognitive performance in dementia. In the neuropsychiatric domain the Neuropsychiatric Inventory (NPI) was applied. Secondary outcome measures included scales to test the improvement or deterioration of daily activities, quality of life and the distress experienced by caregivers. The patients treated with EGb 761 improved throughout the study with a significant advantage of 1.7 points (Alzheimer's disease) and 1.4 points (Vascular

FOR YOUR DOCTOR – ALZHEIMER'S   WORK WITH YOUR DOCTOR

dementia) in the SKT. On the NPI score an advantage of 3.1 points (Alzheimer's disease) and 3.2 points (Vascular dementia) was observed for the patients receiving EGb 761. Similar improvements were found in all other outcome measures. EGb 761 was also very well tolerated with comparable adverse event rates in both treatment groups. *Reference:* *Tribankek, M., et al. A 240-mg Once-daily formulation of ginkgo biloba extract EGB761 is effective in both Alzheimer's disease and vascular dementia: results from a randomized controlled trial. Alzheimer's & Dementia. 4(Supplement 2):T165-T166, 2008.*

Beta Amyloid (Abeta) treatment induced free radical production and increased glucose uptake, apoptosis and cell death in PC12 nerve cells. Addition of the standardized extract of Ginkgo biloba leaves, EGb 761 together with the Abeta protein prevented, in a dose-dependent manner, the Abeta-induced free radical production, increased glucose uptake, apoptosis and cell death. However, pretreatment of the cells with EGb 761 did not rescue the cells from the Abeta-induced toxicity although it prevented the Abeta-induced reactive oxygen species generation. The terpene and flavonoid-free EGb 761 extract, HE 208, although inhibited the Abeta-induced increased glucose uptake, it failed to protect the cells from apoptosis and cytotoxicity induced by Abeta. These results indicate that the terpenoid and flavonoid constituents of EGb 761, acting probably in combination with components present in HE 208, are responsible for rescuing the neuronal cells from Abeta-induced apoptosis and cell death; their mechanism of action being distinct of their antioxidant properties. Because pre- and post-treatment with EGb 761 did not protect the cells from Abeta-induced neurotoxicity, the authors examined whether EGb 761 interacts directly with Abeta. In vitro reconstitution studies demonstrated that EGb 761 inhibits, in a dose-dependent manner, the formation of beta-amyloid-derived diffusible neurotoxic soluble ligands (ADDLs), suggested to be involved in the pathogenesis of Alzheimer's disease. *References:* *Yao, Z. The Ginkgo biloba extract (EGb761) rescues the PC12 neuronal death from beta-amyloid-induced death by inhibiting the formation of beta-amyloid-derived diffusible neurotoxic ligands. Brain Research. 889(1-2):181-190, 2001. -- Division of Hormone Research, Departments of Cell Biology, Pharmacology, and Neuroscience, Georgetown Univ. Medical Center, 3900 Reservoir Rd, NW, Washington, DC, USA.*

Saint John's Wort

The major protein constituent of amyloid deposits in Alzheimer's disease (AD) is the amyloid beta-peptide (Abeta). The authors determined the effect of hyperforin an acylphloroglucinol compound isolated from Hypericum perforatum (St John's Wort), on Abeta-induced spatial memory impairments and on Abeta neurotoxicity. They report here that hyperforin: (1) decreases amyloid deposit formation in rats injected with amyloid fibrils in the hippocampus; (2) decreases the neuropathological changes and behavioral impairments in a rat model of amyloidosis; (3) prevents Abeta-induced neurotoxicity in hippocampal neurons both from amyloid fibrils and Abeta oligomers, avoiding the increase in reactive oxidative species associated with amyloid toxicity. Both effects could be explained by the capacity of hyperforin to disaggregate amyloid deposits in a dose and time-dependent manner and to decrease Abeta aggregation and amyloid formation. Altogether these evidences suggest that hyperforin may be useful to decrease amyloid burden and toxicity in AD patients, and may be a putative therapeutic agent to fight the disease. **Reference:** *Dinamarca, M. C., et al. Hyperforin prevents beta-amyloid neurotoxicity and spatial memory impairments by disaggregation of Alzheimer's amyloid-beta-deposits. Mol Psychiatry. 2006.*

ASTHMA

Astragalus

Asthma is recognized as a common pulmonary disease throughout the world. To date, there has been a growing interest in herbal products in Traditional Chinese Medicine, which is considered to be effective to treat asthma. A Chinese herb Astragalus membranaceus (AM) was found useful in treating allergic diseases. The purpose of this study is to determine whether this herbal injection could suppress allergic-induced AHR and mucus hypersecretion in allergic mice. A mouse model of chronic asthma was used to investigate AM injection on the airway lesions in compared with glucocorticoids. The study was conducted on mice sensitized and challenged with ovalbumin and the whole body plethsmography was performed to assess AHR. The bronchoalveolar lavage (BAL), histopathology were examined. The authors found 28-day AM administration significantly decreased inflammatory infiltration and mucus secretion in the lung tissues of allergic mice. 28-day AM administration enhanced Ova-induced decreased IFN-gamma, and the Ova-induced elevations of IL-5 and IL-13 in BALF were prevented by 28-day injection. They also showed 28-day AM injection markedly suppressed increased AHR in allergic mice. The results indicate Astragalus Membranaceus has a potential role in treating allergic asthma. *Reference: Shen, H. H., et al. Astragalus Membranaceus prevents airway hyperreactivity in mice related to Th2 response inhibition. J Ethnopharmacol. 116(2):363-369, 2008.*

The objective of this study was to explore the effect of Astragalus membranaceus (AM) on T-helper cell type 1 (Thl) specific transcription factor T-box expressed in T cells (T-bet) expression and Thl/Th2 equilibrium. The levels of T-bet mRNA in peripheral blood mononuclear cells (PBMCs) from 15 patients with asthma and 15 healthy subjects were determined by reverse transcription-polymerase chain reaction (RT-PCR). PBMCs in asthma patients were incubated with AM and then the concentration of interferon gamma (IFN-gamma) and interleukin-4 (IL-4) in the supernate before and after AM intervention were determined by ELISA. The numbers of CD4 + CCR3 + and CD4 + CCR5 + cells were counted by flow cytometry. The expression of T-bet mRNA and the level of IFN-gamma were lower, but level of serum IL-4 was higher in asthma patients when compared with those in healthy subjects respectively. After AM (60 microg/ml) intervention, the former two parameters raised and showed a positive correlation between them, while the level of IL-4 was decreased. The mean percentage of CD4 + CCR3 + cells in asthma patients was significantly higher but that of CD4 + CCR5 + cells was lower when compared with those in healthy subjects respectively. After AM intervention, the abnormal change in the two indexes was improved to certain extent, showing a reversing status of Th2 polarization. AM could increase the expression of T-bet mRNA and ThI cytokines such as IFN-Y, and might reverse the Th2 predominant status in asthma patients. **Reference:** *Wang, G., et al. Effects of Astragalus membranaceus in promoting T-helper cell type 1 polarization and interferon-gamma production by up-regulating T-bet expression in patients with asthma. Chin J Integr Med. 12(4):262-267, 2006. – Department of Integrated Traditional Chinese and Western Medicine, West China Hospital, Sichuan University, Chengdu, China.*

Aloe leaves

Aloe vera (10 ml per day consumed orally) for six months produced good results in the treatment of asthma in 40% of patients. It was, however, totally ineffective in patients dependent on corticosteroids. **Reference:** *Shida, T., et al. Effect of Aloe extract on peripheral phagocytosis in adult bronchial asthma. Planta Medica. 51:273-275, 1985.*

Boswellia

This six week double-blind placebo-controlled study of 80 persons with relatively mild asthma found that treatment with boswellia at a dose of 300 mg three times per day reduced the frequency of asthma attacks and improved objective measurements of breathing capacity (dyspnea and wheezing) in 70% of subjects. **Reference:** *Gupta, I., et al. Effects of Boswellia serrata gum resin in patients with bronchial asthma: results of a double-blind, placebo-controlled, 6-week clinical study. Eur J Med Res. 3:511–514, 1998.*

Ginger

It is well documented that compounds from rhizomes of Zingiber officinale, commonly called ginger, have anti-inflammatory properties. The authors demonstrate that ginger can exert such functions in vivo, namely in a mouse model of Th2-mediated pulmonary inflammation. The preparation of ginger aqueous extract (Zo.Aq) was characterized by mass spectrometry as an enriched fraction of n-gingerols. Intraperitoneal injections of this extract before airway challenge of ovalbumin (OVA)-sensitized mice resulted in a marked decrease in the recruitment of eosinophils to the lungs as attested by cell counts in bronchoalveolar lavage (BAL) fluids and histological examination. Resolution of airway inflammation induced by Zo.Aq was accompanied by a suppression of the Th2 cell-driven response to allergen in vivo. Thus, IL-4, IL-5 and eotaxin levels in the lungs as well as specific IgE titres in serum were clearly diminished in ginger-treated mice relative to their controls after allergen sensitization and challenge. The authors found that [6]-gingerol, a major constituent of ginger, was sufficient to suppress eosinophilia in our model of inflammation. This is the first evidence that ginger can suppress Th2-mediated immune responses and might thus provide a possible therapeutic application in allergic asthma. **Reference:** *Berthe Ahui, M. L., et al. Ginger prevents Th2-mediated immune responses in a mouse model of airway inflammation. Int Immunopharmacol. 2008.*

It is well documented that compounds from rhizomes of Zingiber officinale, commonly called ginger, have anti-inflammatory properties. The authors demonstrate that ginger can exert such functions in vivo, namely in a mouse model of Th2-mediated pulmonary inflammation. The preparation of ginger aqueous extract (Zo.Aq) was characterized by mass spectrometry as an enriched fraction of n-gingerols. Intraperitoneal injections of this extract before airway challenge of ovalbumin (OVA)-sensitized mice resulted in a marked decrease in the recruitment of eosinophils to the lungs as attested by cell counts in bronchoalveolar lavage (BAL) fluids and histological examination. Resolution of airway inflammation induced by Zo.Aq was accompanied by a suppression of the Th2 cell-driven response to allergen in vivo. Thus, IL-4, IL-5 and eotaxin levels in the lungs as well as specific IgE titres in serum were clearly diminished in ginger-treated mice relative to their controls after allergen sensitization and challenge. The authors found that [6]-gingerol, a major constituent of ginger, was sufficient to suppress eosinophilia in our model of inflammation. This is the first evidence that ginger can suppress Th2-mediated immune responses and might thus provide a possible therapeutic application in allergic asthma. **Reference:** *Berthe Ahui, M. L., et al. Ginger prevents Th2-mediated immune responses in a mouse model of airway inflammation. Int Immunopharmacol. 2008.*

Asthma is a chronic disease characterized by inflammation and hypersensitivity of airway smooth muscle cells (ASMCs) to different spasmogens. The past decade has seen increased use of herbal treatments for many chronic illnesses. Ginger (Zingiber officinale) is a common food plant that has been used for centuries in treating respiratory illnesses. In this study, the authors report the effect of its 70% aqueous methanolic crude extract (Zo.Cr) on acetylcholine (ACh)-induced airway contraction and Ca2+ signalling in ASMCs using mouse lung slices. Airway contraction and Ca2+ signalling, recorded via confocal microscopy, were induced with ACh, either alone or after pretreatment of slices with Zo.Cr and (or) verapamil, a standard Ca2+ channel blocker. ACh (10 μmol/L) stimulated airway contraction, seen as decreased airway diameter, and also stimulated Ca2+ transients (sharp rise in [Ca2+]i) and oscillations in ASMCs, seen as increased fluo-4-induced fluorescence intensity. When Zo.Cr (0.3-1.0

mg/mL) was given 30 min before ACh administration, the ACh-induced airway contraction and Ca2+ signalling were significantly reduced. Similarly, verapamil (1 μmol/L) also inhibited agonist-induced airway contraction and Ca2+ signalling, indicating a similarity in the modes of action.   When Zo.Cr (0.3 mg/mL) and verapamil (1 μmol/L) were given together before ACh, the degree of inhibition was the same as that observed when each of these blockers was given alone, indicating absence of any additional inhibitory mechanism in the extract.   In Ca2+-free solution, both Zo.Cr and verapamil, when given separately, inhibited Ca2+ (10 mmol/L)-induced increase in fluorescence and airway contraction.   This shows that ginger inhibits airway contraction and associated Ca2+ signalling, possibly via blockade of plasma membrane Ca2+ channels, thus reiterating the effectiveness of this age-old herb in treating respiratory illnesses. *Reference: Ghayur, M. N., et al.   Ginger attenuates acetylcholine-induced contraction and Ca2+ signalling in murine airway smooth muscle cells. Can J Physiol Pharmacol. 86(5):264-271, 2008.*

Mullein

Common mullein (Verbascum thapsus L.) is a medicinal plant readily found in roadsides, meadows and pasture lands and has been used to treat pulmonary problems, inflammatory diseases, asthma, spasmodic coughs, diarrhoea and migraine headaches.   Although it has been used medicinally since ancient times, the popularity of common mullein has been increasing commercially for the past few years. Today, the dried leaves and flowers, swallow capsules, alcohol extracts and the flower oil of this plant can easily be found in health stores in the United States.   The use of common mullein extracts in folk medicine begun recently to be supported by an increasing number of research studies. This paper thoroughly reviews all the scientific research related to Verbascum thapsus L. including plant tissue cultures and the biological properties of this plant. *Reference: Turker, A. U., et al.   Common (Verbascum thapsus L.): recent advances in research. Phytother Res. 19(9):733-739, 2005. --   Abant Izzet Baysal University, Faculty of Science and Arts, Department of Biology, Bolu, Turkey.*

Passion fruit peel

In this study, the effect of oral administration of an extract of purple passion fruit peel (PFP) on asthmatic symptoms was examined.   42 asthmatic patients without other medical problems were given 150 mg/day of PFP or a placebo for four weeks in this randomized, double-blind study.   During the four weeks, they were not to use any other asthma or anti-inflammatory medicine. At the beginning and at the end of the study, the amount of wheezing, coughing and shortness of breath were assessed.   Also the amount of air exhaled in one second and total lung capacity were measured.   The results showed that PFP

243

administration significantly improved wheezing (~ 80%, p < 0.001), coughing (~76%, p < 0.001), and shortness of breath (~88%, p < 0.05) as compared to baseline and placebo. Placebo treated patients did have a marked but not statistically significant improvement in symptoms: wheezing (~20%), coughing (~47%), and shortness of breath (~55%). (The method of assessment of asthma symptoms was not clear and may have been self-reported resulting in a higher than usual placebo effect. Placebo effects can occur when patients expect to improve, underscoring the importance of accounting for them.) Although the total lung capacity of the PFP group improved ~15%, the one-second exhaled volume did not and the placebo group showed some slight improvement in both of these tests. Thus PFP did not measurably improve lung capacity. Although these results should be confirmed by larger, longer term studies, they suggest that PFP may be a viable nutraceutical in the effort to control asthma. **Reference:** *Watson, R. R., et al. Oral administration of the purple passion fruit peel extract reduces wheeze and cough and improves shortness of breath in adults with asthma. Nutrition Research. 28:166–171, 2008.*

Skullcap

The baicalein content of skullcap inhibits type I and II hypersensitivity reactions, confirming its traditional use in asthma. **Reference:** *Nagai, H., et al. Inhibition of hypersensitivity reactions by soluble derivatives of baicalin. Japan J Pharmacol. 25:763-772, 1945. -- van Loon, I. M. The golden root: clinical applications of Scutellaria baicalensis GEORGI flavonoids as modulators of the inflammatory response. Alternative Medicine Review. 2(6):472-480, 1997.*

The baicalin and baicalein content of skullcap has demonstrated anti-asthmatic activity. This is likely to occur from baicalin and baicalein inhibiting histamine release from mast cells. **Reference:** *Baical skullcap - an important herb for allergies and inflammation. Mediherb Professional Newsletter. 34:1-2, 1993.*

CARDIOVASCULAR DISEASE

Hypertension

Hibiscus

In order to compare the antihypertensive effectiveness and tolerability of a standardized extract from Hibiscus sabdariffa with captopril, a controlled and randomized clinical trial was done. Patients from 30 to 80 years old with diagnosed hypertension and without antihypertensive treatment for at least 1 month before were included. The experimental procedure consisted of the administration of an infusion prepared with 10 g of dry calyx from H. sabdariffa on 0.51 water (9.6 mg anthocyanins content), daily before breakfast, or captopril 25 mg twice a day, for 4 weeks. The outcome variables were tolerability, therapeutic effectiveness (diastolic reduction > or = 10 mm Hg) and, in the experimental group, urinary electrolytes modification. Ninety subjects were included, 15 withdrew from the study due to non-medical reasons; so, the analysis included 39 and 36 patients from the experimental and control group, respectively. The results showed that H. sabdariffa was able to decrease the systolic blood pressure (BP) from 139.05 to 123.73mm Hg (ANOVA $p < 0.03$) and the diastolic BP from 90.81 to 79.52mm Hg (ANOVA $p < 0.06$). At the end of the study, there were no significant differences between the BP detected in both treatment groups (ANOVA $p > 0.25$). The rates of therapeutic effectiveness were 0.7895 and 0.8438 with H. sabdariffa and captopril, respectively (chi2, $p > 0.560$), whilst the tolerability was 100% for both treatments. A natriuretic effect was observed with the experimental treatment. The obtained data confirm that the H. sabdariffa extract, standardized on 9.6mg of total anthocyanins, and captopril 50 mg/day, did not show significant differences relative to hypotensive effect, antihypertensive effectiveness, and tolerability. ***Reference: Phytomedicine. 2004 Jul;11(5):375-82. Effectiveness and tolerability of a standardized extract from Hibiscus sabdariffa in patients with mild to moderate hypertension: a controlled and randomized clinical trial. Herrera-Arellano A, Flores-Romero S, Chávez-Soto MA, Tortoriello J. Centro de Investigación Biomédica del Sur, Instituto Mexicano del Seguro Social, Argentina 1 Xochitepec, 62790 Morelos, Mexico.***

Hibiscus sabdariffa L. (Malvaceae) has been used in different countries as an antihypertensive. Pharmacological work has demonstrated that this effect is probably produced by a diuretic activity and inhibition of the angiotensin-converting enzyme (ACE). Two clinical trials have confirmed the antihypertensive effect using watery infusions, in which a natriuretic effect was also detected. To compare therapeutic effectiveness, tolerability, and safety, as well as the effect on serum electrolytes and the ACE inhibitory effect of a herbal medicinal product prepared from the dried extract of H. sabdariffa calyxes (HsHMP) with those of lisinopril on patients with hypertension (HT), a randomized, controlled, and double-blind clinical trial was conducted. Patients of either sex, 25 - 61 years of age, with hypertension stage I or II, were daily treated for 4 weeks with the HsHMP, 250 mg of total anthocyanins per dose (experimental group), or 10 mg of lisinopril (control group). Outcome variables included effectiveness (diastolic blood pressure [DBP] reduction, >or= 10 mmHg), safety (absence of pathological modifications in the biochemical tests of hepatic and renal function), tolerability (absence of intense side effects), effect on serum electrolytes, and effect on ACE activity. Basal analysis included 193 subjects (100 in the experimental group), while outcome variable analysis integrated 171. Results showed that the experimental treatment decreased blood pressure (BP) from 146.48/97.77 to 129.89/85.96 mmHg, reaching an absolute reduction of 17.14/11.97 mmHg (11.58/12.21%, $p < 0.05$). The experimental treatment showed therapeutic effectiveness of 65.12 % as well as tolerability and safety of 100 %. BP reductions and therapeutic effectiveness were lower than those obtained with lisinopril ($p < 0.05$). Under the experimental treatment, the serum chlorine level increased from 91.71 to 95.13 mmol/L ($p = 0.0001$), the sodium level showed a tendency to decrease (from 139.09 to 137.35, $p = 0.07$), while potassium level was not modified. ACE plasmatic activity was inhibited by HsHMP from 44.049 to 30.1 Units (Us; $p = 0.0001$). In conclusion, the HsHMP exerted important antihypertensive effectiveness with a wide margin of tolerability and safety, while it also significantly reduced plasma ACE activity and demonstrated a tendency to reduce serum sodium (Na) concentrations without modifying potassium (K) levels. Further studies are necessary for evaluating the dose-dependency of HsHMP and for detecting lower effective doses. *Reference: Herrera-Arellano, A., et al. Clinical effects produced by a standardized herbal medicinal product of Hibiscus sabdariffa on patients with hypertension. A randomized, double-blind, lisinopril-controlled clinical trial. Planta Medica. 73(1):6-12, 2007.*

Cardamom

Elettaria cardamomum (L.) Maton. (Small cardamom) fruit powder was evaluated for its antihypertensive potential and its effect on some of the cardiovascular risk factors in individuals with stage 1 hypertension. Twenty, newly diagnosed individuals with primary hypertension of stage 1 were administered 3 g of cardamom powder in two divided doses for 12 weeks. Blood pressure was recorded initially and at 4 weeks interval for 3 months. Blood samples were also collected initially and at 4 weeks interval for estimation of lipid profile, fibrinogen and fibrinolysis. Total antioxidant status, however, was assessed initially and at the end of the study. Administration of 3 g cardamom powder significantly ($p<0.001$) decreased systolic, diastolic and mean blood pressure and significantly ($p<0.05$) increased fibrinolytic activity at the end of 12th week. Total antioxidant status was also significantly ($p<0.05$) increased by 90% at the end of 3 months. However, fibrinogen and lipid levels were not significantly altered. All study subjects experienced a feeling of well being without any side-effects. Thus, the present study demonstrates that small cardamom effectively reduces blood pressure, enhances fibrinolysis and improves antioxidant status, without significantly altering blood lipids and fibrinogen levels in stage 1 hypertensive individuals. **Reference:** *Indian J Biochem Biophys. 2009 Dec;46(6):503-6. Blood pressure lowering, fibrinolysis enhancing and antioxidant activities of cardamom (Elettaria cardamomum). Verma SK, Jain V, Katewa SS. Indigenous Drug Research Center, Department of Medicine, RNT Medical College, Udaipur 313 001, Rajasthan, India.*

Testosterone

The aim of this study was to compare sexual activity and plasma testosterone levels of hypertensive men with those of healthy normotensive controls. The authors investigated 110 newly diagnosed, never treated hypertensive (blood pressure [BP] =140/95 mm Hg) men and 110 healthy normotensive (diastolic BP <90 mm Hg) men. All of them were aged 40 to 49 years, married, without any previous sexual dysfunction, nondiabetic, nonobese (body mass index <28 kg/m2), nonsmoking, and not taking any drug. All subjects were evaluated in the morning after an overnight fast. Clinical evaluation included BP, body weight, and height measurements, determination of testosterone, and an interview about sexual activity, assessed as number of sexual intercourse episodes per month. Hypertensive men presented a 25% reduction in sexual activity as compared to normotensive men (5.9 ± 2.6 v 7.9 ± 2.5 sexual intercourse episodes per month, respectively, P < .01) and a 12% reduction in testosterone levels (510.6 ± 151.9 ng/dL v 578.6 ± 146.8 ng/dL, P < .01). In both normotensive and hypertensive men Pearson's correlation analysis showed a significant positive correlation between testosterone levels and sexual activity and a significant negative correlation between testosterone and age and between testosterone and BP values. Multiple regression analysis confirmed a significant inverse relationship between testosterone and age in normotensive men, whereas only a nonsignificant trend was found in the hypertensive ones. In addition, a significant inverse correlation between testosterone and blood pressure levels was confirmed in hypertensive men limited to systolic blood pressure, whereas a nonsignificant trend was observed in the normotensive controls. These findings suggest a relationship between essential hypertension and impaired testosterone levels in men. **Reference:** *Fogari, R., et al. Sexual activity and plasma testosterone levels in hypertensive males. American Journal of Hypertension. 15(3):217-221, 2002.*

The aim of this study was to evaluate the relationship between serum testosterone levels and arterial blood pressure (BP) in the elderly. The authors studied 356 non-diabetic, non-smoking, non-obese men aged 60 to 80 years and untreated for hypertension. All subjects were evaluated in the morning after an overnight fast. Evaluation included measurements of the following: BP (by mercury sphygmomanometer, Korotkoff I and V), body weight, height and free testosterone (T) plasma levels (by radioimmunoassay). According to the BP values, the subjects were classified as normotensives (NT; n=112; SBP/DBP<140/90 mmHg), systolic and diastolic hypertensives (HT; n=127; SBP/DBP>140/90 mmHg), and isolated systolic hypertensives (ISH; n=117; SBP>140 mmHg and DBP<90 mmHg). T values decreased with increasing age in all 3 groups and was significantly lower in HT (-15%) and ISH men (-21%) than in NT men (p<0.05). In each group, the T levels showed a highly significant negative correlation with BMI (p<0.001). A significant negative correlation was also found between T levels and SBP in NT (r=-0.35, p<0.001), ISH (r=-0.67, p<0.001), and HT (r=-0.19, p<0.05) men, whereas a negative correlation with DBP was observed only in the NT men (r=-0.19, p<0.05). Adjusting for the BMI confirmed a significant difference in plasma T levels between ISH and NT men, but not between HT and NT men. Multiple regression analysis employing BP as a dependent variable confirmed a strong relationship between T levels and SBP in all 3 groups, whereas a significant relationship between T levels and DBP was found only in NT men. In conclusion, although further studies are needed to clarify the relationship between plasma T levels and BP, these findings suggest that in elderly men with ISH, the reduced plasma levels of testosterone might contribute to the increased arterial stiffness typical of these subjects. *Reference: Fogari, R., et al. Serum testosterone levels and arterial blood pressure in the elderly. Hypertension Research. 28(8):625-630, 2005. -- Department of Internal Medicine and Therapeutic, Clinica Medica 11, IRCCS Policlinico S. Matteo, University of Pavia, Pavia, Italy.*

Exogenous sex hormone use, including oral contraceptives, post-menopausal hormonal therapy and anabolic steroids, has been associated with blood pressure changes in both sexes, but little is known about the relationship between blood pressure and endogenous sex hormones. The authors examined this relationship in men in the Rancho Bernardo population study. Out of 1132 men aged 30-79 years, those with hypertension, categorically defined as systolic blood pressure (SBP) greater than 160 mmHg and/or diastolic blood pressure (DBP) greater than 95 mmHg had significantly lower testosterone levels than non-hypertensives. Systolic and diastolic blood pressure inversely correlated with testosterone levels (r = 0.17, P less than 0.001 for systolic; r = -0.15, P less than 0.001 for diastolic) in the whole cohort. This association was present over the whole range of blood pressures and sex hormone levels with a stepwise decrease in mean SBP and DBP per increasing quartile of testosterone. Obesity accounted for some, but not all, of this relationship, which was reduced, but still apparent after adjusting for age and body mass index. No other hormone (androstenedione, estrone, estradiol) nor sex hormone-binding globulin showed a consistent relationship with blood pressure. The clinical and physiological significance of this relationship merits further investigation. *Reference: Khaw, K. T., et al. Blood pressure and endogenous testosterone in men: an inverse relationship. Journal of Hypertension. 6(4):329-332, 1988. -- Department of Community and Family Medicine, School of Medicine, University of California, San Diego, La Jolla, USA.*

It has been hypothesized that risk factors for coronary heart disease in men are linked and that the underlying factor linking them may be an alteration in the sex hormone milieu. As a test of this hypothesis, sex hormones and fibrinogen, factor VII and plasminogen activator inhibitor (PAI-1), hemostatic factors recently shown to be risk factors for myocardial infarction, were measured in men with hypertension and in healthy control subjects. The fasting serum testosterone and free testosterone levels were decreased and the plasma factor VII and PAI-1 levels increased in the men with hypertension. **Reference:** *Phillips, G. B., et al. Sex hormones and hemostatic risk factors for coronary heart disease in men with hypertension. Journal of Hypertension. 11(7):699-702, 1993. -- Department of Medicine, Columbia University College of Physicians and Surgeons, St Luke's-Roosevelt Hospital Center, New York, New York.*

Exogenous testosterone may reduce elevated blood sugar levels in men. **Reference:** *Barrett-Connor, E. L. Testosterone & risk factors for cardiovascular disease in men. Diabete Metab. 21:156-161, 1995.*

Garlic

A popular garlic preparation containing 1.3% allicin at a large dose (2400 mg) was evaluated in this open-label study in nine patients with rather severe hypertension (diastolic blood pressure > or = 115 mm Hg). Sitting blood pressure fell 7/16 (+/- 3/2 SD) mm Hg at peak effect approximately 5 hours after the dose, with a significant decrease in diastolic blood pressure (p < 0.05) from 5-14 hours after the dose. No significant side effects were reported. Our results indicate that this garlic preparation can reduce blood pressure. Further controlled studies are needed, particularly with more conventional doses (e.g., < or = 900 mg/day), in patients with mild to moderate hypertension and under placebo-controlled, double-blind conditions. **Reference:** *Pharmacotherapy. 1993 Jul-Aug;13(4):406-7. Can garlic lower blood pressure? A pilot study. McMahon FG, Vargas R. Clinical Research Center, New Orleans, LA 70112.*

In this study, we compared the cardioprotective effects of freshly crushed garlic vis-a-vis that of processed garlic. Two groups of rats were gavaged with respective garlic preparations while the control group received vehicle only. After 30 days, all of the rats were sacrificed and isolated the hearts were subjected to 30 min ischemia followed by 2 h of reperfusion. Both of the garlic preparations provided cardioprotection, but superior cardiac performance was noticed for those fed with freshly crushed garlic. Consistent with these results, the freshly crushed garlic group displayed significantly greater phosphorylation of antiapoptotic ERK1/2 proteins, reduced Bax/Bcl-2 ratio, and reduced phosphorylation of proapoptotic p-

38MAPK and JNK. Moreover, the survival signaling network consisting of Akt-FoxO1 was increased in the freshly crushed garlic treated hearts. Freshly crushed garlic, but not the processed garlic, showed enhanced redox signaling as evident by increased level of p65 subunit of NFkappaB, Nrf2, and enhanced GLUT 4, PPARalpha, and PPARdelta. The results thus show that although both freshly crushed garlic and processed garlic provide cardioprotection, the former has additional cardioprotective properties presumably due to the presence of H2S. *Reference: J Agric Food Chem. 2009 Aug 12;57(15):7137-44. Freshly crushed garlic is a superior cardioprotective agent than processed garlic. Mukherjee S, Lekli I, Goswami S, Das DK. Cardiovascular Research Center, University of Connecticut School of Medicine, Farmington, Connecticut 06030-1110, USA.*

Atherosclerosis

Lead

Lead exposure is a well known cause of cardiovascular damage, including atherosclerosis. Paraoxonase 1 (PON1), a high-density lipoprotein-associated antioxidant enzyme, is capable of hydrolyzing oxidized lipids and thus it protects against atherosclerosis. The mechanism by which heavy metals inhibit serum PON1 activity is still not clear. Our aim was to detect the association between lead exposure and serum PON1 activity and lipid profile and also to study the polymorphism of the PON1 gene. A case-control, cross-sectional study conducted from June 2008 until May 2009. Male workers (n=100) in a lead battery manufactory were recruited for this study. They were compared with 100 male age-matched workers not exposed to lead (control group). Serum lipid profile, paraoxonase activity and lead were measured in blood samples. The DNA was extracted for detecting the Q192R polymorphism of the PON1 gene by polymerase chain reaction followed by restriction fragment length polymorphism. There was significant difference in triglycerides, total cholesterol and high-density lipoprotein cholesterol (HDL-C) (P=.01,.05 and.04, respectively) between cases and controls. Multiple linear regression analysis showed that blood lead levels were significantly associated with decreased serum paraoxonase activity (P=.03) in lead workers. The paraoxonase genotype QR was the most prevalent in 34/53 subjects (64%) among the lead-exposed groups, while the genotype QQ was more prevalent in the control group, in 15/25 subjects (60%), with a significant difference between the control and other groups (P<.05). *Reference: Ann Saudi Med. 2011 Sep-Oct; 31(5): 481–487. doi: 10.4103/0256-4947.84625. PMCID: PMC3183682. Assessment of the role of paraoxonase gene polymorphism (Q192R) and paraoxonase activity in the susceptibility to atherosclerosis among lead-exposed workers. Manal Kamal,a Mona M. Fathy,a Eman Taher,b Manal Hasan,c and May Tolbad.*

Lead is a ubiquitous environmental toxin that is capable of causing numerous acute and chronic illnesses. Population studies have demonstrated a link between lead exposure and subsequent development of hypertension (HTN) and cardiovascular disease. In vivo and in vitro studies have shown that chronic lead exposure causes HTN and cardiovascular disease by promoting oxidative stress, limiting nitric oxide availability, impairing nitric oxide signaling, augmenting adrenergic activity, increasing endothelin production, altering the renin-angiotensin system, raising vasoconstrictor prostaglandins, lowering vasodilator prostaglandins, promoting inflammation, disturbing vascular smooth muscle $Ca2+$ signaling, diminishing endothelium-dependent vasorelaxation, and modifying the vascular response to vasoactive agonists. Moreover, lead has been shown to cause endothelial injury, impede endothelial repair, inhibit angiogenesis, reduce endothelial cell growth, suppress proteoglycan production, stimulate vascular smooth muscle cell proliferation and phenotypic transformation, reduce tissue plasminogen activator, and raise plasminogen activator inhibitor-1 production. Via these and other actions, lead exposure causes HTN and promotes arteriosclerosis, atherosclerosis, thrombosis, and cardiovascular disease. In conclusion, studies performed in experimental animals, isolated tissues, and cultured cells have provided compelling evidence that chronic exposure to low levels of lead can cause HTN, endothelial injury/dysfunction, arteriosclerosis, and cardiovascular disease. More importantly, these studies have elucidated the cellular and molecular mechanisms of lead's action on cardiovascular/renal systems, a task that is impossible to accomplish using clinical and epidemiological investigations alone. *Reference:* Am J Physiol Heart Circ Physiol. 2008 August; 295(2): H454–H465. Published online 2008 June 20. doi: 10.1152/ajpheart.00158.2008. PMCID: PMC2519216. Mechanisms of lead-induced hypertension and cardiovascular disease, Nosratola D. Vaziri.

Mercury

Exposure to mercury is known to increase cardiovascular risk but the underlying mechanisms are not well explored. We analysed whether chronic exposure to low mercury doses affects endothelial modulation of the coronary circulation. Left coronary arteries and hearts from Wistar rats treated with either HgCl2 (first dose 4.6 µg·kg−1, subsequent doses 0.07 µg·kg−1 day−1, 30 days) or vehicle were used. Endothelial cells from pig coronary arteries incubated with HgCl2 were also used. Mercury treatment increased 5-HT-induced vasoconstriction but reduced acetylcholine-induced vasodilatation. It also reduced nitric oxide (NO) production and the effects of NO synthase inhibition with L-NAME (100 µmol·L−1) on 5-HT and acetylcholine responses. Superoxide anion production and mRNA levels of NOX-1 and NOX-4 were all increased. The superoxide anion scavenger tiron (1 mmol·L−1) reduced 5-HT responses and increased acetylcholine responses only in vessels from mercury-treated rats. In isolated hearts from mercury-treated rats, coronary perfusion and diastolic pressure were unchanged, but developed isovolumetric systolic pressure was reduced. In these hearts, L-NAME increased coronary perfusion pressure and diastolic pressure while it further reduced developed systolic pressure. Chronic exposure to low doses of mercury promotes endothelial dysfunction of coronary arteries, as shown by decreased NO bioavailability induced by increased oxidative stress. These effects on coronary function increase resistance to flow, which under overload conditions might cause ventricular contraction and relaxation impairment. These findings provide further evidence that mercury, even at low doses, could be an environmental risk factor for cardiovascular disease. *Reference: Br J Pharmacol. 2011 April; 162(8): 1819–1831. doi: 10.1111/j.1476-5381.2011.01203.x. PMCID: PMC3081124. Endothelial dysfunction of rat coronary arteries after exposure to low concentrations of mercury is dependent on reactive oxygen species. Lorena B Furieri, María Galán, María S Avendaño, Ana B García-Redondo, Andrea Aguado, Sonia Martínez, Victoria Cachofeiro, M Visitación Bartolomé, María J Alonso, Dalton V Vassallo, and Mercedes Salaices.*

Cadmium

Cadmium is a toxic heavy metal which has been shown to be a possible risk factor of atherosclerosis in epidemiological and experimental studies. Since intimal hyperplasia in vascular tissue is an important component of atherosclerosis, the authors examined the effect of cadmium on the proliferation of vascular smooth muscle cells cultured in a serum-free medium. It was found that cadmium at 100 nM or less can increase the incorporation of [3H]thymidine into the acid-insoluble fraction of growing bovine and rabbit aortic smooth muscle cells but not of growing bovine aortic endothelial cells. Although vascular smooth muscle cells are sensitive to cadmium cytotoxicity, no increase in the leakage of lactate dehydrogenase from the cells was caused by the metal at 200 nM or less in bovine aortic smooth muscle cells. Intracellular accumulation of radioactive calcium in bovine aortic smooth muscle cells was significantly increased by cadmium. It was therefore suggested that low levels of cadmium may promote the proliferation of vascular smooth muscle cells through intracellular calcium-dependent signalling pathway. The present study supports the hypothesis that cadmium can be a risk factor of atherosclerosis through dysfunction of vascular smooth muscle cells as well as vascular endothelial cells under certain conditions. *Reference: Fujiwara, Y., et al. Promotion of cultured vascular smooth muscle cell proliferation by low levels of cadmium. Toxicol Lett. 94(3):175-180, 1998. Department of Environmental Science, Faculty of Pharmaceutical Sciences, Hokuriku University, Kanazawa, Japan.*

It is unclear whether environmental cadmium exposure is associated with cardiovascular disease, although recent data suggest associations with myocardial infarction and peripheral arterial disease. The objective of this study was to evaluate the association of measured cadmium exposure with stroke and heart failure (HF) in the general population. We analyzed data from 12,049 participants, aged 30 years and older, in the 1999–2006 National Health and Nutrition Examination Survey (NHANES) for whom information was available on body mass index, smoking status, blood cotinine level, alcohol consumption, and socio-demographic characteristics. At their interviews, 492 persons reported a history of stroke, and 471 a history of HF. After adjusting for demographic and cardiovascular risk factors, a 50% increase in blood cadmium corresponded to a 35% increased odds of prevalent stroke [OR: 1.35; 95% confidence interval (CI): 1.12–1.65] and a 50% increase in urinary cadmium corresponded to a 9% increase in prevalent stroke [OR: 1.09; 95% CI: 1.00–1.19]. This association was higher among women [OR: 1.38 95% CI: 1.11–1.72] than men [OR: 1.30; 95% CI: 0.93–1.79] (p-value for interaction=0.05). A 50% increase in blood cadmium corresponded to a 48% increased odds of prevalent HF [OR: 1.48; 95% CI: 1.17–1.87] and a 50% increase in urinary cadmium corresponded to a 12% increase in prevalent HF [OR: 1.12; 95% CI: 1.03–1.20], with no difference in sex-specific associations. Environmental exposure to cadmium was associated with significantly increased stroke and heart failure prevalence. Cadmium exposure may increase these important manifestations of cardiovascular disease. There has been increasing interest in the potential adverse cardiovascular effects of environmental exposures, including heavy metals (Bhatnagar 2006; Houston 2007; Weinhold 2004). Cadmium is a ubiquitous environmental toxin which may plausibly contribute to cardiovascular disease (CVD), although existing literature is limited. The major known sources of exposure for the U.S. general population are emissions from industrial activity and waste management operations, intake of certain foods (e.g. leafy vegetables, grains, organ meats, and crustaceans) and exposure to cigarette smoke. Previous studies found an association between blood cadmium and peripheral arterial disease (Navas-Acien et al. 2004) and between urinary cadmium and peripheral arterial disease and myocardial infarction (Everett and Frithsen 2008; Navas-Acien et al. 2005). Blood cadmium is thought to be a marker of current exposure but also appears to reflect body burden from long-term retention of cadmium in the liver and kidney; urinary cadmium is thought to more specifically be a marker of cumulative exposure (ATSDR 2008; Olsson et al. 2002). Cadmium may exert its adverse cardiovascular effects by promoting atherosclerosis and by inducing disadvantageous cardiac functional and metabolic changes (Houtman 1993; Kopp et al. 1983). We sought to examine the association of community-level cadmium exposure with two aspects of CVD for which there is little to no information: stroke and heart failure (HF). Stroke is the third leading cause of death in the U.S., and a leading cause of adult disability. The data addressing the association of cadmium with stroke is rather limited. In the English village of Shipham, where soil levels and dietary intake of cadmium were very high, researchers found no evidence of adverse effects on blood pressure and hepatic, renal and skeletal systems (Morgan and Simms 1988; Strehlow and Barltrop 1988). However, in research based in the same geographical area, a 40-year cohort study found significant excess mortality from stroke, and a follow-up ecological study reported borderline significant excess stroke mortality (Elliott et al. 2000; Inskip et al. 1982). HF is a disabling and deadly disease whose prevalence continues to rise in the U.S. despite a decline in general cardiovascular disease morbidity and mortality (Bahrami et al. 2008). To our knowledge, the possible association of cadmium exposure with HF has not been examined. Associations between cadmium exposure and these outcomes would potentially be important, because cadmium exposure is pervasive but modifiable, and stroke and HF are important sources of morbidity and mortality. *Reference: Cadmium exposure in association with history of stroke and heart failure. Junenette L. Peters, ScD, Todd S. Perlstein, MD, Melissa J. Perry, PhD, Eileen McNeely, PhD, and Jennifer Weuve, ScD.*

L-Arginine

Ten men (average age 41) with atherosclerosis were given 21 grams of l-arginine per day (orally) for three days. After a washout period they were given a placebo. Arginine treatment was found to result in a 2.6-fold greater increase in arterial dilatation compared with the placebo. Arginine treatment resulted in a 16% reduction in the adhesion of monocytes to epithelial cells. *Reference: Oral L-arginine improves endothelium-dependent dilatation and reduces monocyte adhesion to endothelial cells in young men with coronary artery disease. Atherosclerosis. Adams, R. R., et al. 129(2):261-269, 1997.*

L-Arginine completely blocked the progression of carotid intimal plaques, reduced aortic intimal thickening, and preserved endothelium-dependent vasodilator function. *Reference: Dietary L-arginine reduces the progression of atherosclerosis in cholesterol-fed rabbits: comparison with lovastatin. Boger, R. H., et al. Circulation. . 96(4):1282-1290, 1997.*

Atherogenesis is enhanced in arterial segments exposed to disturbed blood flow, indicating the active participation of the hemodynamic environment in lesion formation. Turbulent shear stress selectively regulates responsive genes in the endothelium and increases the damage induced by free radicals. The purpose of the present study was to evaluate the effects of intervention with antioxidants and l-arginine on endothelial NO synthase (eNOS) and oxidation-sensitive gene perturbation induced by disturbed flow in vitro and in vivo. Both human endothelial cells exposed to shear stress and high atherosclerosis-prone areas of hypercholesterolemic low-density lipoprotein receptor knockout (LDLR(-/-)) mice showed increased activities of redox-transcription factors (ELK-1, p-Jun, and p-CREB) and decreased expression of eNOS. Intervention with antioxidants and l-arginine reduced the activation of redox-transcription factors and increased eNOS expression in cells and in vivo. These results demonstrate that atherogenic effects induced by turbulent shear stress can be prevented by cotreatment with antioxidants and l-arginine. The therapeutic possibility to modulate shear stress-response genes may have important implications for the prevention of atherosclerosis and its clinical manifestations. **Reference:** *Arginine: NO more than a simple amino acid? Lancet. Chowienczyk, P., et al. 350(9082):901-902, 1997. Beneficial effects of antioxidants and L-arginine on oxidation-sensitive gene expression and endothelial NO synthase activity at sites of disturbed shear stress. de Nigris, F., et al. Proc Natl Acad Sci U S A. 100(3):1420-1425, 2003. Department of Medicine, University of California, San Diego, CA, USA.*

The objective of this study was to evaluate the influence of ingested l-arginine, l-citrulline, and antioxidants (vitamins C and E) on the progression of atherosclerosis in rabbits fed a high-cholesterol diet. The fatty diet caused a marked impairment of endothelium-dependent vasorelaxation in isolated thoracic aorta and blood flow in rabbit ear artery in vivo, the development of atheromatous lesions and increased superoxide anion production in thoracic aorta, and increased oxidation-sensitive gene expression [Elk-1 and phosphorylated cAMP response element-binding protein]. Rabbits were treated orally for 12 weeks with l-arginine, l-citrulline, and/or antioxidants. l-arginine plus l-citrulline, either alone or in combination with antioxidants, caused a marked improvement in endothelium-dependent vasorelaxation and blood flow, dramatic regression in atheromatous lesions, and decrease in superoxide production and oxidation-sensitive gene expression. These therapeutic effects were associated with concomitant increases in aortic endothelial NO synthase expression and plasma $NO(2)(-)+NO(3)(-)$ and cGMP levels. These observations indicate that ingestion of certain NO-boosting substances, including l-arginine, l-citrulline, and antioxidants, can abrogate the state of oxidative stress and reverse the progression of atherosclerosis. This approach may have clinical utility in the treatment of atherosclerosis in humans. **Reference:** *l-Citrulline and l-arginine supplementation retards the progression of high-cholesterol-diet-induced atherosclerosis in rabbits. Proc Natl Acad Sci U S A. 102(38):13681-13686, 2005. Hayashi, T., et al. Department of Geriatrics, Nagoya University Graduate School of Medicine, 65 Tsuruma-cho, Showa-ku, Nagoya, Japan.*

Nitric oxide-dependent factors (serotonin, activated platelets, acetylcholine) cause vasodilation in normal coronary arteries but vasoconstrict atherosclerotic vessels. This experiment tested the hypothesis that intravenous systemic infusions of L-arginine, a precursor for nitric oxide production, dilate the coronary vascular bed of patients undergoing coronary artery bypass graft surgery. Twenty patients scheduled for coronary artery bypass graft surgery surgery were studied in a prospective, blinded, randomized clinical trial. Saphenous vein graft blood flow was measured with a transit time flow probe, and coronary vascular resistance was calculated. After weaning from bypass, patients were given a venous infusion (placebo or 10% arginine hydrochloride [30 g]) over 15 min. Arterial blood samples for the determination of L-arginine and L-citrulline levels were drawn before, 10 min after starting infusion, and 10 min after end of infusion. The placebo group experienced an increase in mean arterial pressure and coronary vascular resistance and a decrease in graft blood flow. Patients in the L-arginine group maintained their baseline values. Mean arterial pressure (L-arginine, 88+/-17 to 92+/-13 mmHg vs. placebo, 80+/-12 to 92+/-9 mmHg, P = 0.021), coronary vascular resistance (L-arginine, 97,000+/-60,000 to 99,600+/-51,000 dynes x s x cm(-5) vs. placebo, 81,000+/-69,000 to 117,000+/-64,000 dynes x s x cm(-5), P = 0.05), and graft blood flow (L-arginine, 55+/-25 to 50+/-19 ml/min vs. placebo, 60+/-34 to 46+/-18, P = 0.05) remained more stable in the L-arginine-treated patients. Systemic L-arginine infusion reduced postbypass coronary vasoconstriction. There were no adverse events associated with the drug infusion. *Reference:* L-Arginine infusion *dilates coronary vasculature in patients undergoing coronary bypass surgery. Anesthesiology. 90(6):1577-1586, 1999. Wallace, A. W., et al.*

Berberine (active constituent of Golden Seal)

Vascular smooth muscle cell (SMC) proliferation plays an important role in the pathogenesis of atherosclerosis and post-angioplasty restenosis. Berberine is a well-known component of the Chinese herb medicine Huanglian (Coptis chinensis), and is capable of inhibiting SMC contraction and proliferation, yet the exact mechanism is unknown. We therefore investigated the effect of berberine on SMC growth after mechanic injury in vitro. DNA synthesis and cell proliferation assay were performed to show that berberine inhibited serum-stimulated rat aortic SMC growth in a concentration-dependent manner. Mechanical injury with sterile pipette tip stimulated the regrowth of SMCs. Treatment with berberine prevented the regrowth and migration of SMCs into the denuded trauma zone. Western blot analysis showed that activation of the MEK1/2 (mitogen-activated protein kinase kinase 1/2), extracellular signal-regulated kinase (ERK), and up-regulation of early growth response gene (Egr-1), c-Fos and Cyclin D1 were observed sequentially after mechanic injury in vitro. Semi-quantitative reverse-transcription PCR assay further confirmed the increase of Egr-1, c-Fos, platelet-derived growth factor (PDGF) and Cyclin D1 expression in a transcriptional level. However, berberine significantly attenuated MEK/ERK activation and downstream target (Egr-1, c-Fos, Cyclin D1 and PDGF-A) expression after mechanic injury in vitro. Our study showed that berberine blocked injury-induced SMC regrowth by inactivation of ERK/Egr-1 signaling pathway thereby preventing early signaling induced by injury in vitro. The anti-proliferative properties of berberine may be useful in treating disorders due to inappropriate SMC growth. *Reference: Biochem Pharmacol. 2006 March 14; 71(6): 806–817. Published online 2006 January 31. doi: 10.1016/j.bcp.2005.12.028. PMCID: PMC2639653. NIHMSID: NIHMS89185. Berberine suppresses MEK/ERK-dependent Egr-1 signaling pathway and inhibits vascular smooth muscle cell regrowth after in vitro mechanical injury. Kae-Woei Liang, Chih-Tai Ting, Sui-Chu Yin, Ying-Tsung Chen, Shing-Jong Lin, James K. Liao, and Shih-Lan Hsua.*

To investigate the effects and molecular mechanisms of berberine on improving insulin resistance induced by free fatty acids (FFAs) in 3T3-L1 adipocytes. The model of insulin resistance in 3T3-L1 adipocytes was established by adding palmic acid (0.5 mmol/L) to the culture medium. Berberine treatment was performed at the same time. Glucose uptake rate was determined by the 2-deoxy-[3H]-D-glucose method. The levels of IkB kinase beta (IKKβ) Ser181 phosphorylation, insulin receptor substrate-1(IRS-1) Ser307 phosphorylation, expression of IKKβ, IRS-1, nuclear transcription factor kappaB p65 (NF-κB p65), phosphatidylinositol-3-kinase p85 (PI-3K p85) and glucose transporter 4 (GLUT4) proteins were detected by Western blotting. The distribution of NF-κB p65 proteins inside the adipocytes was observed through confocal laser scanning microscopy (CLSM). After the intervention of palmic acid for 24 h, the insulin-stimulated glucose transport in 3T3-L1 adipocytes was inhibited by 67%. Meanwhile, the expression of IRS-1 and PI-3K p85 protein was reduced, while the levels of IKKβ Ser181 and IRS-1 Ser307 phosphorylation, and nuclear translocation of NF-κB p65 protein were increased. However, the above indexes, which indicated the existence of insulin resistance, were reversed by berberine although the expression of GLUT4, IKKβ and total NF-κB p65 protein were not changed during this study. Insulin resistance induced by FFAs in 3T3-L1 adipocytes can be improved by berberine. Berberine reversed free-fatty-acid-induced insulin resistance in 3T3-L1 adipocytes through targeting IKKβ. *Reference: World J Gastroenterol. 2008 February 14; 14(6): 876–883. Published online 2008 February 14. doi: 10.3748/wjg.14.876. PMCID: PMC2687054. Berberine reverses free-fatty-acid-induced insulin resistance in 3T3-L1 adipocytes through targeting IKKβ. Ping Yi, Fu-Er Lu, Li-Jun Xu, Guang Chen, Hui Dong, and Kai-Fu Wang. Ping Yi, Department of Integrated Traditional Chinese and Western Medicine, Tongji Hospital, Tongji Medical College, Huazhong University of Science and Technology, Wuhan 430030, Hubei Province, China.*

Berberine (BBR) is a natural alkaloid isolated from the Coptis Chinensis. While this plant has been used in Ayurvedic and Chinese medicine for more than 2500 years, interest in its effects in metabolic and cardiovascular disease has been growing in the Western world in the last decade. Many papers have been published in these years reporting beneficial effects in carbohydrate and lipid metabolism, endothelial function and the cardiovascular system. In this review, we report a detailed analysis of the scientific literature regarding this topic, describing the effects and the underlying mechanisms of BBR on carbohydrate and lipid metabolism, endothelial function and the cardiovascular system. Berberine (BBR) is a natural alkaloid isolated from the Coptis Chinensis. This plant has been used for medicinal purposes for more than 2500 years in Ayurvedic and Chinese medicine. Although routinely prescribed in Asian countries for its antimicrobial activity in the treatment of gastrointestinal infections and diarrhoea, and usually used for the treatment of diabetes mellitus, an interest in its beneficial effects in metabolic and cardiovascular diseases has been growing in the Western world over the last decade. Recent literature suggests BBR is a drug with multiple target characteristics, which are already known in traditional medicine. Its activity in carbohydrate and lipid metabolisms, diabetes mellitus treatment, endothelial function and the cardiovascular system has been investigated in the last decade with interesting results both in animals and clinical studies. This review analyzes the scientific literature on the effects and the underlying mechanisms of BBR on carbohydrate and lipid metabolism, endothelial function and the cardiovascular system. BBR's effects on glucidic metabolism are well known in China, where it has been used as an oral hypoglycemic agent in the treatment of type 2 diabetes mellitus for many years. There are many clinical reports on the hypoglycaemic action of BBR in the Chinese literature, which were confirmed by controlled clinical trials. Several studies have only recently investigated how it may exert its action on glucose metabolism and insulin sensitivity. Insulin resistance is a major metabolic abnormality leading not only to type 2 diabetes, but also to a group of metabolic disorders known as the metabolic syndrome. In 2006, Lee et al investigated the mechanisms underlying the effects of BBR in the treatment of diabetes and obesity and on insulin resistance. Their experiments in vivo and in vitro paved the way to future understanding. They focused interest on a heterotrimeric protein that plays a key role in the regulation of whole-body energy homeostasis; i.e. adenosine mono-phosphate kinase (AMPK), showing that part of the effects exerted by BBR on diabetes and obesity was due to the stimulation of this protein kinase. The administration of BBR to db/db mice led to a significant body weight reduction with both a significant reduction in fasting blood glucose and improvement in glucose tolerance. Similar effects were also observed in high fat fed Whistar rats, in which BBR administration reduced triglycerides (TG), body weight and improved insulin action in comparison to chow fed rats. The mechanisms that were the basis of these results were detected in the expression of genes involved in energy metabolism. BBR downregulated the expression of genes involved in lipogenesis and upregulated those involved in energy expenditure in adipose tissue and in muscle. Particularly, 11β-hydroxysteroid dehydrogenase, a key enzyme linked to visceral obesity and metabolic syndrome, decreased, and the expression of most genes involved in carbohydrate metabolism was also reduced. In contrast, the transcript level of enzymes related to energy dissipation, including glycerol kinase and acyl-CoA dehydrogenase, increased. These results implied that BBR treatment in vivo resulted in a modulation of the gene expression profile that would promote catabolism of high energy intermediates. Others mechanisms involved in BBR actions were clarified by Zhou et al and subsequently confirmed by other authors. They reported that BBR promotes glucose uptake in 3T3-L1 preadipocytes through a mechanism distinct from insulin. Insulin increases cellular glucose uptake by promoting GLUT4 expression on the cell surface through the activation of phosphatidylinositol 3-kinase (PI3K). On the contrary, BBR's effect on glucose uptake was insensitive to wortmannin, an inhibitor of PI3K. It seemed that BBR could induce glucose transport by activating GLUT1; particularly BBR increases glucose transport by enhancing GLUT1 gene expression. These effects are mediated by the activation of AMPK, which coordinates both short and long term metabolic changes, leading to an improvement in energy production and a reduction of energy storage. Specifically, its activation results in an increase in the uptake of glucose from the blood to target organs. Further, AMPK inhibits the accumulation of fat by modulating down-stream-signaling components like acetil CoA carbossilase (ACC). AMPK inhibits ACC activity by direct phosphorylation, which leads to a blockage of fatty acid synthesis pathways. AMPK phosphorylation and ACC phosphorylation were increased in myoblasts and adipocytes in vitro after short-term treatment with BBR, and in liver after long-term BBR treatment of db/db mice. The results of various recent studies have pointed out a possible mechanism of activation of AMPK, mediated by BBR. It was observed that BBR reduced oxygen-dependent glucose oxidation through inhibition of the respirator mitochondrial complex I. To compensate for the reduction in aerobic respiration, it was observed that there was an increase in glycolysis, a biochemical pathway that requires more glucose than aerobic respiration for the production of the same amount of ATP. As a consequence, glucose uptake and its utilization were increased, and associated with a persistent elevation in the AMP/ATP ratio, which induced the activation of AMPK. Also metformin and rosiglitazone, in a dose-dependent manner, inhibited respiration; rosiglitazone displayed similar potency to BBR, while metformin was substantially less potent. These data highlighted the importance of complex I of the mitochondrial respiratory chain as a major target for BBR in order to obtain an activation of AMPK. In obese hyperinsulinemic rats, BBR treatment significantly decreased lipid levels, plasma glucose and insulin levels. Oral glucose tolerance tests revealed a decrease of plasma glucose and insulin levels; in addition, the results of insulin tolerance suggested a marked improvement in insulin resistance. According to these in vivo results, it was observed that BBR acutely decreased glucose-stimulated insulin secretion in pancreatic β-cells isolated from rats through the AMPK signalling pathway. This evidence was clinically confirmed by a double-blind, placebo-controlled trial, in which BBR administration decreased fasting and postprandial plasma glucose with slightly decreasing postprandial insulin and body weight reduction in type 2 diabetic patients. Another important mechanism underlying the effects of BBR on insulin sensitivity is increases insulin-receptor (InsR) expression in a dose and time-dependent manner. BBR enhancement of InsR expression improves cellular glucose consumption only in the presence of insulin. Silencing the InsR gene reduces this effect. BBR induces InsR gene expression, with a mechanism of transcriptional regulation through protein kinase C (PKC). In type 2 diabetic mice, treatment with BBR lowered fasting blood glucose and fasting serum insulin, increased insulin sensitivity and elevated InsR mRNA, as well as PKC activity in the liver. In addition, it was observed that BBR did not lower blood glucose in type 1 diabetic mice, because of their insulin deficiency. The same results were obtained in a variety of human cell lines and were confirmed in a randomized clinical trial, in which BBR treatment significantly lowered fasting blood glucose, hemoglobin A1c, TG and insulin levels in patients with type 2 diabetes mellitus. In this study, metformin and rosiglitazone were used as references. The effects of BBR on fasting glucose and hemoglobin A1c were similar to those of metformin and rosiglitazone; moreover, BBR showed an important activity in reducing the serum levels of TG. Serum insulin levels declined significantly. Consistent with the in vitro experiments, the mean percentage of peripheral blood lymphocytes that express InsR on the surface, isolated from the patients treated with BBR, was significantly elevated in comparison to that before BBR treatment. These finding confirmed the activity of BBR on the up-regulation of InsR in type 2 diabetes mellitus patients and its relationship with the glucose-lowering effect. Contrary to thiazolidinediones (TZDs), it has been shown that BBR reduces the expression levels of peroxisome proliferator activated receptor γ, suppresses the differentiation of preadipocytes and reduces the accumulation of lipid droplets. Thus, unlike TZDs, which may lead to weight gain, BBR may be more suitable for insulin-resistant and diabetic patients with obesity. The insulin-sensitizing and glucose-lowering mechanisms of BBR are of great interest in this field. In conclusion, we can summarize that, although all the mechanisms underlying BBR's action on glucidic metabolism are not yet completely clarified and continue to be under investigation, its properties, namely reducing fasting blood glucose, hemoglobin A1c, and insulin levels in patients with type 2 diabetes mellitus, reduction of fat mass and TG, improvement of insulin resistance, and reduction of body weight, make BBR a promising molecule for future development in the treatment of glucidic disorders. *Reference: Cardiovascular and metabolic effects of Berberine, Flora Affuso, Valentina Mercurio, Valeria Fazio, and Serafino Fazio. This article has been cited by other articles in PMC.*

Green Tea

Epidemiological, clinical and experimental studies have established a positive correlation between green tea consumption and cardiovascular health. Catechins, the major polyphenolic compounds in green tea, exert vascular protective effects through multiple mechanisms, including antioxidative, anti-hypertensive, anti-inflammatory, anti-proliferative, anti-thrombogenic, and lipid lowering effects. (1) Tea catechins present antioxidant activity by scavenging free radicals, chelating redox active transition-metal ions, inhibiting redox active transcription factors, inhibiting pro-oxidant enzymes and inducing antioxidant enzymes. (2) Tea catechins inhibit the key enzymes involved in lipid biosynthesis and reduce intestinal lipid absorption, thereby improving blood lipid profile. (3) Catechins regulate vascular tone by activating endothelial nitric oxide. (4) Catechins prevent vascular inflammation that plays a critical role in the progression of atherosclerotic lesions. The anti-inflammatory activities of catechins may be due to their suppression of leukocyte adhesion to endothelium and subsequent transmigration through inhibition of transcriptional factor NFkB-mediated production of cytokines and adhesion molecules both in endothelial cells and inflammatory cells. (5) Catechins inhibit proliferation of vascular smooth muscle cells by interfering with vascular cell growth factors involved in atherogenesis. (6) Catechins suppress platelet adhesion, thereby inhibiting thrombogenesis. Taken together, catechins may be novel plant-derived small molecules for the prevention and treatment of cardiovascular diseases. This review highlights current developments in green tea extracts and vascular health, focusing specifically on the role of tea catechins in the prevention of various vascular diseases and the underlying mechanisms for these actions. In addition, the possible structure-activity relationship of catechins is discussed. *Reference:*   *Curr Med Chem. 2008; 15(18): 1840–1850. PMCID: PMC2748751. NIHMSID: NIHMS145237. Green Tea Catechins and Cardiovascular Health: An Update. Pon Velayutham, Anandh Babu, and Dongmin Liu. Department of Human Nutrition, Foods and Exercise, College of Agriculture and Life Sciences, Virginia Polytechnic Institute and State University, Blacksburg, Virginia 24061, USA.*

Tea polyphenols known as catechins are key components with many biological functions, including anti-inflammatory, antioxidative, and anticarcinogenic effects. These effects are induced by the suppression of several inflammatory factors including nuclear factor-kappa B (NF-κB). While these characteristics of catechins have been well documented, actions of catechins as mediators on inflammation-related cardiovascular diseases have not yet been well investigated. In this article, we reviewed recent papers to reveal the anti-inflammatory effects of catechins in cardiovascular diseases. In our laboratory, we performed oral administration of catechins into murine and rat models of cardiac transplantation, myocarditis, myocardial ischemia, and atherosclerosis to reveal the effects of catechins on the inflammation-induced ventricular and arterial remodeling. From our results, catechins are potent agents for the treatment and prevention of inflammation-related cardiovascular diseases because they are critically involved in the suppression of proinflammatory signaling pathways. *Reference:*   *Tea Polyphenols Regulate Key Mediators on Inflammatory Cardiovascular Diseases. Jun-ichi Suzuki, Mitsuaki Isobe, Ryuichi Morishita, and Ryozo Nagai. Department of Advanced Clinical Science and Therapeutics, Graduate School of Medicine, University of Tokyo, 7-3-1 Hongo, Bunkyo, Tokyo 113-8655, Japan.*

Green tea is manufactured from the leaves of the plant Camellia sinensis Theaceae and has been regarded to possess anti-cancer, anti-obesity, anti-atherosclerotic, anti-diabetic, anti-bacterial, and anti-viral effects. Many of the beneficial effects of green tea are related to the activities of (−)-epigallocatechin gallate (EGCG), a major component of green tea catechins. For about 20 years, we have engaged in studies to reveal the biological activities and action mechanisms of green tea and EGCG. This review summarizes several lines of evidence to indicate the health-promoting properties of green tea mainly based on our own experimental findings. In the book "Yojokun" published in the Edo period, Ekiken Kaibara described that according to the ancient Chinese medical doctor, long-term drinking of green tea would result in a lean body by removing body fat. Evidence has accumulated to show that the ingestion of green tea and tea catechins leads to a reduction in body fat as described in recent reviews. The stimulation of hepatic lipid metabolism might be a factor responsible for the anti-obesity effects of tea catechins. Tea catechins are suggested to inhibit cell growth by suppressing lipogenesis in human MCF-7 breast cancer cells through down-regulation of fatty acid synthase gene expression in the nucleus and stimulation of cell energy expenditure in the mitochondria. The experimental data indicated that the suppression of fatty acid synthase gene expression by tea polyphenols may lead to down-regulation of EGFR/PI3K/Akt/Sp-1 signal transduction. In addition to EGCG's effects described above, we observed that oral administration of an EGCG-free green tea fraction reduced the hepatic gene expression of PEPCK and G6Pase. This fraction also reduced the hepatic gene expression of lipogenic enzymes such as fatty acid synthase, 4-hydroxymethylglutaryl CoA reductase, acetyl CoA carboxylase α, and ATP-citrate lyase in association with the reduced gene expression of sterol response element-binding factor (SREBF)-1 and SREBF-2, key transcription factors for the gene expression of lipogenic enzymes). In accordance with the results for these changes in hepatic gene expression of lipogenic enzymes, the plasma levels of triglycerides and cholesterol of mice given a diet containing the EGCG-free fraction were significantly reduced. The plasma glucose levels were not altered significantly, but tended to be reduced. Thus, green tea contains some component(s) other than catechins which may have anti-obesity and anti-atherosclerotic effects. **Reference:** *Proc Jpn Acad Ser B Phys Biol Sci. 2012 March 9; 88(3): 88–101. doi: 10.2183/ pjab.88.88. PMCID: PMC3365247. Health-promoting effects of green tea. Yasuo SUZUKI, Noriyuki MIYOSHI, and Mamoru ISEMURA.*

Vitamin C

This study sought to assess the effect of cigarette smoking on adhesion of human monocytes to human endothelial cells and to measure the effect of L-arginine and vitamin C supplementation on this interaction. Cigarette smoking has been associated with abnormal endothelial function and increased leukocyte adhesion to endothelium, both key early events in atherogenesis. Supplementation with both oral L-arginine (the physiologic substrate for nitric oxide) and vitamin C (an aqueous phase antioxidant) may improve endothelial function; however, their benefit in cigarette smokers is not known. Serum was collected from eight smokers (mean [+/-SD] age 33 +/- 5 years) with no other coronary risk factors and eight age- and gender-matched lifelong nonsmokers. The serum was added to confluent monolayers of human umbilical vein endothelial cells and incubated for 24 h. Human monocytes obtained by counterflow centrifugation elutriation were then added to these monolayers for 1 h, and adhesion then was measured by light microscopy. To assess reversibility, monocyte/ endothelial cell adhesion was then measured for each subject 2 h after 2 g of oral vitamin C and 2 h after 7 g of oral L-arginine. In smokers compared with control subjects, monocyte/ endothelial cell adhesion was increased (46.4 +/- 4.5% vs. 27.0 +/- 5.2%, p < 0.001), endothelial expression of intercellular adhesion molecule (ICAM)-1 was increased (0.31 +/- 0.02 vs. 0.22 +/- 0.03, p = 0.004), and vitamin C levels were reduced (33.7 +/- 24.1 vs. 53.4 +/- 11.5 mumol/liter, p = 0.028). After oral L-arginine, monocyte/ endothelial cell adhesion was reduced in smokers (from 46.4 +/- 4.5% to 35.1 +/- 4.0%, p = 0.002), as was endothelial cell expression of ICAM-1 (from 0.31 +/- 0.02 to 0.27 +/- 0.01, p = 0.001). After vitamin C, there was no significant change in monocyte/ endothelial cell adhesion or ICAM-1 expression from baseline in the smokers despite an increase in vitamin C levels (to 115 +/- 7 mumol/liter). Cigarette smoking is associated with increased monocyte-endothelial cell adhesion when endothelial cells are exposed to serum from healthy young adults. This abnormality is acutely reversible by oral L-arginine but not by vitamin C. *Reference: Cigarette smoking is associated with increased human monocyte adhesion to endothelial cells: reversibility with oral L-arginine but not vitamin C. Journal of the American College of Cardiology. Adams, M. R., et al. 29(3):491-497, 1997.*

High plasma concentrations of ascorbic acid, a marker of fruit and vegetable intake, are associated with low risk of coronary artery disease. Whether this relationship is explained by a reduction in systemic inflammation is unclear. The authors investigated the relationship between ascorbic acid plasma concentration and coronary artery disease risk, and in addition whether this relationship depended on classical risk factors and C-reactive protein (CRP) concentration. They used a prospective nested case-control design. The study consisted of 979 cases and 1794 controls (1767 men and 1006 women). Increasing ascorbic acid quartiles were associated with lower age, BMI, systolic and diastolic blood pressure, and CRP concentration, but with higher HDL-cholesterol concentration. No associations existed between ascorbic acid concentration and total cholesterol concentration or LDL-cholesterol concentration. When data from men and women were pooled, the risk estimates decreased with increasing ascorbic acid quartiles such that people in the highest ascorbic acid quartile had an odds ratio for future coronary artery disease of 0.67 (95 % CI 0.52, 0.87) compared with those in the lowest quartile (P for linearity=0.001). This relationship was independent of sex, age, diabetes, smoking, BMI, LDL-cholesterol, HDL-cholesterol, systolic blood pressure and CRP level. These data suggest that the risk reduction associated with higher ascorbic acid plasma concentrations, a marker of fruit and vegetable intake, is independent of classical risk factors and also independent of CRP concentration. *Reference: Plasma concentrations of ascorbic acid and C-reactive protein, and risk of future coronary artery disease, in apparently healthy men and women: the EPIC-Norfolk prospective population study. British*

Journal of Nutrition. 96(3):516-522, 2006. Boekholdt, S. M., et al. Department of Vascular Medicine, Academic Medical Center, Amsterdam, The Netherlands.

The notion that oxidation of lipids and propagation of free radicals may contribute to the pathogenesis of atherosclerosis is supported by a large body of evidence. To circumvent the damage caused by oxygen free radicals, antioxidants are needed which provide the much needed neutralization of free radical by allowing the pairing of electrons. In this study the authors investigated the effect of ascorbic acid, a water soluble antioxidant on the development of hypercholesterolemia induced atherosclerosis in rabbits. Rabbits were made hypercholesterolemic and atherosclerotic by feeding 100 mg cholesterol/day. Different doses of ascorbic acid were administered to these rabbits. Low dose of ascorbic acid (0.5 mg/100 g body weight/day) did not have any significant effect on the percent of total area covered by atherosclerotic plaque. However, ascorbic acid when fed at a higher dose (15 mg/100 g body weight/day) was highly effective in reducing the atherogenecity. With this dose the percent of total surface area covered by atherosclerotic plaque was significantly less (p < 0.001). This suggests that use of ascorbic acid may have great promise in the prevention of hypercholesterolemia induced atherosclerosis. *Reference: Effect of ascorbic acid on prevention of hypercholesterolemia induced atherosclerosis. Mol Cell Biochem. 285(1-2):143-147, 2006. Das, S., et al. Department of Biochemistry, Sir Ganga Ram Hospital, New Delhi, India.*

Periodontitis has been causally linked to cardiovascular disease, which is mediated through the oxidative stress induced by periodontitis. Since vitamin C has been suggested to limit oxidative damage, the authors hypothesized that vitamin C intake may reduce endothelial oxidative stress induced by periodontitis in the aorta. The aim of this study was to investigate the effects of vitamin C intake on the initiation of atherosclerosis in a ligature-induced rat periodontitis model. Eighteen 8-week-old-male Wistar rats were divided into three groups of six rats and all rats received daily fresh water and powdered food through out the 6-week study. In the vitamin C and periodontitis groups, periodontitis was ligature-induced for the first 4 weeks. In the vitamin C group, rats were given distilled water containing 1g/L vitamin C for the 2 weeks after removing the ligature. In the periodontitis group, there was lipid deposition in the descending aorta and significant increases of serum level of hexanoyl-lysine (HEL), and aortic levels of nitrotyrosine expression, HEL expression and 8-hydroxydeoxyguanosine (8-OHdG) compared to the control group. Vitamin C intake significantly increased plasma vitamin C level and GSH:GSSG ratio (178% and 123%, respectively), and decreased level of serum HEL and aortic levels of nitrotyrosine, HEL and 8-OHdG (23%, 87%, 84%, and 38%, respectively). These results suggest that vitamin C intake attenuates the degree of experimental atherosclerosis induced by periodontitis in the rat by decreasing oxidative stress. *Reference: Vitamin*

C intake attenuates the degree of experimental atherosclerosis induced by periodontitis in the rat by decreasing oxidative stress. Arch Oral Biol. 2009. Ekuni, D., et al. Department of Preventive Dentistry, Okayama University Graduate School of Medicine, Dentistry and Pharmaceutical Sciences, Okayama, Japan.

Hyperlipidemia is associated with endothelial dysfunction, an early event in atherosclerosis and predictor of risk for future coronary artery disease. Epidemiological studies suggest that increased dietary intake of antioxidants reduces the risk of coronary artery disease. The purpose of this study was to determine whether antioxidant vitamin therapy improves endothelial function and affects surrogate biomarkers for oxidative stress and inflammation in hyperlipidemic children. In a randomized, double-blind, placebo-controlled trial, the effects of antioxidant vitamins C (500 mg/d) and E (400 IU/d) for 6 weeks and the National Cholesterol Education Program Step II (NCEP-II) diet for 6 months on endothelium-dependent flow-mediated dilation (FMD) of the brachial artery were examined in 15 children with familial hypercholesterolemia (FH) or the phenotype of familial combined hyperlipidemia (FCH). Antioxidant vitamin therapy improved FMD of the brachial artery compared with baseline (P<0.001) without an effect on biomarkers for oxidative stress (autoantibodies to epitopes of oxidized LDL, F2-isoprostanes, 8-hydroxy-2'-deoxyguanosine), inflammation (C-reactive protein), or levels of asymmetric dimethylarginine, an endogenous inhibitor of nitric oxide. Antioxidant therapy with vitamins C and E restores endothelial function in hyperlipidemic children. Early detection and treatment of endothelial dysfunction in high-risk children may retard the progression of atherosclerosis. ***Reference:*** *Antioxidant vitamins C and E improve endothelial function in children with hyperlipidemia. Endothelial Assessment of Risk from Lipids in Youth (EARLY) Trial. Circulation. 2003. Engler, M. M., et al.*

Oxidative stress has been implicated as an important etiologic factor in atherosclerosis and vascular dysfunction. Antioxidants may inhibit atherogenesis and improve vascular function by two different mechanisms. First, lipid-soluble antioxidants present in low-density lipoprotein (LDL), including alpha-tocopherol, and water-soluble antioxidants present in the extracellular fluid of the arterial wall, including ascorbic acid (vitamin C), inhibit LDL oxidation through an LDL-specific antioxidant action. Second, antioxidants present in the cells of the vascular wall decrease cellular production and release of reactive oxygen species (ROS), inhibit endothelial activation (i.e., expression of adhesion molecules and monocyte chemoattractants), and improve the biologic activity of endothelium-derived nitric oxide (EDNO) through a cell- or tissue-specific antioxidant action. alpha-Tocopherol and a number of thiol antioxidants have been shown to decrease adhesion molecule expression and monocyte-endothelial interactions. Vitamin C has been demonstrated to potentiate EDNO activity and normalize vascular function in patients with coronary artery disease and associated risk factors, including hypercholesterolemia, hyperhomocysteinemia, hypertension, diabetes, and smoking. *Reference: On the role of vitamin C and other antioxidants in atherogenesis and vascular dysfunction. Proc Soc Exp Biol Med. 222(3):196-204, 1999. Frei, B*

Loss of endothelium-derived nitric oxide (EDNO) contributes to the clinical expression of atherosclerosis. Increased oxidative stress has been linked to impaired endothelial vasomotor function in atherosclerosis, and recent studies demonstrated that short-term ascorbic acid treatment improves endothelial function. This randomized, double-blind, placebo-controlled study, examined the effects of single-dose (2 grams PO) and long-term (500 mg per day) ascorbic acid treatment on EDNO-dependent flow-mediated dilation of the brachial artery in patients with angiographically established atherosclerosis. Flow-mediated dilation was examined by high-resolution vascular ultrasound at baseline, 2 hours after the single dose, and 30 days after long-term treatment in 46 patients with atherosclerosis. Flow-mediated dilation improved from 6.6+/-3.5% to 10.1+/-5.2% after single-dose treatment, and the effect was sustained after long-term treatment (9. 0+/-3.7%), whereas flow-mediated dilation was 8.6+/-4.7% at baseline and remained unchanged after single-dose (7.8+/-4.4%) and long-term (7.9+/-4.5%) treatment with placebo. Plasma ascorbic acid concentrations increased from 41.4+/-12. 9 to 115.9+/-34.2 micromol/L after single-dose treatment and to 95. 0+/-36.1 micromol/L after long-term treatment. In patients with atherosclerosis, long-term ascorbic acid treatment has a sustained beneficial effect on EDNO action. Because endothelial dysfunction may contribute to the pathogenesis of cardiovascular events, this study indicates that ascorbic acid treatment may benefit patients with atherosclerosis. *Reference: Effect of ascorbic acid in the regulation of cholesterol metabolism and the pathogenesis of atherosclerosis. Int J Vit Nutr Res. 47:1-18, 1977. Ginter, E. Long-term ascorbic acid administration reverses endothelial vasomotor dysfunction in patients with coronary artery disease. Circulation. 99:3234-3240, 1999. Gokce, N., et al.*

Chronic smoking is associated with endothelial dysfunction, an early stage of atherosclerosis. It has been suggested that endothelial dysfunction may be a consequence of enhanced degradation of nitric oxide secondary to formation of oxygen-derived free radicals. To test this hypothesis, the authors investigated the effects of the antioxidant vitamin C on endothelium dependent responses in chronic smokers. Forearm blood flow responses to the endothelium-dependent vasodilator acetylcholine and the endothelium-independent vasodilator sodium nitroprusside were measured by venous occlusion plethysmography in 10 control subjects and 10 chronic smokers. Drugs were infused into the brachial artery, and forearm blood flow was measured for each drug before and during concomitant intra-arterial infusion of the antioxidant vitamin C (18 mcg per minute). In control subjects, vitamin C had no effect on forearm blood flow in response to acetylcholine and sodium nitroprusside. In chronic smokers, the attenuated forearm blood flow responses to acetylcholine were markedly improved by concomitant administration of vitamin C, whereas the vasodilator responses to sodium nitroprusside were not affected. The authors concluded that vitamin C markedly improves endothelium dependent responses in chronic smokers. This observation supports the concept that endothelial dysfunction in chronic smokers is at least in part mediated by enhanced formation of oxygen-derived free radicals. **Reference:** *Antioxidant vitamin C improves endothelial dysfunction in chronic smokers. Circulation. 94(1):6-9, 1996. Heitzel, T., et al.*

Strong clinical and experimental evidence suggests that chronic latent vitamin C deficiency leads to hypercholesterolaemia and the accumulation of cholesterol in certain tissues. Ascorbic acid supplementation of the diet of hypercholesterolaemic humans and animals generally results in a significant reduction in plasma cholesterol concentration. While most studies relating ascorbic acid to atherosclerosis have used the rabbit as a model, those concerned with elucidating the role of ascorbic acid in the regulation of cholesterol metabolism have generally used the guinea pig. Comparatively little use has been made of the non-human primates. A significant advance in recent years has been the development of a model of chronic latent scurvy in the guinea pig. Chronic dietary inadequacy of vitamin C may influence the pathogenesis of atherosclerosis as it affects not only plasma cholesterol and triglyceride concentrations but also the integrity of the vascular wall. Ascorbic acid is involved in the regulation of cholesterol metabolism in several ways. Dietary inadequacy of vitamin C is associated indirectly with a lowering of cholesterol absorption, this effect resulting from a reduction in the availability of bile acids, monoglycerides and fatty acids. The excretion of cholesterol as neutral steroids, however, appears not to be affected by ascorbic acid. Although much of the evidence for the involvement of ascorbic acid in cholesterol synthesis is equivocal, it seems likely that cholesterol synthesis is decreased in vitamin C deficiency. A series of studies using guinea pigs with chronic latent vitamin C deficiency has provided clear evidence that bile acid synthesis is reduced in this condition. Indirect evidence strongly suggests that this results from a decrease in the activity of the microsomal enzyme cholesterol 7 alpha-hydroxylase. However, some evidence suggests that the mitochondrial reactions of bile acid synthesis require ascorbic acid. The role of ascorbic acid in the regulation of steroidogenesis appears to involve selective inhibitory and stimulatory effects on the desmolase, hydroxylase and dehydrogenase reactions which lead to the formation of pregnenolone and its subsequent conversion to steroid hormones. **Reference:** *The role of ascorbic acid in the regulation of cholesterol metabolism and in the pathogenesis of artherosclerosis. Atherosclerosis. 24(1-2):1-18, 1976. Turley, S. D., et al.*

Atherosclerosis is associated with stiffening of conduit arteries and increased platelet activation, partly as a result of reduced bioavailability of nitric oxide (NO), a mediator that normally has a variety of protective effects on blood vessels and platelets. Increased levels of oxygen free radicals are a feature of atherosclerosis that contributes to reduced NO bioavailability and might lead to increased arterial stiffness and platelet activation. Vitamin C is a dietary antioxidant that inactivates oxygen free radicals. This placebo-controlled, double-blind, randomized study was designed to establish whether acute oral administration of vitamin C (2 g), would reduce arterial stiffness and in vitro platelet aggregation in healthy male volunteers. Plasma vitamin C concentrations increased from 42+/-8 to 104+/-8 microM at 6 h after oral administration, and were associated with a significant reduction in augmentation index, a measure of arterial stiffness (by 9.6+/-3.0%; p = 0.016), and ADP-induced platelet aggregation (by 35+/-13%; p = 0.046). There was no change in these parameters after placebo. Vitamin C, therefore, appears to have beneficial effects, even in healthy subjects. The mechanism responsible is likely to involve protection of NO from inactivation by oxygen free radicals, but this requires confirmation. If similar effects are observed in patients with atherosclerosis or risk factors, vitamin C supplementation might prove an effective therapy in cardiovascular disease. *Reference: Role of ascorbic acid in the regulation of cholesterol metabolism and the pathogenesis of atherosclerosis. American Journal of Clinical Nutrition. 27:866-876, 1974. Turley, S., et al. Oral vitamin C reduces arterial stiffness and platelet aggregation in humans. Journal Of Cardiovascular Pharmacology. 34(5):690-693, 1999. Wilkinson, I. B., et al. Clinical Pharmacology Unit & Research Centre, University of Edinburgh, Western General Hospital, Scotland.*

Fish Oil

Omega-3 fatty acids, which are found abundantly in fish oil, are increasingly being used in the management of cardiovascular disease. It is clear that fish oil, in clinically used doses (typically 4 g/d of eicosapentaenoic acid and docosahexaenoic acid) reduce high triglycerides. However, the role of omega-3 fatty acids in reducing mortality, sudden death, arrhythmias, myocardial infarction, and heart failure has not yet been established. This review will focus on the current clinical uses of fish oil and provide an update on their effects on triglycerides, coronary artery disease, heart failure, and arrhythmia. We will explore the dietary sources of fish oil as compared with drug therapy, and discuss the use of fish oil products in combination with other commonly used lipid-lowering agents. We will examine the underlying mechanism of fish oil's action on triglyceride reduction, plaque stability, and effect in diabetes, and review the newly discovered anti-inflammatory effects of fish oil. Finally, we will examine the limitations of current data and suggest recommendations for fish oil use. The addition of omega-3 FA to a healthy diet appears to be safe when used for the primary and secondary prevention of CAD. The potential benefits are not limited to a reduction in triglycerides. However, the incremental benefits to modern therapy and a prudent diet are yet to be fully evaluated. *Reference: Cardiol Rev. 2010 Sep-Oct; 18(5): 258–263. doi: 10.1097/CRD.0b013e3181ea0de0. Fish Oil for the Treatment of Cardiovascular Disease. Daniel Weitz, MD, Howard Weintraub, MD, Edward Fisher, MD, and Arthur Z. Schwartzbard, MD. Department of Medicine, Leon H. Charney Division of Cardiology, NYU Langone Medical Center, New York, NY*

Uptake of oxidized low-density lipoprotein (ox-LDL) by endothelial cells is a critical step for the initiation and development of atherosclerosis. Adhesion molecules are inflammatory makers, which are upregulated by ox-LDL and play a pivotal role in atherogenesis. A number of studies suggest that fish and its constituents can reduce inflammation and decrease atherosclerosis. The authors hypothesized that fish oil constituents namely docosahexaenoic acid (DHA) and eicosapentaenoic acid (EPA) may reduce expression of adhesion molecules induced by ox-LDL. Cultured human coronary artery endothelial cells (HCAECs) were incubated with ox-LDL for 24 h. Parallel groups of cells were pretreated with DHA or EPA (10 or 50 &mgr;M) overnight before incubation with ox-LDL. Ox-LDL markedly increased the expression of P-selectin and intracellular adhesion molecule-1 (ICAM-1) (both protein and mRNA) in HCAECs, and enhanced the adhesion of monocytes to the cultured HCAECs. Both EPA and DHA decreased ox-LDL-induced upregulation of expression of P-selectin and ICAM-1, and the enhanced adhesion of monocytes to HCAECs. To determine the role of protein kinase B (PKB) as an intracellular-signaling pathway, HCAECs were treated with the PKB upstream inhibitor wortmannin (100 nM) or transfected with plasmids encoding dominant-negative mutants of PKB (PKB-DN) before treatment with DHA. Ox-LDL alone downregulated the activity of PKB; DHA attenuated this effect of ox-LDL, and both wortmannin and PKB-DN blocked the effect of DHA. The present study in human coronary endothelial cells suggests that both EPA and DHA attenuate ox-LDL-induced expression of adhesion molecules, and the adhesion of monocytes to HCAECs by modulation of PKB activation. These effects may be important mechanisms of anti-atherosclerotic effects of fish and fish oils. *Reference: J Mol Cell Cardiol. 35(7):769-775, 2003. Chen, H., et al. Department of Medicine and Physiology and Biophysics, University of Arkansas for Medical Sciences and Central Arkansas Veterans Health Care System, AR, Little Rock, USA.*

The omega-3 fatty acids of fish and fish oil have great potential for the prevention and treatment of patients with coronary artery disease. Unlike many of the pharmaceutical agents used in patients with coronary artery disease that have just a single mechanism of action, the eicosapentaenoic and docosahexaenoic acids of fish oil have multifaceted actions. One of their most important effects is the prevention of arrhythmias, with documentation derived from experiments in cultured myocytes, experiments in animals, epidemiologic correlations, and clinical trials.

Especially important is the ability of these n-3 fatty acids to inhibit ventricular fibrillation and consequent cardiac arrest. Eicosapentaenoic acid has several antithrombotic actions, particularly in inhibiting the synthesis of thromboxane A2, the prostaglandin that causes platelet aggregation and vasoconstriction. Fish oil retards the growth of the atherosclerotic plaque by inhibiting both cellular growth factors and the migration of monocytes. The omega-3 fatty acids promote the synthesis of the beneficial nitric oxide in the endothelium. Experiments in humans indicate a profound hypolipidemic effect of fish oil, especially lowering of plasma triglycerides. Both very-low-density lipoprotein production and apolipoprotein B synthesis are inhibited by fish oil. Fish oils also have a mild blood pressure- lowering effect in both normal and mildly hypertensive individuals. These composite effects suggest a prominent therapeutic role for fish oil in the prevention and treatment of coronary artery disease. *Reference: Are fish oils beneficial in the prevention and treatment of coronary artery disease? American Journal of Clinical Nutrition. 66(4 Supplement):1020S-1031S, 1997. Connor, S. L., et al.*

Dietary intake of long-chain n-3 polyunsaturated fatty acids (PUFA) reduces the risk for atherosclerosis. The authors examined the effect of a fish oil (FO)-rich diet on the development of atherosclerotic lesions in apolipoprotein E-deficient (apoE(-/-)) mice, which are vulnerable because of their high plasma cholesterol and triacylglycerol levels, focusing on the expression of endothelial adhesion molecules. Mice were fed semi-purified diets containing 5% corn oil (CO), rich in n-6 PUFA or menhaden oil as FO, rich in long-chain n-3 PUFA and 0.15% cholesterol after reaching 4 weeks of age, and they were killed when they were 4 weeks, 12 weeks, 18 weeks or 24 weeks old. Oxidative stress in plasma and aortic tissue was not increased in mice fed the FO-rich diet, despite its high peroxidizability index. A reduction of stenosis and intrusion at the aortic root, a decrease in the surface area of atherosclerotic lesions at the aorta and a decrease in P-selectin, vascular cellular adhesion molecule-1 (VCAM-1) and intercellular adhesion molecule-1 (ICAM-1) expression were observed in FO-fed mice compared to CO-fed mice. It seems likely that the reduced expression of VCAM-1 and ICAM-1 could be transcriptionally regulated by nuclear factor-kappaB in the aortic root. The protective effect of FO against atherosclerosis was more evident at early ages. Fish oil reduces adhesion molecule expression in lesions in apoE(-/-) mice. Because these molecules are involved in lesion progression the effect of FO may explain the observed decrease in atherogenesis. *Reference: Atherosclerosis prevention by a fish oil-rich diet in apoE(-/-) mice is associated with a reduction of endothelial adhesion molecules. Atherosclerosis. 2008. Casos, K., et al.*

Epidemiological studies have shown an inverse relationship between intake of N-3 fatty acids and incidence of stroke. And, there is a high incidence of stroke in patients with carotid atherosclerosis. The authors investigated the relationship between intake of N-3 fatty acids and carotid atherosclerosis in the cross-sectional study. A total of 1920 Japanese, aged over 40 years, received a population-based health examination in 1999. They underwent B-mode carotid ultrasonography to evaluate the carotid intimal-medial thickness (IMT). Eating patterns were evaluated by a 105 items food frequency questionnaire. A complete data set was available for 1902 subjects (785 men and 1117 women). With multiple linear regression analysis, after adjustments for age, sex, and total energy intake, intakes of EPA (P < 0.05), DHA (P < 0.05), and docosapentaenoic acid (P < 0.05) were significantly and inversely related to IMT. These data indicate that dietary N-3 fatty acid, especially very long chain N-3 fatty acids, may protect against carotid atherosclerosis. *Reference: Very long chain N-3 fatty acids intake and carotid atherosclerosis; An epidemiological study evaluated by ultrasonography. Atherosclerosis. 176(1):145-149, 2004. Hino, A., et al. The Third Department of Internal Medicine, Kurume University School of Medicine, Kurume, Japan.*

Eicosapentaenoic acid, which is one of the n-3 polyunsaturated fatty acids (PUFA), is reported to exert its antithrombotic and anti-atherogenic effect partly through the modulation of vascular cell functions. Vascular smooth muscle cell (VSMC) proliferation plays an important role in the pathogenesis of atherosclerosis. The authors reported the differential effect of various PUFA on VSMC proliferation. First we established a method for preparing PUFA rich cells in culture to mimic the in vivo situation using PUFA triacylglycerol emulsion. Using these fatty acid rich cells, the authors found that only EPA and docosahexaenoic acid, although less potent than EPA, inhibited the proliferation of VSMC among the fatty acids tested. This effect of EPA was reversed by the addition of anti-oxidants. It is suggested that production of the oxidized species at a low concentration from EPA inhibited the proliferation of VSMC. This anti-proliferative effect of EPA and DHA on VSMC could partly explain the anti-atherosclerotic effect of marine lipids. *Reference: Eicosapentaenoic acid and docosahexaenoic acid suppress the proliferation of vascular smooth muscle cells. Atherosclerosis. 104(1-2):95-103, 1993. Shiina, T., et al.*

This study involved 223 patients with confirmed atherosclerosis affecting the arteries of the heart. Half of the participants received 6,000 mg of omega-3 fish oil capsules containing 3,300 mg EPA + DHA per day for the first three months of this study. For a further 21 months these same participants received 3,000 mg of omega-3 fish oil capsules containing 1,650 mg EPA + DHA. The other half of the participants in this study received a placebo. Participants were examined after two years (3 months + 21 months). Of the subjects receiving fish oils capsules, 59 experienced changes in their condition. 36 of these patients showed mild progression of athersclerosis. 19 patients experienced some form of regression of atherosclerosis - 17 experienced mild regression and 2 experienced moderate improvement. Of the subjects receiving placebo, 51 experienced change in their condition: 44 patients experienced mild or moderate progression of atherosclerosis and 7 experienced mild regression. The researchers concluded that the difference in favour of fish oils supplementation was statistically significant. *Reference: The effect of dietary omega-3 fatty acids on coronary atherosclerosis. Ann Intern Med. 130(7):554-562, 1999. von Schacky, C., et al.*

The molecular and cellular mechanisms that fish oil (FO) exerts its physiological function are complicated. The present study brings evidence on the in vivo effect of FO on the development of atherosclerosis in apolipoprotein E knockout (apoE(-/-)) mice. The authors also test the hypothesis that the modulation of the cellular oxidative stress and antioxidant status contributes to the anti-atherosclerotic effect of FO. ApoE(-/-) mice were fed a diet rich either in FO or corn oil (CO) for 10 weeks. Both FO and CO had a plasma triacylglycerol-raising effect in apoE(-/-) mice, whereas aortic atherosclerotic lesions were significantly reduced in the mice that had consumed a high FO diet compared to those fed a high CO diet. The levels of hepatic superoxide dismutase (SOD) and catalase (CAT) activities were remarkably higher in the mice fed the FO diet than in mice fed the CO diet and the control diet. The authors then investigated the effects of FO and CO on the production of superoxide anion (O(2)(z.rad;-)) and reactive oxygen species (ROS) in cultured J774 macrophages. Antioxidant status was assessed by the determination of antioxidant enzyme activities. Both FO and CO induced high levels of O(2)(z.rad;-) and total ROS at a short time in macrophages. However, only the FO group restored the induction of O(2)(z.rad;-) and ROS to near basal levels after oil treatment for 24 h. Throughout the time course experiments, antioxidant enzyme activities in the FO group mostly displayed a greater increase than in the corresponding CO group after the same time period of oil treatment. In the present study, FO reduced the formation of atherosclerotic lesions in the aortic arteries of apoE(-/-) mice not through any lipid-lowering effect. The protective role of FO in the development of atherosclerosis may result from its antioxidative defense mechanism through the induction of antioxidant enzyme activities. *Reference: Fish oil increases antioxidant enzyme activities in macrophages and reduces atherosclerotic lesions in apoE-knockout mice. Cardiovasc Res. 61(1):169-176, 2004. Wang, H. H., et al.*

Lycopene

High circulating levels of carotenoids have been thought to exhibit a protective function in the development of atherosclerosis. The authors investigated whether aortic atherosclerosis was associated with lower levels of the major serum carotenoids in alpha-carotene, beta-carotene, beta-cryptoxanthin, lutein, lycopene, and zeaxanthin-in a subsample of the elderly population of the Rotterdam Study. Aortic atherosclerosis was assessed by presence of calcified plaques of the abdominal aorta. The case-control analysis comprised 108 subjects with aortic atherosclerosis and controls. In an age- and sex-adjusted logistic regression model, serum lycopene was inversely associated with the risk of atherosclerosis. The odds ratio for the highest compared to the lowest quartile of serum lycopene was 0.55 (95% CI 0.25-1.22; p(trend)=0.13).   Multivariate adjustment did not appreciably alter these results.   Stratification by smoking status indicated that the inverse association between lycopene and aortic calcification was most evident in current and former smokers (OR=0.35; 95% CI 0.13-0.94; p(trend)=0.04).   No association with atherosclerosis was observed for quartiles of serum concentrations of alpha-carotene, beta-carotene, lutein, and zeaxanthin.   This study provides evidence for a modest inverse association between levels of serum lycopene and presence of atherosclerosis, the association being most pronounced in current and former smokers. These findings suggest that lycopene may play a protective role in the development of atherosclerosis. *Reference: Serum carotenoids and atherosclerosis. The Rotterdam Study.   Atherosclerosis.   148(1):49-56, 2000. Klipstein-Grobusch, K., et al.*

Menopause is a pro-atherogenic state with a sharp rise in the incidence of coronary artery disease. This pilot study was designed as an equivalence randomized clinical trial to explore the potential of LycoRed (containing 2 mg lycopene) as an alternative to hormone replacement therapy (HRT) for the prevention of coronary artery disease in postmenopausal women. 41 healthy postmenopausal women were randomly allocated to receive either continuous combined HRT (n = 21) or LycoRed (n = 20) for six months. Serum lipid profile, marker of lipid peroxidation (malondialdehyde), and the level of endogenous antioxidant (glutathione) were measured at the baseline, and 3 and 6 months after the intervention in both groups. At 6 months, HRT resulted in a significant decrease in total cholesterol (TC) level by 23.5%, low-density lipoproteins (LDL) by 19.6%, and an increase in high-density lipoproteins (HDL) by 38.9%. The LycoRed group showed similar changes in TC (-24.2%), LDL (-14.9%) and HDL (+26.1%). Triglyceride levels showed a smaller though significant increase at 6 months, but not at 3 months, in both groups.   There was no significant change in the very LDL (VLDL) level in either group.   Malondialdehyde levels decreased significantly by 16.3% and 13.3%, whereas glutathione levels increased significantly by 5.9% and 12.5% in HRT and LycoRed groups, respectively.   Both HRT and LycoRed had a favorable effect on serum lipids and oxidative stress markers which were comparable. LycoRed can be used as an alternative to HRT to reduce the risk of atherosclerosis in postmenopausal women. *Reference: LycoRed as an alternative to hormone replacement therapy in lowering serum lipids and oxidative stress markers: A randomized controlled clinical trial. J Obstet Gynaecol Res.   32(3):299-304, 2006. Misra, R., et al. Departments of Obstetrics and Gynecology, All India Institute of Medical Sciences, Ansari Nagar, New Delhi, India.*

It is now well accepted that oxysterols play important roles in the formation of atherosclerotic plaque, involving cytotoxic, pro-oxidant and proinflammatory processes. It has been recently suggested that tomato lycopene may act as a preventive agent in atherosclerosis, although the exact mechanism of such a protection is not clarified. The main aim of this study was to investigate whether lycopene is able to counteract oxysterol-induced proinflammatory cytokines cascade in human macrophages, limiting the formation of atherosclerotic plaque. Therefore, THP-1 macrophages were exposed to two different oxysterols, such as 7-keto-cholesterol (4-16 muM) and 25-hydroxycholesterol (2-4 muM), alone and in combination with lycopene (0.5-2 muM). Both oxysterols enhanced pro-inflammatory cytokine [interleukin (IL)-1beta, IL-6, IL-8, tumor necrosis factor alpha) secretion and mRNA levels in a dose-dependent manner, although at different extent. These effects were associated with an increased reactive oxygen species (ROS) production through an enhanced expression of NAD(P)H oxidase. Moreover, a net increment of phosphorylation of extracellular regulated kinase 1/2, p-38 and Jun N-terminal kinase and of nuclear factor kB (NF-kappaB) nuclear binding was observed. Lycopene prevented oxysterol-induced increase in pro-inflammatory cytokine secretion and expression. Such an effect was accompanied by an inhibition of oxysterol-induced ROS production, mitogen-activated protein kinase phosphorylation and NF-kappaB activation. The inhibition of oxysterol-induced cytokine stimulation was also mimicked by the specific NF-kappaB inhibitor pyrrolidine dithiocarbamate. Moreover, the carotenoid increased peroxisome proliferator-activated receptor gamma levels in THP-1 macrophages. Taken all together, these data bring new information on the anti-atherogenic properties of lycopene, and on its mechanisms of action in atherosclerosis prevention. *Reference: Lycopene prevention of oxysterol-induced proinflammatory cytokine cascade in human macrophages: inhibition of NF-kappaB nuclear binding and increase in PPARgamma expression. J Nutr Biochem. 2010. Palozza, P., et al. Institute of General Pathology, Catholic University- School of Medicine, Rome, Italy.*

Increasing evidence suggests that lycopene may protect against atherosclerosis, although, the exact mechanism(s) is still unknown. Because lycopene is an efficient antioxidant, it has been proposed for a long time that this property may be responsible for its beneficial effects. Consistent with this, the carotenoid has been demonstrated to inhibit ROS production in vitro and to protect LDL from oxidation. However, recently, other mechanisms have been evoked and include: prevention of endothelial injury; modulation of lipid metabolism through a control of cholesterol synthesis and oxysterol toxic activities; reduction of inflammatory response through changes in cytokine production; inhibition of smooth muscle cell proliferation through regulation of molecular pathways involved in cell proliferation and apoptosis. Focusing on cell culture studies, this review summarizes the experimental evidence for a role of lycopene in the different phases of atherosclerotic process. *Reference: Lycopene in atherosclerosis prevention: an integrated scheme of the potential mechanisms of action from cell culture studies. Arch Biochem Biophys. 2010. Palozza, P., et al. Institute of General Pathology, Catholic University, School of Medicine, Rome, Italy.*

Coronary heart disease (CHD) is one of the primary causes of death in the Western world. The emphasis so far has been on the relationship between serum cholesterol levels and the risk of CHD. More recently, oxidative stress induced by reactive oxygen species (ROS) is also considered to play an important part in the etiology of this disease. Oxidation of the circulating low-density lipoprotein (LDL(ox)) is thought to play a key role in the pathogenesis of atherosclerosis and CHD. According to this hypothesis, macrophages inside the arterial wall take up the LDL(ox) and initiate the process of plaque formation. Dietary antioxidants such as vitamin E and beta-carotene have been shown in in vitro studies to prevent the formation of LDL(ox) and their uptake by microphages. In a recent study, healthy human subjects ingesting lycopene, a carotenoid antioxidant, in the form of tomato juice, tomato sauce, and oleoresin soft gel capsules for 1 week had significantly lower levels of LDL(ox) compared with controls. The antioxidant effects of lycopene have also been shown in four other human trials, including one where lycopene consumption reduced the levels of breath pentane. However, in one recent study, dietary supplementation with beta-carotene but not with lycopene was shown to inhibit LDL oxidation. The sources of lycopene used in most of these studies were either tomato products or lycopene extracted from tomatoes containing other carotenoids in various proportions. Therefore, it is not possible to attribute the effects solely to lycopene. Mechanisms other than the antioxidant properties of lycopene have also been shown to reduce the risk of CHD. Lycopene was shown to inhibit the activity of an essential enzyme involved in cholesterol synthesis in an in vitro and a small clinical study suggesting a hypocholesterolemic effect. Other possible mechanisms include enhanced LDL degradation, LDL particle size and composition, plaque rupture, and altered endothelial functions. Recent epidemiological studies have also shown an inverse relationship between tissue and serum levels of lycopene and mortality from CHD, cerebrovascular disease, and myocardial infraction. However, the most impressive population-based evidence comes from a multicenter case-control study where subjects from 10 European countries were evaluated for relationship between antioxidant status and acute myocardial infarctions. After adjusting for a range of dietary variables, only lycopene levels but not beta-carotene were found to be protective. At present, the role of lycopene in the prevention of CHD is strongly suggestive. Although the antioxidant property of lycopene may be one of the principal mechanism for its effect, other mechanisms may also be responsible. Controlled clinical and dietary intervention studies using well-defined subject populations and disease end points must be undertaken in the future to provide definitive evidence for the role of lycopene in the prevention of CHD. **Reference:** *Lycopene, tomatoes, and the prevention of coronary heart disease. Exp Biol Med (Maywood). 227(10):908-913, 2002. Rao, A. V. Department of Nutritional Sciences, Faculty of Medicine, University of Toronto, Toronto, Ontario, Canada.*

Although a number of epidemiological studies have evaluated the association between ss-carotene and the risk of cardiovascular diseases, there has been little research on the role of lycopene, an acyclic form of ss-carotene, with regard to the risk of cardiovascular disease. The authors investigated the relationship between plasma concentrations of lycopene and intima-media thickness of the common carotid artery wall (CCA-IMT) in 520 middle-aged men and women (aged 45 to 69 years) in eastern Finland. They were examined from 1994 to 1995 at the baseline of the Antioxidant Supplementation in Atherosclerosis Prevention (ASAP) study, a randomized trial concerning the effect of vitamin E and C supplementation on atherosclerotic progression. The subjects were classified into 2 categories according to the median concentration of plasma lycopene (0.12 micromol/L in men and 0.15 micromol/L in women). Mean CCA-IMT of the right and left common carotid arteries was 1.18 mm in men and 0.95 mm in women with plasma lycopene levels lower than the median and 0.97 mm in men (P:<0.001 for difference) and 0.89 mm in women (P:=0.027 for difference) with higher levels of plasma lycopene. In ANCOVA adjusting for cardiovascular risk factors and intake of nutrients, in men, low levels of plasma lycopene were associated with a 17.8% increment in CCA-IMT (P:=0.003 for difference). In women, the difference did not remain significant after the adjustments. The authors conclude that low plasma lycopene concentrations are associated with early atherosclerosis, manifested as increased CCA-IMT, in middle-aged men living in eastern Finland. *Reference: Low plasma lycopene concentration is associated with increased intima-media thickness of the carotid artery wall. Arterioscler Thromb Vasc Biol. 20(12):2677-2681, 2000. Rissanen, T., et al. Research Institute of Public Health, University of Kuopio, Kuopio, Finland.*

Vitamin E

Vitamin E, a naturally occurring antioxidant, has been found to reduce atherosclerotic lesion formation in animal models as well as cardiovascular morbidity in several observational studies. However, a number of case-control and prospective cohort studies failed to confirm its value in the primary and secondary prevention of morbidity and mortality from coronary artery disease. Several small or larger randomized interventional trials completed to date failed to resolve the conflict. Notably, even in large, well-conducted prospective epidemiologic studies, the potential effects of residual confounding may be on the same order of magnitude as the reported benefit. The response to vitamin E supplementation in specific patient subpopulations with chronic inflammation and/or higher degrees of oxidative stress has not been studied as yet. Therefore, further large randomized interventional trials are warranted to clarify accurately the role of vitamin E in the primary and secondary prevention of atherosclerotic coronary disease in these patient groups. Several in vitro and in vivo studies have provided solid evidence regarding the antiatherogenic effects of α-T. The discrepancy between the findings in the observational and intervention studies could be well attributed to inherent difficulties in the study of the beneficial effects of α-T but also to deficiencies in the design of the studies performed until now. Further even more prolonged studies especially in specific patient subpopulations, ie, patients with increased oxidative stress and/or chronic inflammation, with the use of more delicate determination of the oxidative status of the patients and probably more efficient pharmacologic forms, are warranted in order to permit a more accurate estimation of the cardiovascular efficacy of α-T. *Reference: Vasc Health Risk Manag. 2009; 5: 767–774. Published online 2009 September 18. PMCID: PMC2747395. Antiatherogenic effects of vitamin E: the search for the Holy Grail. Dimitrios Kirmizis and Dimitrios Chatzidimitriou.*

The authors studied the effects of alpha-tocopheryl acetate supplementation on the development of fatty streaks and its ability to modulate the expression of monocyte chemoattractant protein (MCP)-1 in aortic lesions of apoliprotein E knockout mice. For this purpose, 16-week-old apolipoprotein E knockout mice received alpha-tocopherol supplemention (800 mg)/kg diet) for 6 weeks. After this time, total and lipoprotein cholesterol in the serum, hepatic tocopherol, aortic lesion area and MCP-1 (protein and mRNA) expression were analysed. The dietary supplementation with alpha-tocopherol did not reduce serum cholesterol nor change lipoprotein profile, but it reduced the area of the aortic lesion by 55 %. The reduction in the lesion size was correlated with the reduced expression of MCP-1 mRNA and protein, as detected by real-time quantitative polymerase chain reaction and immunohistochemistry respectively. The results obtained here are relevant to the study of atherosclerosis, as they correlate the effectiveness of vitamin E supplementation in inhibiting the plaque formation with diminished expression of MCP-1 at the aortic lesion. *Reference: Monocyte chemoattractant protein-1 involvement in the alpha-tocopherol-induced reduction of atherosclerotic lesions in apolipoprotein E knockout mice. British Journal of Nutrition. 90(1):3-11, 2003. Alvarez-Leite, J. I., et al.*

A role of oxidative stress in atherosclerosis lies on experimental results carried out in vitro and in animal models. In humans, the supplementation with the antioxidant vitamin E has given in some cases supportive results and in others no effects. From in vitro studies, a large amount of data has shown that alpha-tocopherol (the major component of vitamin E) regulates key events in the cellular pathogenesis of atherosclerosis. The authors first described the inhibition of protein kinase C (PKC) activity by alpha-tocopherol to be at the basis of the vascular smooth muscle cell growth inhibition by this compound. Subsequently, PKC was recognized to be the target of alpha-tocopherol in different cell types, including monocytes, macrophages, neutrophils, fibroblasts and mesangial cells. Inhibiting the activity of protein kinase C by alpha-tocopherol results in different events in different cell types: inhibition of platelet aggregation, of nitric oxide production in endothelial cells, of superoxide production in neutrophils and macrophages as well as impairment of smooth muscle cell proliferation.

Adhesion molecule expression and inflammatory cell cytokine production are also influenced by alpha-tocopherol. Scavenger receptors, particularly important in the formation of atherosclerotic foam cells, are also modulated by alpha-tocopherol. The oxidized LDL scavenger receptors SR-A and CD36 are down regulated at the transcriptional level by alpha-tocopherol. The relevance of CD36 expression in the onset of atherosclerosis has been indicated by the protection against atherosclerosis by CD36 knockout mice. The effect of alpha-tocopherol against atherosclerosis is not due only to the prevention of LDL oxidation but also to the down regulation of the scavenger receptor CD36 and to the inhibition of PKC activity. *Reference: The role of alpha-tocopherol in preventing disease. Eur J Nutr. 43(Supplement 1):118-125, 2004 Azzi, A., et al. .*

Much experimental evidence suggests that lipid oxidation is important in atherogenesis and in epidemiological studies dietary antioxidants appear protective against cardiovascular events. However, most large clinical trials failed to demonstrate benefit of oral antioxidant vitamin supplementation in high-risk subjects. This paradox questions whether ingestion of antioxidant vitamins significantly affects lipid oxidation within established atherosclerotic lesions. This placebo-controlled, double blind study of 104 carotid endarterectomy patients determined the effects of short-term alpha-tocopherol supplementation (500 IU/day) on lipid oxidation in plasma and advanced atherosclerotic lesions. In the 53 patients who received alpha-tocopherol there was a significant increase in plasma alpha-tocopherol concentrations (from 32.66 +/- 13.11 at baseline to 38.31 +/- 13.87 (mean +/- SD) micromol/l, $p < 0.01$), a 40% increase (compared with placebo patients) in circulating LDL-associated alpha-tocopherol ($p < 0.0001$), and their LDL was less susceptible to ex vivo oxidation than that of the placebo group (lag phase 115.3 +/- 28.2 and 104.4 +/- 15.7 min respectively, $p < 0.02$). Although the mean cholesterol-standardised alpha-tocopherol concentration within lesions did not increase, alpha-tocopherol concentrations in lesions correlated significantly with those in plasma, suggesting that plasma alpha-tocopherol levels can influence lesion levels. There was a significant inverse correlation in lesions between cholesterol-standardised levels of alpha-tocopherol and 7beta-hydroxycholesterol, a free radical oxidation product of cholesterol. These results suggest that within plasma and lesions alpha-tocopherol can act as an antioxidant. They may also explain why studies using < 500 IU alpha-tocopherol/day failed to demonstrate benefit of antioxidant therapy. Better understanding of the pharmacodynamics of oral antioxidants is required to guide future clinical trials. *Reference: Oral alpha-tocopherol supplementation inhibits lipid oxidation in established human atherosclerotic lesions. Free Radic Res. 37(11):1235-1244, 2003. Carpenter, K. L., et al. Department of Pathology, University of Cambridge, Tennis Court Road, Cambridge, UK.*

Although the cardioprotective effects of supplemental doses of vitamin E have been investigated in several conditions, its role in gonadectomyinduced fatty lesion formation is unclear. The present study was designed to examine the efficacy of vitamin E in a dose-dependent manner on indices of oxidative stress and preventing the formation of aortic fatty lesions in orchidectomized (Orx) aged rats. Forty 12-month old male Sprague-Dawley rats were either sham-operated (Sham) or Orx and fed a semi-purified control diet for 120 days. Thereafter, rats were assigned to four treatment groups (n=10): Sham and one Orx group received 75 IU vitamin E and served as controls, and the other two Orx groups received either 250 or 500 IU vitamin E per kg diet for 90 days. Vitamin E at the highest dose (500 IU) was able to lower serum total cholesterol by 16% and significantly increase superoxide dismutase by 9% compared to Orx controls. Similarly, this dose was able to significantly reduce the development of atherosclerotic lesion formation and aortic fatty streak area by 93% compared to Orx controls. The findings of this study suggest that dietary vitamin E supplementation in Orx aged rats provide anti-atherogenic effects, in part, due to vitamin E's antioxidative properties. Clinical studies are needed to confirm whether supplemental doses of vitamin E can prevent the development of atherosclerosis in older men particularly with low testosterone level. *Reference: Vitamin E dose-dependently reduces aortic fatty lesion formation in orchidectomized aged rats. Aging Clin Exp Res. 2009. Chai, S. C., et al. Department of Nutrition, Food & Exercise Sciences, Florida State University, Tallahassee, FL, USA.*

Decreased antioxidant status may increase lipid peroxidation and the susceptibility of low-density lipoprotein to oxidiation. This study of 41 patients with coronary artery disease (atherosclerosis) and 41 controls evaluated plasma levels of vitamins A, C and E and coronary artery disease risk. There was a significant decrease in plasma levels of vitamins A, C and E in patients with coronary artery disease compared to controls. The authors concluded that decreased plasma concentrations of vitamins A and E are independently associated with increased vascular disease risk and that vitamin supplementation should be considered for the primary and secondary prevention of coronary artery disease. *Reference: Antioxidant vitamins and coronary artery disease risk in South African males. Clin Chim Acta. 278:55-60, 1998. Delport, R., et al.*

Oxidative stress and inflammation play a crucial role in atherosclerosis. However, prospective clinical trials of dietary antioxidants with anti-inflammatory properties, such as alpha-tocopherol (AT), have not yielded positive results. AT supplementation decreases gamma-tocopherol (GT) levels. GT is an antioxidant with potent anti-inflammatory activity, and plasma GT levels are inversely associated with cardiovascular diseases. Thus, studies using pure GT, alone or in conjunction with AT, will elucidate its utility in cardiovascular disease prevention. *Reference: Failure of vitamin E in clinical trials: is gamma-tocopherol the answer? Nutr Rev. 63(8):290-293, 2005. Devaraj, S., et al. Laboratory for Atherosclerosis and Metabolic Research, Department of Pathology and Laboratory*

Medicine, University of California-Davis Medical Center, Sacramento, USA.

Data from the 1970s first suggested that vitamin E may be effective in decreasing mortality from cardiovascular disease. As the understanding of the antioxidant effect of this vitamin evolved, researchers began to further study the biologic effects of vitamin E. In vitro studies have shown vitamin E to have several potentially cardioprotective effects, including antagonizing the oxidation of low-density lipoproteins, inhibiting platelet aggregation and adhesion, preventing smooth muscle proliferation, and preserving normal coronary dilation. Several prospective studies, including the US Nurses' Health Study and the US Health Professionals' Follow-up Study, found a 34% and 39% reduction, respectively, in the risk of having a cardiac event for those taking vitamin E supplements. The Iowa Women's Health Study found a 47% reduction in cardiac mortality. Results of randomized, controlled clinical trials have not found consistent benefit, however. The best known of these trials, the Cambridge Heart Antioxidant Study, found a 47% reduction in fatal and nonfatal myocardial infarction in patients with proven coronary atherosclerosis who were given 400 or 800 IU of vitamin E daily. There was, however, no effect on mortality. While emerging and promising data suggest the potential benefit of vitamin E for high-risk cardiac patients, physicians should be alert to the results of randomized, controlled clinical trials already in progress. **Reference:** *The role of vitamin E in the prevention of heart disease. Arch Fam Med. 8(6):537-542, 1999. Emmert, D. H.,et al.*

Hyperlipidemia is associated with endothelial dysfunction, an early event in atherosclerosis and predictor of risk for future coronary artery disease. Epidemiological studies suggest that increased dietary intake of antioxidants reduces the risk of coronary artery disease. The purpose of this study was to determine whether antioxidant vitamin therapy improves endothelial function and affects surrogate biomarkers for oxidative stress and inflammation in hyperlipidemic children. In a randomized, double-blind, placebo-controlled trial, the effects of antioxidant vitamins C (500 mg/d) and E (400 IU/d) for 6 weeks and the National Cholesterol Education Program Step II (NCEP-II) diet for 6 months on endothelium-dependent flow-mediated dilation (FMD) of the brachial artery were examined in 15 children with familial hypercholesterolemia (FH) or the phenotype of familial combined hyperlipidemia (FCH). Antioxidant vitamin therapy improved FMD of the brachial artery compared with baseline (P<0.001) without an effect on biomarkers for oxidative stress (autoantibodies to epitopes of oxidized LDL, F2-isoprostanes, 8-hydroxy-2'-deoxyguanosine), inflammation (C-reactive protein), or levels of asymmetric dimethylarginine, an endogenous inhibitor of nitric oxide. Antioxidant therapy with vitamins C and E restores endothelial function in hyperlipidemic children. Early detection and treatment of endothelial dysfunction in high-risk children may retard the progression of atherosclerosis. **Reference:** *Antioxidant vitamins C and E improve* *endothelial function in children with hyperlipidemia. Endothelial Assessment of Risk from Lipids in Youth (EARLY) Trial. Circulation. 2003. Engler, M. M., et al.*

Alpha-tocopherol supplementation (1200 IU/day) has been shown to decrease the adhesion of monocytes to the endothelium of blood vessels. **Reference:** *The roles of vitamin E and oxidized lipids in atherosclerosis. International Clinical Nutrition Review. 8(3)134 -139, 1988. Hennig, B. et al. The effect of alpha-tocopherol on monocyte proatherogenic activity. Journal of Nutrition. 131(2 Supplement):389S-394S, 2001. Jia lal, I., et al.*

The development of atherosclerosis is a multifactorial process in which both elevated plasma cholesterol levels and proliferation of smooth muscle cells play a central role. Numerous studies have suggested the involvement of oxidative processes in the pathogenesis of atherosclerosis and especially of oxidized low density lipoprotein. Some epidemiological studies have shown an association between high dietary intake and high serum concentrations of vitamin E and lower rates of ischemic heart disease. Cell culture studies have shown that alpha-tocopherol brings about inhibition of smooth muscle cell proliferation. This takes place via inhibition of protein kinase C activity. alpha-Tocopherol also inhibits low density lipoprotein induced smooth muscle cell proliferation and protein kinase C activity. The following animal studies showed that vitamin E protects development of cholesterol induced atherosclerosis by inhibiting protein kinase C activity in smooth muscle cells in vivo. Elevated plasma levels of homocysteine have been identified as an important and independent risk factor for cerebral, coronary and peripheral atherosclerosis. However the mechanisms by which homocysteine promotes atherosclerotic plaque formation are not clearly defined. Earlier reports have been suggested that homocysteine exert its effect via H_2O_2 produced during its metabolism. To evaluate the contribution of homocysteine in the pathogenesis of vascular diseases, the authors examined whether the homocysteine effect on vascular smooth muscle cell growth is mediated by H_2O_2. The authors show that homocysteine induces DNA synthesis and proliferation of vascular smooth muscle cells in the presence of peroxide scavenging enzyme, catalase. The data suggest that homocysteine induces smooth muscle cell growth through the activation of an H_2O_2 independent pathway and accelerate the progression of atherosclerosis. The results indicate a cellular mechanism for the atherogenicity of cholesterol or homocysteine and protective role of vitamin E in the development of atherosclerosis. **Reference:** *Molecular mechanisms of cholesterol or homocysteine effect in the development of atherosclerosis: Role of vitamin E. Biofactors. 19(1-2):63-70, 2003. Kartel Ozer, N., et al. Department of Biochemistry, Faculty of Medicine, Marmara University, Haydarpasa, Istanbul, Turkey.*

Suppression of cell adhesion molecule expression and macrophage accumulation by the endothelium is believed to play an important role in preventing the development of atherosclerosis. Earlier, the authors have shown that in vitro supplementation of human aortic endothelial cells with Vitamin E dose-dependently reduced expression of adhesion molecules and monocyte adhesion. Here, they report the in vivo down-regulation of endothelial cell adhesion molecules expression and macrophage accumulation in the aortas of hypercholesterolemic rabbits supplemented with Vitamin E. To this end, New Zealand White rabbits were fed a semi-purified diet containing 30 (control) or 1000IU/kg Vitamin E. After 4 weeks, both groups' diets were switched to an atherogenic diet (0.3% cholesterol, 9% hydrogenated coconut oil, and 1% corn oil) containing the respective levels of Vitamin E and fed for 2, 4, and 6 weeks. Vitamin E supplemented rabbits had significantly higher levels of Vitamin E in their plasma and aortas. Frozen aorta sections were fixed and stained by an avidin-biotin complex method using Rb2/3 and Rb1/9 monoclonal antibodies against rabbit ICAM-1 and VCAM-1, respectively, and with RAM-11 for macrophage and von Willebrand factor for endothelial cells, followed by staining with secondary antibodies and counterstaining and evaluation under the microscope. At 6 weeks on atherogenic diet treatment, a trend ($P = 0.08$) toward a lower score of ICAM-1 expression by endothelial cells was observed in the aorta of Vitamin E treated rabbits compared to the control. However, a decrease in the score of VCAM-1 expression by endothelial cells in Vitamin E treated rabbits did not reach to a statistical significance. At 4 and 6 weeks on atherogenic diet, Vitamin E supplementation also significantly ($P = 0.003$) inhibited the accumulation of macrophages in the aorta. These results support the concept that down-regulation of adhesion molecule expression and suppression of monocyte/macrophage activation by Vitamin E in vivo is one of the potential mechanisms by which Vitamin E may suppress the development of aortic lesions in a rabbit model of atherosclerosis. *Reference: Vitamin E supplementation suppresses macrophage accumulation and endothelial cell expression of adhesion molecules in the aorta of hypercholesterolemic rabbits. Atherosclerosis. 176(2):265-272, 2004. Koga, T., et al. Vascular Biology Laboratory, Jean Mayer USDA Human Nutrition Research Center on Aging at Tufts University, Boston, MA, USA.*

Oxysterols as oxidation products of cholesterol are considered an atherogenic factor in the development of atherosclerosis in the arteries of cholesterol-fed rabbits. The authors compared the atherogenic effects of diets enriched either with 0.5% oxidized cholesterol (OC; characterized by high amounts of oxysterols) or with pure cholesterol (PC). The effects of antioxidant vitamins E and C added to the PC diet were also evaluated in view of their antioxidative properties for lipoproteins and cholesterol and how this could affect the severity of atherosclerosis. Four groups of rabbits were fed the following for 11 wk: 1) a nonpurified stock diet, 2) this stock diet plus 0.5% OC, 3) the stock diet plus 0.5% PC, and 4) the stock diet plus 0.5% PC and 1000 mg vitamin E and 500 mg vitamin C/kg diet (PC + antioxidants). The OC and PC diets were equally hyperlipidemic and hypercholesterolemic. The severity of atherosclerotic lesions was highest with the OC diet and lowest with the PC + antioxidants diet. The plasma oxysterol concentration was proportional to the severity of atherosclerosis in all three groups of cholesterol-fed rabbits. beta-Very-low-density-lipoprotein modification was minimized by vitamins E and C as indicated by its polyacrylamide gel electrophoretic pattern and its increased binding to the rabbit liver membrane in vitro. This study indicated that OC and PC were equally atherogenic but that the addition of antioxidants to the PC diet significantly reduced its severity, even when hypercholesterolemia persisted. This indicated that atherogenesis can result from an excessive accumulation of oxidation products of cholesterol in the plasma. *Reference: Effect of cholesterol-rich diets with and without added vitamins E and C on the severity of atherosclerosis in rabbits. American Journal of Clinical Nutrition. 66(5):1240-1249, 1997. Mahfouz, M. M., et al.*

Observational and experimental studies indicate that dietary vitamin E supplementation is associated with reduced risk of atherosclerosis. Evidence indicates that vitamin E, in addition to inhibition of oxidative modification of LDL, may inhibit atherogenesis through several other mechanisms at the molecular and cellular levels, which also include its nonantioxidant functions. Six-year effect of combined vitamin C and E supplementation on atherosclerotic progression: the Antioxidant Supplementation in Atherosclerosis Prevention (ASAP) Study. *Reference: Vitamin E and atherosclerosis: beyond prevention of LDL oxidation.   Journal of Nutrition.   131(2 Supplement):366S-368S, 2001. Meydani, M.*

Male New Zealand White rabbits were made hypercholesterolemic by feeding an atherogenic diet (0.5% cholesterol, 3% peanut oil, and 3% coconut oil) with or without (control) antioxidants for 8 weeks. The antioxidant treatments were intravenous injection of beta-carotene (25 mg/kg/BW, twice weekly), dietary supplementation of alpha-tocopherol (0.5%), and a combination of both. Antioxidant treatments significantly increased plasma and LDL antioxidant levels in the above three groups. Intravenous injection of beta-carotene significantly decreased total and LDL cholesterol concentrations, thoracic atherosclerotic lesion area, and intimal thickness, but had no effects on LDL oxidation ex vivo as compared to control. Added dietary alpha-tocopherol significantly decreased the susceptibility of LDL to oxidation ex vivo, aortic atherosclerotic lesion area and intimal thickness, but had no effects on plasma cholesterol levels as compared to control. Combination of both antioxidants significantly decreased total and LDL cholesterol concentrations, susceptibility of LDL to oxidation ex vivo, as well as atherosclerotic lesion area and intimal thickness at aortic arch and thoracic aorta as compared to control, but not beta-carotene or alpha-tocopherol groups. These data suggest that the antihypercholesterolemic effects of beta-carotene and antioxidant effects of alpha-tocopherol may benefit rabbits fed an atherogenic diet by inhibiting the development of atherosclerotic lesions. *Reference: Beta-*

carotene and alpha-tocopherol inhibit the development of atherosclerotic lesions in hypercholesterolemic rabbits. Int J Vitam Nutr Res. 67(3):155-163, 1997. Sun, J., et al.

Prevention and regression of induced atherosclerosis by d-alpha-tocopherol was investigated in 24 male M. fascicularis. One group received a basal diet, while three others consumed an atherogenic diet. Two of the latter groups also received tocopherol, one at the onset of the study (prevention) and the other after atherosclerosis was established by ultrasound evaluation (regression). Atherosclerosis was monitored over a 36-month period by duplex ultrasound imaging of the common carotid arteries. At termination, 24 arterial sites were examined for histopathology. In those animals receiving an atherogenic diet, mean percent ultrasound stenosis at 36 months posttreatment was lower in the tocopherol-supplemented groups (61 and 18%) than in the unsupplemented group (87%). Plasma tocopherol concentration was negatively correlated with percent ultrasound stenosis (p less than 0.002). Percent stenosis in the regression group decreased from 33 to 8% (p less than 0.05) 8 months after tocopherol supplementation. Although not consistently significant, histopathological changes were greater in untreated compared to treated animals. D-alpha-tocopherol may be prophylactically and therapeutically effective in atherosclerosis. **Reference:** *Effects of D-alpha-tocopherol supplementation on experimentally induced primate atherosclerosis. Journal of the American College of Nutrition. 11(2):131-8, 1992. Verlangieri, A. J., et al.*

Epidemiologic studies have suggested that vitamin E (alpha-tocopherol) may play a preventive role in reducing the incidence of atherosclerosis. The authors conducted a cost- effectiveness analysis of vitamin E supplementation in patients with coronary artery disease using data from the Cambridge Heart Antioxidant Study (CHAOS). The main clinical outcome used in the economic evaluation was the incidence of acute myocardial infarction (AMI) which was nonfatal. Utilization of health care resources was estimated by conducting a survey of Australian clinicians and published Australian and US cost data. Cost savings of $127 (A$181) and $578/patient randomized to vitamin E therapy compared with patients receiving placebo were found for Australian and US settings, respectively. Savings in the vitamin E group were due primarily to reduction in hospital admissions for AMI. This occurred because the vitamin E group had a 4.4% lower absolute risk of AMI than did the placebo group. Less than 10% of health care costs in the Australian evaluation was due to vitamin E ($150 (A$214/patient]). This economic evaluation indicates that vitamin E therapy in patients with angiographically proven atherosclerosis is cost-effective in the Australian and US settings. **Reference:** *Cost-effectiveness of vitamin E therapy in the treatment of patients with angiographically proven coronary narrowing (CHAOS trial) - Cambridge Heart Antioxidant Study. American Journal of Cardiology. 82(4):414-417, 1998.*

The hypothesis that oxidative stress has a role in atherosclerosis rests on a large body of experimental work carried out in animal models of heart disease. The situation is more complex in humans, in that the results from vitamin E supplementation trials have been conflicting. There is emerging information that alpha-tocopherol may play a critical role in maintaining the function of key cellular components in the atherosclerotic process through its ability to inhibit the activity of protein kinase C, a key player in many signal transduction pathways. alpha-Tocopherol modulates pathways of platelet aggregation, endothelial cell nitric oxide production, monocyte/macrophage superoxide production and smooth muscle cell proliferation. Regulation of adhesion molecule expression and inflammatory cell cytokine production by alpha-tocopherol has also been reported. **Reference:** *Does vitamin E decrease heart attack risk? Journal of Nutrition. 131(2 Supplement):395S-397S, 2001.*

1,200 IU per day of vitamin E was found to significantly lower C-reactive protein levels and interleukin 6 levels within three months. This would be be expected to result in a reduced risk of atherosclerosis as both substances are involved in the mechanisms of atherosclerosis. The study involved 25 non-diabetics, 24 diabetics without cardiovascular complications and 23 diabetics with cardiovascular complications. IL-6 and C-reactive protein levels fell in all three groups. **Reference:** *Free Radical Biology and Medicine. 29(8):790-792, 2000.*

CELIAC DISEASE

Copper

Celiac disease was diagnosed in two unrelated infants aged 7 and 7.5 months with severe malnutrition. They showed typical clinical, biological, and histological signs of the disease. Moreover, accompanying copper deficiency was suggested by severe hypocupremia and persistent neutropenia; bone radiographs were also compatible with this diagnosis. Rapid and complete correction of these anomalies could only be obtained after addition of oral copper sulfate to the gluten-free diet. Mechanisms possibly involved in the development of copper deficiency in young infants with celiac disease are: chronic malabsorption; high copper needs in rapidly growing infants; and possibly increased biliary and digestive losses. It is therefore suggested that young children with severe celiac disease should be monitored for their copper status. *Reference: Goyens, P., et al. Copper deficiency in infants with active celiac disease. J Pediatr. Gastroenterol. Nutr. 4(4):677-680, 1985.*

Copper uptake during three hours from an oral test dose of copper sulphate solution giving three mg Cu++, close to the recommended daily dietary intake, was significantly reduced in patients with proximal intestinal disease, compared with normal subjects. Three out of ten patients had abnormal and otherwise unexplained blood counts compatible with the known haematological effects of copper deficiency and were restored to normal levels on a gluten-free diet. Copper deficiency and proximal intestinal disease should be suspected in patients with otherwise unexplained anaemia, especially neutropenia. *Reference: Jameson, S., et al. Copper malabsorption in coeliac disease. Sci Total Environ. 42(1-2):29-36, 1985.*

Selenium & Carnitine

Celiac disease (CD) is a gluten-induced enteropathy that results in malabsorption of nutrients. The authors studied the serum levels of carnitine and selenium in children with CD. Serum levels of free carnitine and selenium were studied in 30 children (mean age 8.1 [4.4] years) with CD and 30 age- and gender-matched healthy children. All patients had type 3 duodenal lesions. The mean (SD) serum levels of free carnitine and selenium were lower among patients with CD (24.5 [7.7] micromol/mL and 52.1 (12.9) micromol/mL, respectively) than among healthy controls (29.4 [9.2] and 65.1 [17.2] micromol/mL; $p < 0.05$ each). Levels were similar in children with and without diarrhea. Serum carnitine and selenium levels are decreased in children with CD, probably due to malabsorption. *Reference: Yuce, A., et al. Serum carnitine and selenium levels in children with celiac disease. Indian J Gastroenterol. 23(3):87-88, 2004. -- Section of Gastroenterology, Hepatology and Nutrition, Department of Pediatrics, Faculty of Medicine, Hacettepe University, Ankara, Turkey.*

Zinc

This study was done to determine the zinc levels in 30 children with celiac disease. Serum zinc level was estimated at inclusion and zinc supplementation was given for 3 months. Zinc levels were repeated at 3 and 6 months after inclusion. The serum zinc levels of newly diagnosed CD cases (0.64 +/- 0.34 ug/mL) versus controls (0.94+/- 0.14 ug/mL) were significantly lower (95% CI -0.44 to -1.4), whereas in the old cases this difference was non-significant. The serum zinc level among severely malnourished and stunted celiac cases was also significantly lower irrespective of their treatment status. The authors conclude that serum zinc levels are low in newly diagnosed and severely malnourished children with celiac disease. *Reference: Singhal, N., et al. Serum zinc levels in celiac disease. Indian Pediatr. 45(4):319-321, 2008.*

Vitamin A

A 64 year old man presented with a 6 week history of sudden progressive redness of his right eye associated with blurring of vision. His left eye was asymptomatic and he had no ocular history of note. He had a history of diet controlled coeliac disease proved by jejunal biopsy. Several weeks earlier he had complained of persistent diarrhoea despite adherence to his gluten-free diet. On examination visual acuity was counting fingers on the right and 6/6 on the left. The left eye was normal except for multiple fluorescein staining scattered fine superficial punctate erosions. The right eye was diffusely injected and the cornea showed filamentary changes with multiple underlying punctate staining epithelial defects. There were no other pathological features. A provisional diagnosis of filamentary keratitis was made and he was treated with topical acetylcysteine to the right eye and topical lubricants to the left eye. Two weeks later he reported a marked deterioration in symptoms. Visual acuity remained unchanged. Corneal examination revealed a large central full thickness epithelial defect. Regular topical lubricants were applied and a botulinum toxin injection was administered. Full physical examination at this stage revealed a thin man but no other relevant findings. After 1 week there was complete failure of re-epithelialisation. The suspicion of a keratomalacia secondary to vitamin A deficiency was raised and an intramuscular injection of 100 000 units of vitamin A was immediately administered. Subsequent serum vitamin A levels were 13 (normal 330–1100). Six days later there was a dramatic symptomatic improvement. Visual acuity had improved to 6/18. The cornea was almost completely healed with only a few areas of superficial epithelial deficit remaining. The patient was referred back to the gastroenterologists who investigated his continuing malabsorptive symptoms and administered standard dietary supplementation including regular vitamin A injections. *Reference: Alwitry, A. Vitamin A deficiency in coeliac disease. Br J Ophthalmol. 84(9):1079-1080, 2000.*

Vitamin B6

Signs of mental depression are typical in adults presenting with celiac disease. The response to treatment was evaluated in 12 consecutive patients by means of the Minnesota Multiphasic Personality Inventory (MMPI), with surgical patients serving as controls. The celiacs reported no change in depressive symptoms after 1 year's gluten withdrawal despite evidence of improvement in the small intestine. When retested after 3 years, however, after 6 months of 80 mg/day of oral pyridoxine (vitamin B6) therapy, they showed a fall in the score of scale 2 ('depression') from 70 to 56 (p less than 0.01), which became normalized like other pretreatment abnormalities in the MMPI. Cholecystectomy in the control subjects produced no alterations in the MMPI profile. The results indicate a causal relationship between adult celiac disease and concomitant depressive symptoms which seems to implicate metabolic effects from pyridoxine deficiency influencing central mechanisms regulating mood. *Reference: Hallert, C., et al. Reversal of psychopathology in adult celiac disease with the aid of pyridoxine (vitamin B6). Scand J Gastroenterol. 18(2):299, 1983.*

The concentration of serum pyridoxal phosphate was determined before and 15, 30, 60, 90, and 120 minutes following an oral load test with 5 mg pyridoxine hydrochloride/kg body weight in 14 children with acute celiac disease and in 15 control subjects. Children with acute celiac disease suffer from a biochemical vitamin B6 deficiency. The increase in pyridoxal phosphate of children with acute celiac disease after loading was significantly decreased when compared with that of control subjects. In children with celiac disease maximal concentration of serum pyridoxal phosphate appeared later (after 60 minutes) and was decreased in comparison to control subjects (after 30 minutes). A positive correlation existed between the net increase of pyridoxal phosphate 60 minutes following pyridoxine loading and the net increase of blood xylose 60 minutes after oral loading. The results are compatible both with a malabsorption of pyridoxine in childhood celiac disease and a shifting of the site of pyridoxine absorption from the upper part of jejunum into the more distal parts of intestine. *Reference: Reinken, L., et al. Vitamin B6 absorption in children with acute celiac disease and in control subjects. Journal of Nutrition. 108(10):1562-1565, 1978.*

Vitamin B12

Iron and folate malabsorption are common in untreated celiac disease as the proximal small intestine is predominantly affected. Vitamin B12 deficiency is thought to be uncommon, as the terminal ileum is relatively spared. This study investigated the prevalence of vitamin B12, deficiency in patients with untreated celiac disease. A prospective study of 39 consecutive biopsy-proven celiac disease patients (32 women, seven men; median age 48 yr, range 22-77 yr) between September 1997 and February 1999 was undertaken. The full blood count, serum vitamin B12, red blood cell folate, and celiac autoantibodies (IgA antigliadin and IgA antiendomysium antibodies) were measured before and after a median of

4 months (range 2-13 months) of treatment with a gluten-free diet. In vitamin B12-deficient patients, intrinsic factor antibodies and a Schilling test, part 1, were performed. A total of 16 (41%) patients were vitamin B12 deficient (<220 ng/L) and 16 (41%) patients (11 women and live men) were anemic. Concomitant folate deficiency was present in only 5/16 (31%) of the vitamin B12 patients. The Schilling test, performed in 10 of the vitamin B12-deficient patients, showed five low and five normal results. Although only five patients received parenteral vitamin B12, at follow-up the vitamin B12 results had normalized in all patients. Acral paraesthesia at presentation in three vitamin B12-deficient patients resolved after vitamin B12 replacement. Vitamin B12 deficiency is common in untreated celiac disease, and concentrations should be measured routinely before hematinic replacement. Vitamin B12 concentrations normalize on a gluten-free diet alone, but symptomatic patients may require supplementation. **Reference:** *Dahele, A., et al. Vitamin B12 deficiency in untreated celiac disease. Am J Gastroenterol. 96(3):745-750, 2001.*

Gastric acid secretion in nineteen children with celiac disease remained almost unchanged and the level of fasting serum gastrin was comparable with that of a control group of the same age. The absorption of vitamin B12 was significantly decreased, most clearly in the infants with celiac disease as compared with their controls. The serum B12 level, however, was decreased only in the oldest children. The results suggest that the mucosal lesion in the small intestine is most extensive in the youngest children, but the absorption defect of vitamin B12 becomes clinically significant only after a long duration of the disease and not in childhood. **Reference:** *Kokkonen, J., et al. Gastric function and absorption of vitamin B12 in children with celiac disease. Eur J Pediatr. 132(2):71-75, 1979.*

Vitamin D

A 29-year-old wheelchair-bound woman was presented to us by the gastroenterologist with suspected osteomalacia. She had lived in the Netherlands all her life and was born of Moroccan parents. Her medical history revealed iron deficiency, growth retardation, and celiac disease, for which she was put on a gluten-free diet. She had progressive bone pain since 2 years, difficulty with walking, and about 15 kg weight loss. She had a short stature, scoliosis, and pronounced kyphosis of the spine and poor condition of her teeth. Laboratory results showed hypocalcemia, an immeasurable serum 25-hydroxyvitamin D level, and elevated parathyroid hormone and alkaline phosphatase levels. Spinal radiographs showed unsharp, low contrast vertebrae. Bone mineral density measurement at the lumbar spine and hip showed a T-score of −6.0 and −6.5, respectively. A bone scintigraphy showed multiple hotspots in ribs, sternum, mandible, and long bones. A duodenal biopsy revealed villous atrophy (Marsh 3C) and positive antibodies against endomysium, transglutaminase, and gliadin, compatible with active celiac disease. A bone biopsy showed severe osteomalacia but normal bone volume. She was treated with calcium intravenously and later orally. Furthermore, she was treated with high oral doses of vitamin D and a gluten-free diet. After a few weeks of treatment, her bone pain decreased, and her muscle strength improved. *Reference: Bone pain and extremely low bone mineral density due to severe vitamin D deficiency in celiac disease. Noortje M. Rabelink, Hans M. Westgeest, Nathalie Bravenboer, Maarten A. J. M. Jacobs, Paul Lips. Arch Osteoporos. 2011 December; 6(1-2): 209–213. Published online 2011 June 15. doi: 10.1007/s11657-011-0059-7.*

Vitamin E

Celiac disease (CD) is a genetically linked immune-mediated enteropathy triggered by the ingestion of gluten-containing grains food. Deficiencies of trace elements and vitamins may be found in patients with untreated CD. No systematic studies have been carried out on vitamin E status in celiacs. Tocopherol deficiency is implicated in the biological processes leading to malignant cell transformations, neurological complications, brown bowel syndrome and reproductive disorders. Untreated patients with CD have higher incidences of these disorders than in general population. The aim of this study was to investigate vitamin E status in patients with celiac disease. The authors examined retinol plasma level and tocopherol levels both in plasma and in erythrocytes in 18 patients (age: 2-53 years) with active CD and 12 celiacs (age: 3-36 years) on gluten-free diet without antiendomysium antibodies for at least 2 years. Vitamins were measured by high-pressure liquid chromatography according to the procedure of Driskell. In untreated patients levels of plasma tocopherol (13.7 +/-3.8 micromol/L vs. 20 +/-7.1 micromol/L; $p<0.02$), erythrocytes tocopherol (1.7 +/-0.45 micromol/L vs.2.89 +/-0.52 micromol/L; $p<0.001$) and ratio of plasma tocopherol to serum total cholesterol (3.36 +/-0.9 micromol/L vs. 4.24 +/-0.85 micromol/L; $p<0.02$) were significantly lower compared to those on gluten-free diet. In all patients with active CD, concentrations of tocopherol in erythrocytes were below the norm ($N>2.5$ micromol/L). In untreated patients vitamin A levels did not achieve a significant difference in comparison with the celiacs on gluten-free diet (1.75 +/-0.57 micromol/L vs. 1.97 +/-0.72 micromol/L; $p>0.05$). The lowest levels of tocopherol (in plasma: 5.7 micromol/L, in erythrocytes: 0.74 micromol/L) and retinol (0.8 micromol/L; $N>0.7$ micromol/L) were detected in the same patient refusing dietetic treatment for more than 10 years. The conventional treatment of CD is gluten-free diet, but monitoring of tocopherol concentrations, especially in erythrocytes, and correction of its deficiency may offer some benefit for patients who fail to adhere strictly to a gluten free-diet or newly diagnosed celiacs. *References: Neurological disorders in adult celiac disease. Hugh J Freeman. Can J Gastroenterol. 2008 November; 22(11): 909–911. -- Idiopathic cerebellar ataxia associated with celiac disease: lack of distinctive neurological features M. T. Pellecchia, R. Scala, A. Filla, G. De Michele, C. Ciacci, P. Barone. J Neurol Neurosurg Psychiatry. 1999 January; 66(1): 32–35. -- Hozyasz, K. K., et al. [Vitamin E levels in patients with coeliac disease.] Med Wieku Rozwoj. VII(4Part 2):593-604, 2004.*

Vitamin K

A man was admitted with abdominal pain. Treatment for acute diverticulitis was instituted with intravenous antibiotics and oral limitation. Imaging demonstrated a complex inflammatory mass. Prothrombin time (PT), activated partial thromboplastin time (APTT) and fibrinogen were within normal limits. However, repeat preoperative clotting studies demonstrated a severe unexpected coagulopathy to have developed since admission that could have caused fatal intraoperative exsanguination. Direct assays showed severe, isolated deficiency of vitamin K dependent clotting factors, and mixing studies normalized both the PT and APTT, ruling out a coagulation inhibitor. The coagulopathy responded to intravenous vitamin K administration. Dietary insufficiency underlies vitamin K deficiency in the presence of normal biliary and enteral function. A significant coagulopathy can result with additional eradication of intestinal microflora. Hypoprothombinaemia is recognized as a consequence of protracted treatment with broad spectrum antibiotics, and vigilance is required for those at risk. The development of such a rapid and unexpected coagulopathy posed a complex preoperative management issue delaying operative intervention; although avoided by fortuitous preoperative screening, it could have caused significant intraoperative bleeding. The remarkably specific lack of vitamin K dependent clotting factors strongly suggested a vitamin K deficiency and administration of coumarins was ruled out. *Reference: Iatrogenic vitamin K deficiency and life threatening coagulopathy. Samuel John Ford, Alistair Webb, Richard Payne, and Norbert Blesing.*

Lycopene

Oxidative stress plays an important role in inflammatory process of celiac disease. The authors have studied the effect of the lycopene, quercetin and tyrosol natural antioxidants on the inducible nitric oxide synthase (iNOS) and cyclooxygenase-2 (COX-2) gene expression in RAW 264.7 macrophages stimulated by gliadin in association with IFN-gamma. The IFN-gamma plus gliadin combination treatment was capable of enhancing iNOS and COX-2 gene expression and nuclear factor-kappaB (NF-kappaB), interferon regulatory factor-1 (IRF-1) and signal transducer and activator of transcription-1alpha (STAT-1alpha) activation induced by reactive oxygen species generation at 24 h. Lycopene, quercetin and tyrosol inhibited all these effects. The results here reported suggest that these compounds may represent nontoxic agents for the control of pro-inflammatory genes involved in celiac disease. *Reference: De Stefano, D., et al. Lycopene, quercetin and tyrosol prevent macrophage activation induced by gliadin and IFN-gamma. Eur J Pharmacol. 2007.*

Nutritional Study

Celiac disease (CD), a common heritable chronic inflammatory condition of the small intestine caused by permanent intolerance to gluten/gliadin (prolamin), is characterized by a complex interplay between genetic and environmental factors. Developments in proteomics have provided an important contribution to the understanding of the biochemical and immunological aspects of the disease and the mechanisms involved in toxicity of prolamins. It has been demonstrated that some gliadin peptides resistant to complete proteolytic digestion may directly affect intestinal cell structure and functions by modulating gene expression and oxidative stress. In recent years, the creation of the two research fields Nutrigenomics and Nutrigenetics, has enabled the elucidation of some interactions between diet, nutrients and genes. Various dietary components including long chain ω-3 fatty acids, plant flavonoids, and carotenoids have been demonstrated to modulate oxidative stress, gene expression and production of inflammatory mediators. Therefore their adoption could preserve intestinal barrier integrity, play a protective role against toxicity of gliadin peptides and have a role in nutritional therapy of celiac disease. **Conclusions:** Celiac disease is characterized by a complex interaction between genetic and environmental factors. The mucosal damage in celiac patients is considered to be induced by interplay between innate and adaptive immune responses to ingested gluten. Developments in proteomics have provided an important contribution to the understanding of the biochemical and immunological aspects and the mechanisms involved in toxicity of prolamins. Inflammation and oxidative stress due to an increase of reactive oxygen species and a decrease of antioxidant defenses are involved in the molecular mechanisms of celiac disease. This in turn leads to uncontrolled activation of the redox-sensitive, pro-inflammatory transcription factors NF-κB, continued production of ROS and RNS and support of chronic inflammation. Previous studies have demonstrated that several nutrients exert antioxidant effects and influence gene expression, therefore they represent a useful approach for nutritional intervention in CD subjects, as corroborated by recent in vitro studies that have demonstrated that phytonutrients (lycopene, quercetin, vitamin C and tyrosol) protect against the cytotoxic effect of gliadin. A protective effect has also been exerted by DHA. To realize the usefulness of nutritional genomics as a tool for targeted medical nutrition therapy, further basic research, extensive epidemiological studies and controlled intervention trials are needed to investigate whether long chain unsaturated fatty acids , antioxidant vitamins , plant polyphenols and carotenoids modulate in vivo predisposition of chronic inflammatory conditions and thus have a role in the therapy of celiac disease. *Reference: Celiac Disease, Inflammation and Oxidative Damage: A Nutrigenetic Approach. Gianna Ferretti, Tiziana Bacchetti, Simona Masciangelo, and Letizia Saturni.*

Pancreatic enzymes

References:

- *Gullo, L. Indication for pancreatic enzyme treatment in non-pancreatic digestive diseases. Digestion. 54(Supplement 2):43-47, 1993. Institute of Medicine and Gastroenterology, University of Bologna, Italy.*

- *Enzyme replacement therapy for pancreatic insufficiency: present and future. Aaron Fieker, Jessica Philpott, Martine Armand. Clin Exp Gastroenterol. 2011; 4: 55–73. Published online 2011 May 4. doi: 10.2147/CEG.S17634.*
- *Hepatobiliary Disorders in Celiac Disease: An Update. Kaushal K. Prasad, Uma Debi, Saroj K. Sinha, Chander K. Nain, Kartar Singh. Int J Hepatol. 2011; 2011: 438184. Published online 2010 November 14. doi: 10.4061/2011/438184.*
- *Clin Exp Gastroenterol. 2011; 4: 55–73. Published online 2011 May 4. doi: 10.2147/CEG.S17634. PMCID: PMC3132852. Enzyme replacement therapy for pancreatic insufficiency: present and future. Aaron Fieker, Jessica Philpott, and Martine Armand. Division of Digestive Diseases, University of Oklahoma, OKC, OK, USA; INSERM, U476.*

Probiotics

The complex communities of microorganisms that colonise the human gastrointestinal tract play an important role in human health. The development of culture-independent molecular techniques has provided new insights in the composition and diversity of the intestinal microbiota. Here, we summarise the present state of the art on the intestinal microbiota with specific attention for the application of high-throughput functional microbiomic approaches to determine the contribution of the intestinal microbiota to human health. Moreover, we review the association between dysbiosis of the microbiota and both intestinal and extra-intestinal diseases. Finally, we discuss the potential of probiotic microorganism to modulate the intestinal microbiota and thereby contribute to health and well-being. The effects of probiotic consumption on the intestinal microbiota are addressed, as well as the development of tailor-made probiotics designed for specific aberrations that are associated with microbial dysbiosis. It is known for over three decades that the human body contains tenfold more microbial cells (1014) than human cells (Savage 1977). These microorganisms colonise practically every surface of the human body that is exposed to the external environment, including the skin, oral cavity, respiratory, urogenital and gastrointestinal tract. Of these body sites, the gastrointestinal (GI) tract is by far the most densely colonised organ. The complex community of microorganisms residing in or passing through the GI tract is referred to as the intestinal microbiota. The intestinal microbiota plays a role in metabolic, nutritional, physiological and immunological processes in the human body. It exerts important metabolic activities by extracting energy from otherwise indigestible dietary polysaccharides such as resistant starch and dietary fibres. These metabolic activities also lead to the production of important nutrients, such as short-chain fatty acids (SCFA), vitamins (e.g. vitamin K, vitamin B12 and folic acid) and amino acids, which humans are unable to produce themselves (Hamer et al. 2008; Wong et al. 2006). In addition, the intestinal microbiota participates in the defence against pathogens by mechanisms such as colonisation resistance and production of antimicrobial compounds. Furthermore, the intestinal microbiota is involved in the development, maturation and maintenance of the GI sensory and motoric functions, the intestinal barrier and the mucosal immune system. These are just a few examples of the functional contributions of the intestinal microbiota to human health, a subject that is regularly reviewed (Barbara et al. 2005; Cerf–Bensussan and Gaboriau–Routhiau 2010; O'Hara and Shanahan 2006; Sekirov et al. 2010; Zoetendal et al. 2008). In recent years, a sharp increase is seen in the number of publications addressing the intestinal microbiota. They have provided various lines of evidence supporting a close link between the intestinal microbiota and human health. This review aims to summarise the current knowledge on the composition and diversity of the intestinal microbiota. In addition, it is discussed how new molecular approaches have provided novel insights towards the phylogenetic and functional characterisation of the intestinal microbiota. Furthermore, recent insights on the link between the intestinal microbiota and human health are provided. Finally, an overview is presented of ways to modulate the intestinal microbiota with specific attention for the use of probiotics, defined as live microorganisms which, when administered in adequate amounts, confer a health benefit on the host (FAO/WHO 2002). *Reference: Genes Nutr. 2011 August; 6(3): 209–240. Published online 2011 May 27. doi: 10.1007/ s12263-011-0229-7. PMCID: PMC3145058. Intestinal microbiota in human health and disease: the impact of probiotics. Jacoline Gerritsen, Hauke Smidt, Ger T. Rijkers, and Willem M. de Vos.*

Cardiomyopathy

The authors examined 52 patients with idiopathic cardiomyopathy (IDCM) for celiac disease. Three of them had coeliac disease, suggesting that prevalence of celiac disease in IDCM patients is increased. *Reference: Curione, M., et al. Prevalence of coeliac disease in idiopathic dilated cardiomyopathy Lancet. 354:222-223, 1999.*

Diabetes

The association of celiac disease (CD) and type 1 diabetes is now clearly documented. Immunoglobulin A (IgA) antitransglutaminase antibodies were measured to determine the prevalence of celiac disease in a diabetic population of children and to determine the temporal relationship between type 1 diabetes onset and CD. The authors measured IgA antitransglutaminase antibodies using human recombinant antigen in parallel with classical markers (IgA and IgG antigliadin, IgA antiendomysium) in 284 children with diabetes. In the population studied, the prevalence of CD was 3.9% (11 of 284). Two cases of CD were diagnosed before the onset of diabetes, and in 8 patients, the diagnoses of CD and diabetes were concomitant, suggesting that CD was present before the onset of diabetes. In 1 case, a girl who presented with thyroiditis, serology for CD became positive after diabetes had been diagnosed. An excellent correlation was observed between IgA antiendomysium and IgA antitransglutaminase antibodies. The authors propose using IgA antitransglutaminase as a screening test for practical reasons. Furthermore, IgA antitransglutaminase levels and mucosa abnormalities were closely correlated. The presence of antitransglutaminase antibodies should alert pediatricians to the atypical forms of CD. This study indicates that CD is most often present before the onset of diabetes mellitus type 1. *Reference: Peretti, N., et al. The temporal relationship between the onset of type 1 diabetes and celiac disease: a study based on immunoglobulin a antitransglutaminase screening. Pediatrics. 113(5):418-422, 2004.*

The incidence of antibodies to maize using an immunofluorescent technique has been found to be 14% in controls, 33% in Crohn's disease, 50% in ulcerative colitis and 44% in coeliac disease. This result indicates that humoral immunity to maize is probably unimportant in the pathogenesis of Crohn's disease. The similar incidence of antibodies in the inflammatory bowel disease and coeliac groups suggests absorption of dietary antigen secondary to an increased mucosal permeability. *Reference: Gut. 2005 June; 54(6): 769–774. doi: 10.1136/gut.2004. 057174, Clin Exp Immunol. 1979 January; 35(1): 147–148. PMCID: PMC1537589. Antibodies to maize in patients with Crohn's disease, ulcerative colitis and coeliac disease. I W Davidson, R S Lloyd, P J Whorwell, and R Wright.*

Background and aims: To elucidate the dynamics of nitric oxide (NO) production induced by rectal gluten challenge and the relation between NO production and mucosal granulocyte activation. **Subjects and methods:** Release of rectal NO was measured in 13 patients with coeliac disease and in 18 controls before and after rectal wheat gluten challenge. Rectal gas was collected with a rectal balloon using a newly developed instrument/technique, the "mucosal patch technique". The instrument allows simultaneous measurements of concentrations of granulocyte mediators in the rectal mucosa. We measured myeloperoxidase (MPO), eosinophil cationic protein (ECP), and histamine. For comparison, we made similar measurements after corn (maize) gluten challenge. **Results:** In all coeliac patients rectal NO concentration increased after gluten challenge and reached a peak after 15 hours (mean 9464 (SEM 2393) parts per billion (ppb); range 250–24982). The maximum MPO and ECP increase occurred five hours after challenge. A correlation was found between mucosal MPO and NO production at 15 hours. Six of the patients showed an increase in NO production 15 hours after rectal corn gluten challenge but this was much smaller than after gluten challenge. No increases were seen in the control group after either challenge. **Conclusion:** Mucosal activation of neutrophils and eosinophils precedes pronounced enhancement of mucosal NO production after rectal wheat gluten challenge in patients with coeliac disease. Some of our coeliac patients displayed signs of an inflammatory reaction, as measured by NO and granulocyte markers, after rectal corn gluten challenge. **Reference:** *Gut mucosal granulocyte activation precedes nitric oxide production: studies in coeliac patients challenged with gluten and corn. G Kristjánsson, M Högman, P Venge, and R Hällgren. Department of Gastroenterology, Department of Medical Cell Biology, Section of Integrative Physiology, Laboratory for Inflammation Research, Department of Rheumatology, Uppsala University Hospital, Uppsala, Sweden. Correspondence to: Dr G Kristjánsson, Department of Medical Sciences, Uppsala University, Department of Gastroenterology, Uppsala University Hospital, 75185 Uppsala, Sweden; gudjon.kristjansson@medsci.uu.se.*

In this study, we compared corn gluten hydrolyzates, BCAAs, and leucine for their effects on body weight reduction in high fat-induced obese rats in order to determine the major active components in the corn gluten hydrolyzates. After obesity was induced for 13 weeks with high fat diet, the overweight-induced SD rats (n = 64) were stratified according to body weight, randomly blocked into eight treatments, and raised for 8 weeks. Four groups were changed to a normal diet and the other groups remained on the high fat diet. Each of the groups within both diets was fed either casein, corn gluten hydrolyzates, leucine, or branched chain amino acids, respectively. Daily food intake, body weight gain, and food efficiency ratio were significantly lower in the corn gluten hydrolyzate groups compared to the other groups, regardless of the high fat diet or normal fat diet. The rats fed the corn gluten hydrolyzates diet had the lowest perirenal fat pad weights whereas muscle weight was significantly increased in the corn gluten hydrolyzates groups. Plasma triglyceride, hepatic total lipid, and total cholesterol contents were significantly reduced in the corn gluten hydrolyzates groups. Other lipid profile measurements were not significantly changed. Plasma triglyceride and hepatic total lipid were also significantly reduced in the BCAA and leucine groups. Leptin levels were significantly lower and adiponectin was significantly higher in the corn gluten hydrolyzates groups. Fasting blood glucose, insulin, C-peptide, and HOMA-IR levels were also significantly reduced in the corn gluten hydrozylates groups, regardless of fat level. **Reference:** *Nutr Res Pract. 2010 April; 4(2): 106–113. Published online 2010 April 28. doi: 10.4162/nrp.2010.4.2.106. Effects of corn gluten hydrolyzates, branched chain amino acids, and leucine on body weight reduction in obese rats induced by a high fat diet. Ha Yoon Bong, Ji Yeon Kim, Hye In Jeong, Min Sun Moon, Joohee Kim, and Oran Kwon. Department of Nutritional Science and Food Management, Ewha Woman's University, 11-1 Daehyeon-dong, Seodeamun-gu, Seoul 120-750, Korea.*

CHOLESTEROL

References:

- Erasmus, Udo. *Fats that Heal, Fats that Kill. Alive Books, Burnaby, BC, Canada. 1993:66.*

- Papas, Andreas. *The Vitamin E Factor. HarperCollins, New York, USA. 1999:129.*

- Cheraskin, E., et al. *The biologic parabola: A look at serum cholesterol. Journal of the American Medical Association. 247:302, 1982.*

- Neaton, J. D., et al. *Serum cholesterol level and mortality findings for men screened in the Multiple Risk Factor Intervention Trial. Multiple Risk Factor Intervention Trial Research Group. Arch Intern Med. 152(7):1490-1500, 1992.*

With increased efforts to lower serum cholesterol levels, it is important to quantify associations between serum cholesterol level and causes of death other than coronary heart disease, for which an etiologic relationship has been established. For an average of 12 years, 350,977 men aged 35 to 57 years who had been screened for the Multiple Risk Factor Intervention Trial were followed up following a single standardized measurement of serum cholesterol level and other coronary heart disease risk factors; 21,499 deaths were identified. A strong, positive, graded relationship was evident between serum cholesterol level measured at initial screening and death from coronary heart disease. This relationship persisted over the 12-year follow-up period. No association was noted between serum cholesterol level and stroke.   The absence of an association overall was due to different relationships of serum cholesterol level with intracranial hemorrhage and nonhemorrhagic stroke. For the latter, a positive, graded association with serum cholesterol level was evident. For intracranial hemorrhage, cholesterol levels less than 4.14 mmol/L (less than 160 mg/dL) were associated with a two-fold increase in risk. A serum cholesterol level less than 4.14 mmol/L (less than 160 mg/dL) was also associated with a significantly increased risk of death from cancer of the liver and pancreas; digestive diseases, particularly hepatic cirrhosis; suicide; and alcohol dependence syndrome. In addition, significant inverse graded associations were found between serum cholesterol level and cancers of the lung, lymphatic, and hematopoietic systems, and chronic obstructive pulmonary disease.   No significant associations were found of serum cholesterol level with death from colon cancer, with accidental deaths, or with homicides. Overall, the inverse association between serum cholesterol level and most cancers weakened with increasing follow-up but did not disappear. The association between cholesterol level and death due to cancer of the lung and liver, chronic obstructive pulmonary disease, cirrhosis, and suicide weakened little over follow-up. The association of serum cholesterol with specific causes of death varies in direction, strength, gradation, and persistence. Further research on the determinants of low serum cholesterol level in populations and long-term follow-up of participants in clinical trials are necessary to assess whether inverse associations with noncardiovascular disease causes of death are consequences of non-cardiovascular disease, whether serum cholesterol level and noncardiovascular disease are both consequences of other factors, or whether these associations are causal. *Reference: Division of Biostatistics, School of Public Health, University of Minnesota, Minneapolis, USA.*

The authors investigated whether decline over time in serum cholesterol was associated with the risk of death from cancer in French men. They studied 6,230 working men, age 43-52 years in 1967-1972, who had at least three annual measurements of serum cholesterol. They estimated individual change over time in serum total cholesterol using within-person linear regression. During an average of 17 years of follow-up after the last examination, 747 subjects died from cancer. The multivariate-adjusted relative risks for subjects in the fourth (highest increase in serum total cholesterol), third, and second quartiles, compared with men in the first quartile (who had a decrease in serum total cholesterol), were 0.70 [95% confidence interval (CI) = 0.56-0.87], 0.71 (95% CI = 0.57-0.88), and 0.74 (95% CI = 0.61-0.91), respectively. The group with the highest decline in cholesterol displayed an excess risk for most cancer sites. These associations were more pronounced in subjects whose weight remained stable or decreased over time than in those who gained weight. *Reference: Zureik, M., et al. Decline in serum total cholesterol and the risk of death from cancer. Epidemiology. 8(2):137-143, 1997.*

Oxidative modification of LDL is known to elicit an array of pro-atherogenic responses, but it is generally underappreciated that oxidized LDL (OxLDL) exists in multiple forms, characterized by different degrees of oxidation and different mixtures of bioactive components. The variable effects of OxLDL reported in the literature can be attributed in large part to the heterogeneous nature of the preparations employed. In this review, we first describe the various subclasses and molecular composition of OxLDL, including the variety of minimally modified LDL preparations. We then describe multiple receptors that recognize various species of OxLDL and discuss the mechanisms responsible for the recognition by specific receptors. Furthermore, we discuss the contentious issues such as the nature of OxLDL in vivo and the physiological oxidizing agents, whether oxidation of LDL is a prerequisite for atherogenesis, whether OxLDL is the major source of lipids in foam cells, whether in some cases it actually induces cholesterol depletion, and finally the Janus-like nature of OxLDL in having both pro- and anti-inflammatory effects. Lastly, we extend our review to discuss the role of LDL oxidation in diseases other than atherosclerosis, including diabetes mellitus, and several autoimmune diseases, such as lupus erythematosus, anti-phospholipid syndrome, and rheumatoid arthritis. Antioxid. Redox Signal. 13, 39–75. **Introduction**.

There is overwhelming evidence that LDL is oxidatively modified in vivo, and that this modification results in an increase in its proinflammatory and proatherogenic properties. However, despite extensive studies over the last 3 decades from numerous laboratories, the sites of LDL oxidation in vivo, the nature of the physiological oxidizing agents, the nature and composition of oxidized LDL in circulation, and the pathophysiological relevance of LDL oxidation for atherosclerosis and other diseases are all matters of controversy. Because of the heterogeneity of the oxidized LDL preparations, whether prepared in vitro or isolated from the natural sources, there is no consensus on the exact definition or composition of oxidized LDL. In this review, we will briefly summarize the biochemistry and composition of the various preparations of oxidized LDL described in the literature, and discuss their pathophysiological properties and potential therapeutic implications. Special attention will be paid to the relationship between the extent of LDL modification and its biological effects, the specific actions of the bioactive components of oxidized LDL, and the controversial aspects of the role of oxidatively modified LDL in cholesterol loading and atherogenesis. The reader is referred to several excellent articles on the historical aspects of LDL oxidation hypothesis (269, 302, 303), mechanisms of oxidation, composition of oxidized LDL preparations, immunoassays for oxidized LDL (38, 284), clinical trials of antioxidant drugs, and studies with experimental models of atherosclerosis (33, 146, 164, 191, 240, 263, 280). **Definitions, Biochemistry, and Composition.** The term "oxidized LDL" is used to describe a wide variety of LDL preparations that have been oxidatively modified ex vivo under defined conditions, or isolated from biological sources. The major problem in comparing the results of oxidized LDL studies from various laboratories is the heterogeneity of the preparations employed. There is no accepted 'gold standard' for preparing oxidized LDL ex vivo, and the preparations isolated from the tissues differ greatly from lab to lab, both in the composition and biological effects. The oxidized LDL preparations described in literature are broadly (and somewhat arbitrarily) divided into two main categories: "minimally modified LDL" (MM-LDL) and "(fully or extensively) oxidized" LDL (OxLDL). The major difference between the two groups is that the MM-LDL, while chemically different from unmodified LDL, is still recognized by the LDL receptor, but not by most of the known scavenger receptors. On the other hand, the OxLDL preparations are all recognized by a variety of scavenger receptors but not by the LDL receptor. Each of the two categories of oxidized LDL is composed of an array of preparations that differ widely from each other in composition and biological effects. As to be expected, the type of oxidizing agent used and the conditions of oxidation of LDL determine the chemical and biological properties of OxLDL. Unfortunately, most studies do not report the detailed composition of OxLDL used, or even the exact conditions of LDL oxidation, which complicates the comparison of their biological effects. Even when identical conditions are used to oxidize the LDL ex vivo, the products could differ significantly, depending upon the fatty acid composition and antioxidant status of the starting LDL preparation. Minimally modified LDL

(MM-LDL) is a general term used to describe a variety of LDL preparations that are sufficiently modified to be chemically distinguished from unmodified LDL, but retain the ability to bind to LDL receptor, are not recognized by most scavenger receptors, and have distinct biological activity not shown by unmodified LDL, such as the induction of chemotactic or pro-inflammatory proteins by endothelial cells and macrophages. Since the MM-LDL have been prepared by a wide range of methods, they also differ significantly from each other in their chemical and biological properties (Table 1). Furthermore, since LDL itself is composed of several distinct subfractions that differ in density, size, composition, and antioxidant levels, the oxidation of total LDL gives rise to a mixture of OxLDL species even under controlled conditions. The 'average' LDL particle has been calculated to contain 600 molecules of free cholesterol, 1600 molecules of cholesteryl ester, 700 molecules of phospholipid (64% PC, 1.5% PE, 26% SM, and 11% LPC), 180 molecules of TG, and 1 molecule of ApoB (124). In addition, varying amounts of antioxidants (α tocopherol, γ tocopherol, ubiquinol, lycopene, β carotene) are present in the LDL particles (257). Although there are several oxidizable components in LDL, the polyunsaturated fatty acids (mostly arachidonic acid and linoleic acid) of LDL lipids are the major targets of oxidizing agents. The first detectable product of lipid oxidation is the hydroperoxy derivative of a phospholipid (Fig. 1). This also results in the rearrangement of double bonds to form conjugated dienes that are conveniently detected by an increase in absorbance at 235nm (A235). Further oxidation results in the truncation of sn-2 acyl chain, forming short-chain aldehyde or carboxy derivatives. The aldehydes may form adducts with the lysine residues of apo B, either before or after hydrolysis from the phospholipids by phospholipase A2. HNE (4-hydroxynonenal) is one of the most abundant aldehydes in oxidized LDL, which derivatizes thiols and free amino groups of LDL Apo B and cellular proteins. ***Reference:*** *Antioxid Redox Signal. 2010 July 1; 13(1): 39–75. doi: 10.1089/ars.2009.2733. PMCID: PMC2877120. Oxidized LDL: Diversity, Patterns of Recognition, and Pathophysiology. Irena Levitan, Suncica Volkov, and Papasani V. Subbaiah.*

Studies have shown that testosterone levels correlate with mood. There is historic evidence of a strong positive correlation of testosterone with parameters such as mental well being, joyfulness, social interactivity, general arousal reaction, and wakefulness. Negative correlations have been reported with depression, nervousness, irritability, and anxiety. In hypogonadal men receiving Androgel, positive mood parameters, such as sense of well being and energy level improved while negative parameters such as sadness and irritability decreased. The improvement in mood was observed on day 30 and was maintained with continued treatment for six42 and 36 months.26 The improvement in mood parameters was not dependent on the magnitude of increase in serum testosterone levels. In fact, once serum testosterone increased into the low normal range, maximal improvement in mood parameters was seen. Thus, improvement in mood (similar to sexual function) in response to testosterone therapy appears to be dependent on reaching a threshold of serum testosterone that lies in the low normal range. The same results were replicated with the use of Testim where mood improved early after institution of treatment that was maintained for the duration of the treatment up to three months27,29 and one year.30 In a short-term study with Testim, Loizides and colleagues54 showed that measures of positive and negative mood improved significantly, beginning with the first week of therapy and reaching a maximal response at the second week. Kuhnert and colleagues28 have reported similar findings. *Reference: Clin Interv Aging. 2009; 4: 397–412. Published online 2009 November 18. PMCID: 85864. Safety and efficacy of testosterone gel in the treatment of male hypogonadism. Kishore M Lakshman and Shehzad Basaria.*

Community cohort studies and meta-analyses of randomized trials have shown a relation between low or lowered cholesterol and death by violence (homicide, suicide, accident); in primates, cholesterol reduction has been linked to increased behavioral acts of aggression. In this study we test for the first time whether cholesterol level is related to commission of violent crimes against others in a large community cohort. The authors merged one-time cholesterol measurements on 79,777 subjects enrolled in a health screening project in Varmland, Sweden with subsequent police records for arrests for violent crimes in men and women aged 24-70 at enrollment; and with information on covariates. They performed a nested case control comparison of cholesterol in violent criminals - defined as those with two or more crimes of violence against others - to cholesterol in nonoffenders matched on age, enrollment year, sex, education and alcohol, using variable-ratio matching, with a nonparametric sign test. 100 individuals met criteria for criminal violence. Low cholesterol (below the median) was strongly associated with criminal violence in unadjusted analysis (Men: risk ratio 1.94, P=0.002; all subjects risk ratio 2.32, P<0.001). Age emerged as a strong confounder. Adjusting for covariates using a matching procedure, violent criminals had significantly lower cholesterol than others identical in age, sex, alcohol indices and education, using a nonparametric sign test (P=0.012 all subjects; P=0.035 men). Adjusting for other factors, low cholesterol is associated with increased subsequent criminal violence. *Reference: Golomb, B. A., et al. Low cholesterol and violent crime. J Psychiatr Res. 34(4-5):301-309, 2000.*

The authors report on the social behavior of 30 adult male cynomolgus monkeys, maintained in social groups of five animals each and assigned for 22 months to one of two dietary conditions: a) "luxury"--relatively high fat, high cholesterol (43% calories from fat, 0.34 mg cholesterol/Calorie of diet); or b) "prudent"--relatively low fat, low cholesterol (30% calories from fat, 0.05 mg cholesterol/Calorie of diet). The dietary manipulation resulted in higher total serum cholesterol (TSC) and lower high density lipoprotein cholesterol (HDLC) concentrations in luxury diet animals than in their prudent diet counterparts (p's less than 0.05). Additionally, the authors monitored the occurrence of 21 behavioral acts frequently exhibited by this species in captivity. Of these behaviors, only contact aggression differed between dietary conditions (p less than 0.03), with prudent diet monkeys initiating more aggression than luxury diet animals. These results are consistent with studies linking relatively low serum cholesterol concentrations to violent or antisocial behavior in psychiatric and criminal populations and could be relevant to understanding the significant increase in violence-related mortality observed among people assigned to cholesterol-lowering treatment in clinical trials. *Reference: Kaplan, J. R., et al. The effects of fat and cholesterol on social behavior in monkeys. Psychosom Med. 53(6):634-642, 1991. Department of Comparative Medicine, Bowman Gray School of Medicine, Winston-Salem, North Carolina, USA.*

Epidemiologic studies link plasma cholesterol reduction to increased mortality rates as a result of suicide, violence, and accidents. Deficient central serotonergic activity is similarly associated with violence and suicidal behavior. The authors investigated the relationship among dietary and plasma cholesterol, social behavior, and the serotonin system as a possible explanation for these findings. Juvenile cynomolgus monkeys (eight female and nine male) were fed a diet high in fat and either high or low in cholesterol. We then evaluated their behavior over an 8-month period. Plasma lipids and cerebrospinal fluid metabolites of serotonin, norepinephrine, and dopamine were assessed on two occasions, at 4 and 5.5 months after the initiation of behavioral observations. Animals that consumed a low-cholesterol diet were more aggressive, less affiliative, and had lower cerebrospinal fluid concentrations of 5-hydroxyindoleacetic acid than did their high-cholesterol counterparts (p < .05 for each). The association among dietary cholesterol, serotonergic activity, and social behavior was consistent with data from other species and experiments and suggested that dietary lipids can influence brain neurochemistry and behavior; this phenomenon could be relevant to our understanding of the increase in suicide and violence-related death observed in cholesterol-lowering trials. *Reference: Kaplan, J., et al. Demonstration of an association among dietary cholesterol, central serotonergic activity, and social behaviour in monkeys. Psychosom Med. 56(6):479-484, 1994. Department of Comparative Medicine, Bowman Gray School of Medicine, Winston-Salem, NC 27157-1040.*

Low dietary cholesterol intake may result in reduced central serotonergic activity, which itself has been reported in numerous studies of violent individuals. Researchers studied 25 violent psychiatric patients. For 7 days, the patients wore signaling devices that emitted an average of seven signals a day. Following each signal, patients filled out a mood questionnaire. Total serum cholesterol concentration was positively associated with measures of affect, cognitive efficiency, activation, and sociability, suggesting a link between low total serum cholesterol and dysphoria. These findings are consistent with the cholesterol-serotonin hypothesis and with the substantive literature linking both aggression and depression to depressed central serotonergic activity. *Reference: Hillbrand, M., et al. Serum cholesterol concentrations and mood states in violent psychiatric patients: an experience sampling study. Journal of Behavioral Medicine. 2000; 23(6): 519-529, 2000.*

The aim of our study is to evaluate the possible association between lower plasma cholesterol and depression in the elderly. 140 subjects over 65 years old of both sexes were enrolled, of which 60 were affected by depression (DSM-III-R and Hamilton test) and 80 composed a control group homogeneous for sex and age with the previous one. Plasma cholesterol, HLD-cholesterol (HDL-C), LDL-cholesterol (LDL-C) and triglycerides were measured. A statistically significant difference between cholesterol and LDL-C ($p < 0.001$) was noted in the total group, in both males and females. Such modifications were independent of sex. In the group with lower cholesterol (cut-off $< = 160$ mg/dl) a prevalence of depression three times greater than subjects with higher cholesterol was found. The authors recommended a prudent use of lipid-lowering medications in the elderly because of its uncertain benefits. *Reference: Cadeddu, G., et al. Relationship between cholesterol levels and depression in the elderly. Minerva Med. 86(6):251-256, 1995.*

To investigate the possibility that increases in depressive symptoms might occur in patients who have undergone cholesterol-lowering interventions, the authors administered the Center for Epidemiological Studies-Depression scale before and after cholesterol lowering to 6 men who were referred to a lipid clinic. All of the patients' cholesterol levels were reduced after the 6-week intervention, and 4 of the patients' depression scores increased; scores of 2 of the 4 met the criteria for mild clinical depression. Further study of possible links among low cholesterol, depressive symptoms, and serotonergic activity is needed. *Reference: Davidson, K. W., et al. Increases in depression after cholesterol-lowering drug treatment. Behav Med. 22(2):82-84, 1996. Dalhousie University in Halifax, Nova Scotia, USA.*

Polyunsatured fatty acids are made out of a hydrocarbonated chain of variable length with several double bonds. The position of the first double bond (omega) differentiates polyunsatured omega 3 fatty acids (for example: alpha-linolenic acid or alpha-LNA) and polyunsatured omega 6 fatty acids (for example: linoleic acid or LA). These two classes of fatty acids are said to be essential because they cannot be synthetised by the organism and have to be taken from alimentation. The omega 3 are present in linseed oil, nuts, soya beans, wheat and cold water fish whereas omega 6 are present in maize, sunflower and sesame oil. Fatty acids are part of phospholipids and, consequently, of all biological membranes. The membrane fluidity, of crucial importance for its functioning, depends on its lipidic components. Phospholipids composed of chains of polyunsatured fatty acids increase the membrane fluidity because, by bending some chains, double bonds prevent them from compacting themselves perfectly. Membrane fluidity is also determined by the phospholipids/free cholesterol ratio, as cholesterol increases membrane viscosity. A diet based on a high proportion of essential polyunsatured fatty acids (fluid) would allow a higher incorporation of cholesterol (rigid) in the membranes to balance their fluidity, which would contribute to lower blood cholesterol levels. Brain membranes have a very high content in essential polyunsatured fatty acids for which they depend on alimentation. Any dietary lack of essential polyunsatured fatty acids has consequences on cerebral development, modifying the activity of enzymes of the cerebral membranes and decreasing efficiency in learning tasks. The prevalence of depression seems to increase continuously since the beginning of the century. Though different factors most probably contribute to this evolution, it has been suggested that it could be related to an evolution of alimentary patterns in the Western world, in which polyunsatured omega 3 fatty acids contained in fish, game and vegetables have been largely replaced by polyunsatured omega 6 fatty acids of cereal oils. Some epidemiological data support the hypothesis of a relation between lower depression and/or suicide rates and a higher consumption of fish. These data do not however prove a relation of causality. Several cohort studies (on nondepressed subjects) have assessed the relationship between plasma cholesterol and depressive symptoms with contradictory results. Though some results found a significant relationship between a decrease of total cholesterol and high scores of depression, some other did not. Studies among patients suffering from major depression signalled more constantly an association between low cholesterol and major depression. Besides, some trials showed that clinical recovery may be associated with a significant increase of total cholesterol. The hypothesis that a low cholesterol level may represent a suicidal risk factor was discovered accidentally following a series of epidemiological studies which revealed an increase of the suicidal risk among subjects with a low cholesterol level. Though some contradictory studies do exist, this relationship has been confirmed by several subsequent cohort studies. These findings have challenged the vast public health programs aimed at promoting the decrease of cholesterol, and even suggested to suspend the administration of lipid lowering drugs. Recent clinical studies on populations treated with lipid lowering drugs showed nevertheless a lack of significant increase of mortality, either by suicide or accident. In addition, several controlled studies among psychiatric patients revealed a decrease of the concentrations of plasma cholesterol among patients who had attempted suicide in comparison with other patients. In major depression, all studies revealed a significant decrease of the polyunsaturated omega 3 fatty acids and/or an increase of the omega 6/omega 3 ratio in plasma and/or in the membranes of the red cells. In addition, two studies found a higher severity of depression when the level of polyunsaturated omega 3 fatty acids or the ratio omega 3/omega 6 was low. Parallel to these modifications, other biochemical perturbations have been reported in major depression, particularly an activation of the inflammatory response system, resulting in an increase of the pro-inflammatory cytokines (interleukins: IL-1b, IL-6 and interferon g) and eicosanoids (among others, prostaglandin E2) in the blood and the CSF of depressed patients. These substances cause a peroxidation and, consequently a catabolism of membrane phospholipids, among others those containing polyunsaturated fatty acids. The cytokines and eicosanoids derive from polyunsaturated fatty acids and have opposite physiological functions according to their omega 3 or omega 6 precursor. Arachidonic acid (omega 6) is, among others, precursor of pro-inflammatory prostaglandin E2 (PGE2), whereas polyunsaturated omega 3 fatty acids inhibit the formation of PGE2. It has been shown that a dietary increase of polyunsaturated omega 3 fatty acids reduced strongly the production of IL-1 beta, IL-2, IL-6 and TNF-alpha (tumor necrosis factor-alpha). In contrast, diets with a higher supply of linoleic acid (omega 6) increased significantly the production of pro-inflammatory cytokines, like TNF-alpha. Therefore, polyunsaturated omega 3 fatty acids could be associated at different levels in the pathophysiology of major depression, on the one hand through their role in the membrane fluidity which influences diverse steps of neurotransmission and, on the other hand, through their function as precursor of pro-inflammatory cytokines and eicosanoids disturbing neurotransmission. In addition, antidepressants could exhibit an immunoregulating effect by reducing the release of pro-inflammatory cytokines, by increasing the release of endogenous antagonists of pro-inflammatory cytokines like IL-10 and, finally, by acting like inhibitors of cyclo-oxygenase. Data available concerning the administration of supplements of DHA (docosahexanoic acid) or other polyunsaturated fatty acids omega 3 are limited. In a double blind placebo-controlled study on 30 patients with bipolar disorder, the addition of polyunsaturated omega 3 fatty acids was associated with a longer period of remission. Moreover, nearly all the other prognosis measures were better in the omega 3 group. Very recently, a controlled trial showed the benefits of adding an omega 3 fatty acid, eicosopentanoic acid, among depressed patients. After 4 weeks, six of the 10 patients receiving the fatty acid were considered as responders in comparison with only one of the ten patients receiving placebo. Some epidemiological, experimental and clinical data favour the hypothesis that polyunsaturated fatty acids could play a role in the pathogenesis and/or the treatment of depression. More studies however are needed in order to better precise the actual implication of those biochemical factors among the various aspects of depressive illness. **Reference:** *Colin, A., et al. [Lipids, depression and suicide]. Encephale. 29(Part 1):49-58, 2003. Universite de Liege, CUP La Clairiere, Bertrix.*

The objective of this study was to determine whether a correlation exists between lower serum lipid concentrations and increased suicide risk. Serum lipid profiles were pair-matched for 60 patients who had recently experienced failed attempts at suicide and equal numbers of non-suicidal psychiatric patients, and normal controls. Suicide attempt severity was scored using Weisman and Worden's risk-rescue rating scale. Total serum cholesterol and low density lipoprotein levels were found to be lower in the parasuicidal population at statistically significant levels (P < 0.01 and <0.05, respectively). Triglyceride concentrations were lower in suicide attempters with major depression compared with non-suicidal depressed patients. Risk-rescue rating scores were negatively correlated with total serum cholesterol levels (r = -0.347, P = 0.007). Low lipid metabolism may be a potential biological marker in the assessment of suicide risk. Further investigations are necessary to elucidate the biological mechanisms of these findings. *Reference: Lee, H. J., et al. Serum lipid levels and suicide attempts. Acta Psychiatr Scand. 108(3):215-221, 2003. Department of Psychiatry, Korea University, College of Medicine, Ansan City, Korea.*

The objective of this study was to examine for a relationship between serum cholesterol and suicidal behavior. Patients admitted after an overdose (N=120) were compared with controls (N=120) for their serum cholesterol levels. Patients who had overdosed had significantly lower serum cholesterol levels than controls (mean+/-S.D. 171+/-31 vs. 196+/-30 mg/dl, P<0.0001). These results add to a grouping literature reporting that low serum cholesterol is associated with suicidal behavior. *Reference: Sarchiapone, M., et al. Further evidence for low serum cholesterol and suicidal behaviour. J Affect Disord. 61(1-2):69-71, 2000. Institute of Psychiatry/Catholic University of Sacred Heart, Rome, Italy.*

All adrenal steroids are derived from cholesterol by various enzymatically mediated modifications of its structure. *Reference: Kaplan, N. M. The Adrenal Glands. In: Griffin, James E. & Ojeda, Sergio O. Textbook of Endocrine Physiology (3rd Edition). Oxford University Press. New York, USA, 1996:285-286.*

Vitamin D3 can be hydroxylated sequentially by cytochrome P450scc (CYP11A1) producing 20-hydroxyvitamin D3, 20,23-dihydroxyvitamin D3 and 17,20,23-trihydroxyvitamin D3. The aim of this study was to characterize the ability of vitamin D3 to associate with phospholipid vesicles and to determine the kinetics of metabolism of vitamin D3 by P450scc in vesicles and in 2-hydroxypropyl-β-cyclodextrin (cyclodextrin). Gel filtration of phospholipid vesicles showed that the vitamin D3 remained quantitatively associated with the phospholipid membrane. Vitamin D3 exchanged between vesicles at a rate 3.8-fold higher than for cholesterol exchange and was stimulated by N-62 StAR protein. The Km of P450scc for vitamin D3 in vesicles was 3.3 mol vitamin D3/mol phospholipid and the rate of conversion of vitamin D3 to 20-hydroxyvitamin D3 was first order with respect to the vitamin D3 concentration for the range of concentrations of vitamin D3 that could be incorporated into the vesicle membrane. 20-Hydroxyvitamin D3 was further hydroxylated by P450scc in vesicles, producing primarily 20,23-dihydroxyvitamin D3, with Km and kcat values 22- and 6-fold lower than those for vitamin D3, respectively. 20,23-

Dihydroxyvitamin D3 was converted to 17,20,23-trihydroxyvitamin D3 with even lower Km and kcat values. Vitamin D3 and cholesterol were metabolized with comparable efficiencies in cyclodextrin, but the Km for both showed a strong dependence on the cyclodextrin concentration, decreasing with decreasing cyclodextrin. This study shows that vitamin D3 quantitatively associates with phospholipid vesicles, can exchange between membranes, and can be hydroxylated by membrane-associated P450scc but with lower efficiency than for cholesterol hydroxylation. The kcat values for metabolism of vitamin D3 in vesicles and 0.45% cyclodextrin are similar, but the ability to solubilize vitamin D3 at a concentration higher than its Km makes the cyclodextrin system more efficient for producing the hydroxyvitamin D3 metabolites for further characterization. **Reference:** *Int J Biochem Cell Biol. Author manuscript; available in PMC 2009 January 1. Published in final edited form as: Int J Biochem Cell Biol. 2008; 40(11): 2619–2626. Published online 2008 May 20. doi: 10.1016/j.biocel.2008.05.006. PMCID: PMC2575023. NIHMSID: NIHMS51233. Kinetics of vitamin D3 metabolism by cytochrome P450scc (CYP11A1) in phospholipid vesicles and cyclodextrin. Robert C. Tuckey,a,* Minh N. Nguyen,a and Andrzej Slominskib.*

DIABETES MELLITUS

Testosterone

References:
- Central Effects of Estradiol in the Regulation of Adiposity. LM Brown, DJ Clegg. J Steroid Biochem Mol Biol. Published in final edited form as: J Steroid Biochem Mol Biol. 2010 October; 122(1-3): 65–73. Published online 2009 December 24. doi: 10.1016/j.jsbmb.2009.12.005.
- The Link between the Metabolic Syndrome and Cancer. Sandra Braun, Keren Bitton-Worms, Derek LeRoith. Int J Biol Sci. 2011; 7(7): 1003–1015. Published online 2011 August 16.
- Estrogens and the Diabetic Kidney. Christine Maric, Shannon Sullivan. Gend Med. Author manuscript; available in PMC 2011 September 23. Published in final edited form as: Gend Med. 2008; 5(Suppl A): S103–S113. doi: 10.1016/j.genm.2008.03.010.
- Testosterone Concentrations in Diabetic and Nondiabetic Obese Men. Sandeep Dhindsa, Michael G. Miller, Cecilia L. McWhirter, Donald E. Mager, Husam Ghanim, Ajay. Chaudhuri, Paresh Dandona. Diabetes Care. 2010 June; 33(6): 1186–1192. Published online 2010 March 3. doi: 10.2337/dc09-1649

Psyllium

Water-soluble dietary fibers decrease postprandial glucose concentrations and decrease serum cholesterol concentrations. This study examined the effects of administering psyllium to men with type 2 diabetes. The objective was to evaluate the safety and effectiveness of psyllium husk fiber used adjunctively to a traditional diet for diabetes in the treatment of men with type 2 diabetes and mild-to-moderate hypercholesterolemia. After a 2-wk dietary stabilization phase, 34 men with type 2 diabetes and mild-to-moderate hypercholesterolemia were randomly assigned to receive 5.1 g psyllium or cellulose placebo twice daily for 8 wk. Serum lipid and glycemic indexes were evaluated biweekly on an outpatient basis and at weeks 0 and 8 in a metabolic ward. In the metabolic ward, the psyllium group showed significant improvements in glucose and lipid values compared with the placebo group. Serum total and LDL-cholesterol concentrations were 8.9% ($P < 0.05$) and 13.0% ($P = 0.07$) lower, respectively, in the psyllium than in the placebo group. All-day and post lunch postprandial glucose concentrations were 11.0% ($P < 0.05$) and 19.2% ($P < 0.01$) lower in the psyllium than in the placebo group. Both products were well tolerated, with no serious adverse events related to treatment reported in either group. The addition of psyllium to a traditional diet for persons with diabetes is safe, is well tolerated, and improves glycemic and lipid control in men with type 2 diabetes and hypercholesterolemia. ***Reference:*** *Effects of psyllium on glucose and* *serum lipid responses in men with type 2 diabetes and hypercholesterolemia. American Journal of Clinical Nutrition. 70(4):466-473, 1999. Anderson, J. W., et al.*

A study was designed to evaluate the effect of acarbose and Plantago psyllium mucilage on glycemic index (GI) of bread. Twelve patients with non-insulin-dependent diabetes mellitus (NIDDM) and ten healthy volunteers were studied. Three meal tests with an intake of 90 g of white bread (50 g of carbohydrates) were performed on each subject. In one test, 200 mg of acarbose was given, while 15 grams of psyllium mucilage was given in another test, and only bread was ingested in the control test. Serum glucose and insulin concentrations were measured every 30 min from 0-180 min. Net area under curve (AUC) concentrations of glucose and insulin, GI and insulinic index were calculated. In NIDDM patients, AUC-glucose in the test with acarbose (1.9 +/- 0.7 mmol/L) and with psyllium (4.3 +/- 1.2 mmol/L) were significantly lower than in the control test (7.4 +/- 1.5 mmol/L) ($p < 0.01$). GI of bread plus acarbose was 26 +/- 13, and of bread plus psyllium, 59 +/- 10 ($p < 0.05$). AUC-insulin and insulinic index behave similarly. In healthy individuals, AUC-glucose and GI did not significantly change with the treatments; however, insulinic index with acarbose was 17 +/- 16, and with P. psyllium was 68 +/- 15 ($p < 0.05$). Acarbose or P. psyllium decreased GI of bread in NIDDM patients and diminished insulinic index in NIDDM and in healthy subjects. Adding acarbose or psyllium to meals may reduce glycemic index of carbohydrate foods and may help diabetic control. **Reference:** *Lowering glycemic index of food by acarbose and Plantago psyllium mucilage. Arch Med Res. 29(2):137-141, 1998. Frati Munari, A. C., et al. Departamento de Medicina Interna, Hospital de Especialidades, Mexico.*

Plantago ovata has been reported to reduce postprandial glucose concentrations in diabetic patients. In the present study, the efficacy and possible modes of action of hot-water extracts of husk of P. ovata were evaluated. The administration of P. ovata (0.5 g/kg body weight) significantly improved glucose tolerance in normal, type 1 and type 2 diabetic rat models. When the extract was administered orally with sucrose solution, it suppressed postprandial blood glucose and retarded small intestinal absorption without inducing the influx of sucrose into the large intestine. The extract significantly reduced glucose absorption in the gut during in situ perfusion of small intestine in non-diabetic rats. In 28 d chronic feeding studies in type 2 diabetic rat models, the extract reduced serum atherogenic lipids and NEFA but had no effect on plasma insulin and total antioxidant status. No effect of the extract was evident on intestinal disaccharidase activity. Furthermore, the extract did not stimulate insulin secretion in perfused rat pancreas, isolated rat islets or clonal beta cells. Neither did the extract affect glucose transport in 3T3 adipocytes. Aqueous extracts of P. ovata reduce hyperglycaemia in diabetes via inhibition of intestinal glucose absorption and enhancement of motility. These attributes indicate that P. ovata may be a useful source of active components to provide new opportunities for diabetes therapy. *Reference: Aqueous extracts of husks of Plantago ovata reduce hyperglycaemia in type 1 and type 2 diabetes by inhibition of intestinal glucose absorption. British Journal of Nutrition. 96(1):131-137, 2006. Hannan, J. M., et al. School of Biomedical Sciences, University of Ulster, Coleraine, Northern Ireland, UK.*

The beneficial effect of dietary fiber in the management of type II diabetes is still controversial and has not been totally demonstrated. The purpose of this study was to determine the plasma-lowering effects of 5 g t.i.d. of Plantago Psyllium, as an adjunct to dietary therapy, on lipid and glucose levels, in patients with type II diabetes. Patients were randomly selected from an outpatient clinic of primary care to participate in a double-blind placebo-controlled study in which Plantago Psyllium or placebo was given in combination with a low fat diet. 125 subjects were included in the study that consisted in a 6-week period of diet counseling followed by a 6-week treatment period. Fasting plasma glucose, total plasma cholesterol, LDL cholesterol, HDL cholesterol and triglyceride levels were measured every 2 weeks. The test products (Psyllium or placebo) were supplied to subjects in identically labeled foil packets containing a 5-g dose of product, to consume three doses per day (of 5 g each one), before regular meals. There was an excellent tolerance to Psyllium, without significant adverse effects. No significant changes were observed in the patient's weight for both groups (not significant). Fasting plasma glucose, total cholesterol, LDL cholesterol, and triglycerides levels, showed a significant reduction ($p < 0.05$), whereas HDL cholesterol increased significantly ($p < 0.01$) following Psyllium treatment. These results show that 5 g t.i.d. of Psyllium is useful, as an adjunct to dietary therapy, in patients with type II diabetes, to reduce plasma lipid and glucose levels, resolving the compliance conflict associated with the ingestion of a great amount of fiber in customary diet. *Reference: Lipid- and glucose-lowering efficacy of Plantago Psyllium in type II diabetes. J Diabetes Complications. 12(5):273-278, 1998. Rodriguez-Moran, M., et al.*

The aim of this study was to evaluate the effects of psyllium in type 2 diabetic patients. The study included three phases: phase 1 (1 week), phase 2 (treatment, 14 g fibre/day, 6 weeks) and phase 3 (4 weeks). At the end of each phase a clinical evaluation was performed after the ingestion of a test breakfast of 1824.2 kJ (436 kcal). Measurements included concentrations of blood glucose, insulin, fructosamine, GHbA(1c), C-peptide and 24 h urinary glucose excretion. In addition, uric acid, cholesterol and several mineral and vitamin concentrations were also evaluated. The study was performed at the Department of Pharmacology, Toxicology and Nursing at the University of Leon (Spain). Twenty type 2 diabetic patients (12 men and 8 women) participated in the study with a mean age of 67.4 y for men and 66 y for women. The mean body mass index of men was 28.2 kg/m(2) and that of women 25.9 kg/m(2). Glucose absorption decreased significantly in the presence of psyllium (12.2%); this reduction is not associated with an important change in insulin levels (5%). GHbA(1c), C-peptide and 24 h urinary glucose excretion decreased (3.8, 14.9 and 22.5%, respectively) during the treatment with fibre (no significant differences) as well as fructosamine (10.9%, significant differences). Psyllium also reduced total and LDL cholesterol (7.7 and 9.2%, respectively, significant differences), and uric acid (10%, significant difference). Minerals and vitamins did not show important changes, except sodium that increased significantly after psyllium administration. The results obtained indicate a beneficial therapeutic effect of psyllium (Plantaben(R)) in the metabolic control of type 2 diabetics as well as in lowering the risk of coronary heart disease. Consumption of this fiber does not adversely affect either mineral or vitamin A and E concentrations. *Reference: Therapeutic effects of psyllium in type 2 diabetic patients. Eur J Clin Nutr. 56(9):830-842, 2002. Sierra, M., et al. Department of Pharmacology, Toxicology and Nursing, University of Leon, Leon, Spain.*

Psyllium is a bulk-forming laxative and is high in both fiber and mucilage. The beneficial effect of dietary fiber in the management of type II diabetes, has not been totally demonstrated. The purpose of this study was to determine the plasma-lowering effects of 5.1g b.i.d. of psyllium husk fiber, as an adjunct to dietary and drug therapy on lipid and glucose levels, in patients with type II diabetes. Patients were randomly selected from an outpatient clinic of primary care to participate in a double-blind placebo-controlled study in which Plantago ovata Forsk., or placebo was given in combination with their anti-diabetic drugs. Forty-nine subjects were included in the studies that were given diet counseling before the study and then followed for 8 weeks in the treatment period. Fasting plasma glucose (FBS) was measured every 2 weeks, and total plasma cholesterol (TC), LDL-cholesterol (LDL-C), HDL-cholesterol (HDL-C), triglyceride (TG), and insulin levels were measured every 4 weeks. Glycosylated hemoglobin (HbA1c) was also measured at the beginning and ending of the study. The test products (psyllium or placebo) were supplied to subjects in identically labeled foil packets containing a 5.1g dose of product, to consume two doses per day, half an hour before breakfast and dinner. Both products were well tolerated, with no serious adverse events related to treatment was reported in either. Better gastric tolerance to metformin was recorded in the psyllium group. FBS, and HbA1c, showed a significant reduction (p<0.05), whereas HDL-C increased significantly (p<0.05) following psyllium treatment. LDL/HDL ratio was significantly decreased (p<0.05). These results show that 5.1g b.i.d. of psyllium for persons with type II diabetes is safe, well tolerated, and improves glycemic control. *Reference: Psyllium decreased serum glucose and glycosylated hemoglobin significantly in diabetic outpatients. J Ethnopharmacol. 2005. Ziai, S. A., et al. Department of Pharmacology, Institute of Medicinal Plants, ACECR, No. 97 Bozorgmehr Street, Qods Street, Enghelab Avenu, Tehran, Iran.*

Lycium

References:
- *Lycium barbarum Extracts Protect the Brain from Blood-Brain Barrier Disruption and Cerebral Edema in Experimental Stroke. Di Yang, Suk-Yee Li, Chung-Man Yeung, Raymond Chuen-Chung Chang, Kwok-Fai So, David Wong, Amy C. Y. Lo. PLoS One. 2012; 7(3): e33596. Published online 2012 March 16. doi: 10.1371/journal.pone.0033596.*
- *Traditional Chinese Medicine in Treatment of Metabolic Syndrome. Jun Yin, Hanjie Zhang, Jianping Ye. Endocr Metab Immune Disord Drug Targets. Author manuscript; available in PMC 2009 June 1. Published in final edited form as: Endocr Metab Immune Disord Drug Targets. 2008 June; 8(2): 99–111.*
- *Evaluation of the Antidiabetic and Antilipaemic Activities of the Hydroalcoholic Extract of Phoenix Dactylifera Palm Leaves and Its Fractions in Alloxan-Induced Diabetic Rats. Seyyed Ali Mard, Kowthar Jalalvand, Masoumeh Jafarinejad, Hoda Balochi, Mohammad Kazem Gharib Naseri. Malays J Med Sci. 2010 Oct-Dec; 17(4): 4–13.*

The effects of polysaccharide extracted from Lycium barbarum (LBP) on blood glucose, oxidative stress and DNA damage in rats with non-insulin dependent diabetes mellitus (NIDDM) were studied. The results show that LBP treatment (10 mg/kg.d) for 4 weeks led to decreased levels of blood glucose, malondialdehyde (MDA) and nitric oxide (NO) in serum of fasting rats; and to increased serum level of superoxidedismutase (SOD). Furthermore, LBP could reduce cellular DNA damage in peripheral lymphocytes of NIDDM rats. The DNA damage was determined by using the single cell gel (comet) assay with alkaline electrophoresis and was quantified by measuring tail length and tail moment. These results suggest that LBP can control blood glucose and modulate the metabolism of glucose, leading to significant improvement of oxidative stress markers (SOD, MDA) in rats with NIDDM. And that, LBP decreases DNA damage possibly via a decrease in oxidative stress levels. In conclusion, LBP as a dietary supplement may prevent the development of complications or even tendency to carcinogenesis in NIDDM rats. *Reference: Effect of Lycium barbarum polysaccharide on the improvement of antioxidant ability and DNA damage in NIDDM rats. Yakugaku Zasshi. 126(5):365-371, 2006. Wu, H., et al. Department of Nutrition & Food Hygiene, School of Public Health, Fudan University, Shanghai, P. R. China.*

Lycium barbarum is one of the traditional oriental medicines. It has been reported to reduce blood glucose levels. In this study, the effect of Lycium barbarum polysaccharide (LBP) on the improvement of insulin resistance and lipid profile was studied in rats, a model for non-insulin dependent diabetes mellitus (NIDDM). The rats were divided into three groups: control, NIDDM control, and NIDDM+LBP. Diabetes model groups were made by feeding high-fat diet and subjecting to i.p. streptozotocin (50 mg/kg). LBP treatment for 3 weeks resulted in a significant decrease in the concentration of plasma triglyceride and weight in NIDDM rats. Furthermore, LBP markedly decreased the plasma cholesterol levels and fasting plasma insulin levels, and the postprandial glucose level at 30 min during oral glucose tolerance test and significantly increased the Insulin Sensitive Index in NIDDM rats. In the present study, the authors have tested that LBP can alleviate insulin resistance and the effect of LBP is associated with increasing cell-surface level of glucose transporter 4 (GLUT4) in skeletal muscle of NIDDM rats. Under insulin stimulus, GLUT4 content in plasma membrane in NIDDM control rats was significantly lower than that of control ($p<0.01$), and GLUT4 content in the plasma membrane in NIDDM+LBP rats was higher than that of NIDDM control rats ($p<0.01$). LBP can ameliorate insulin resistance, and the mechanism may be involved in increasing cell-surface level of GLUT4, improving GLUT4 trafficking and intracellular insulin signaling. *Reference: Effect of Lycium barbarum polysaccharide on the improvement of insulin resistance in NIDDM rats. Yakugaku Zasshi. 125(12):981-988, 2005 Zhao, R., et al. Department of Biological Engineering, College of Environment & Chemical Engineering, Yanshan University, China.*

Cinnamon

Peroxisome proliferator-activated receptors (PPARs) are transcriptional factors involved in the regulation of insulin resistance and adipogenesis. Cinnamon, a widely used spice in food preparation and traditional antidiabetic remedy, is found to activate PPARγ and α, resulting in improved insulin resistance, reduced fasted glucose, FFA, LDL-c, and AST levels in high-caloric diet-induced obesity (DIO) and db/db mice in its water extract form. In vitro studies demonstrate that cinnamon increases the expression of peroxisome proliferator-activated receptors γ and α (PPARγ/α) and their target genes such as LPL, CD36, GLUT4, and ACO in 3T3-L1 adipocyte. The transactivities of both full length and ligand-binding domain (LBD) of PPARγ and PPARα are activated by cinnamon as evidenced by reporter gene assays. These data suggest that cinnamon in its water extract form can act as a dual activator of PPARγ and α, and may be an alternative to PPARγ activator in managing obesity-related diabetes and hyperlipidemia. *Reference: PPAR Res. 2008; 2008: 581348. Published online 2008 December 11. doi: 10.1155/2008/581348. PMCID: PMC2602825. Improved Insulin Resistance and Lipid Metabolism by Cinnamon Extract through Activation of Peroxisome Proliferator-Activated Receptors. Xiaoyan Sheng, Yuebo Zhang, Zhenwei Gong, Cheng Huang, and Ying Qin Zang. Key Laboratory of Nutrition and Metabolism, Institute for Nutritional Sciences, Shanghai Institutes for Biological Sciences, Graduate School of CAS, Chinese Academy of Sciences, 319 Yue Yang Road, Shanghai 200031, China.*

The causes and control of type 2 diabetes mellitus are not clear, but there is strong evidence that dietary factors are involved in its regulation and prevention. The authors have shown that extracts from cinnamon enhance the activity of insulin. The objective of this study was to isolate and characterize insulin-enhancing complexes from cinnamon that may be involved in the alleviation or possible prevention and control of glucose intolerance and diabetes. Water-soluble polyphenol polymers from cinnamon that increase insulin-dependent in vitro glucose metabolism roughly 20-fold and display antioxidant activity were isolated and characterized by nuclear magnetic resonance and mass spectroscopy. The polymers were composed of monomeric units with a molecular mass of 288. Two trimers with a molecular mass of 864 and a tetramer with a mass of 1152 were isolated. Their protonated molecular masses indicated that they are A type doubly linked procyanidin oligomers of the catechins and/or epicatechins. These polyphenolic polymers found in cinnamon may function as antioxidants, potentiate insulin action, and may be beneficial in the control of glucose intolerance and diabetes. *Reference: Isolation and characterization of polyphenol type-A polymers from cinnamon with insulin-like biological activity. J Agric Food Chem. 52(1):65-70, 2004. Anderson, R. A., et al.*

Multiple trials in the past have shown conflicting results of whether cinnamon lowers glucose or hemoglobin A1C (HbA1C). The purpose of this study was to determine whether cinnamon lowers HbA1C in patients with type 2 diabetes. The author performed a randomized, controlled trial to evaluate whether daily cinnamon plus usual care versus usual care alone lowers HbA1c. The author randomized 109 type 2 diabetics (HbA1C >7.0) from 3 primary care clinics caring for pediatric, adult, and geriatric patients at a United States military base. Participants were randomly allocated to either usual care with management changes by their primary care physician or usual care with management changes plus cinnamon capsules, 1 gram daily for 90 days. HbA1c was drawn at baseline and 90 days and compared with intention-to-treat analysis. This study was approved by an institutional review board. Cinnamon lowered HbA1C 0.83% (95% CI, 0.46-1.20) compared with usual care alone lowering HbA1C 0.37% (95% CI, 0.15-0.59). Taking cinnamon could be useful for lowering serum HbA1C in type 2 diabetics with HbA1C >7.0 in addition to usual care. *Reference: Effectiveness of cinnamon for lowering hemoglobin A1C in patients with type 2 diabetes: a randomized, controlled trial. J Am Board Fam Med Crawford, P., . 22(5):507-512, 2009. Nellis Family Medicine Residency, Mike O'Callaghan Federal Hospital, Las Vegas, NV, USA.*

The objective of this study was to determine whether cinnamon improves blood glucose, triglyceride, total cholesterol, HDL cholesterol, and LDL cholesterol levels in people with type 2 diabetes. A total of 60 people with type 2 diabetes, 30 men and 30 women aged 52.2 +/- 6.32 years, were divided randomly into six groups. Groups 1, 2, and 3 consumed 1, 3, or 6 g of cinnamon daily, respectively, and groups 4, 5, and 6 were given placebo capsules corresponding to the number of capsules consumed for the three levels of cinnamon. The cinnamon was consumed for 40 days followed by a 20-day washout period. After 40 days, all three levels of cinnamon reduced the mean fasting serum glucose (18-29%), triglyceride (23-30%), LDL cholesterol (7-27%), and total cholesterol (12-26%) levels; no significant changes were noted in the placebo groups. Changes in HDL cholesterol were not significant. The results of this study demonstrate that intake of 1, 3, or 6 g of cinnamon per day reduces serum glucose, triglyceride, LDL cholesterol, and total cholesterol in people with type 2 diabetes and suggest that the inclusion of cinnamon in the diet of people with type 2 diabetes will reduce risk factors associated with diabetes and cardiovascular diseases. *Reference: Cinnamon improves glucose and lipids of people with type 2 diabetes. Diabetes Care. 26(12):3215-3218, 2003. Khan, A., et al.*

The anti-diabetic effect of Cinnamomi cassiae extract (Cinnamon bark: Lauraceae) in a type II diabetic animal model (C57BIKsj db/db) was studied. Cinnamon extract was administered at different dosages (50, 100, 150 and 200mg/kg) for 6 weeks. It was found that blood glucose concentration is significantly decreased in a dose-dependent manner ($P<0.001$) with the most in the 200mg/kg group compared with the control. In addition, serum insulin levels and HDL-cholesterol levels were significantly higher ($P<0.01$) and the concentration of triglyceride, total cholesterol and intestinal alpha-glycosidase activity were significantly lower after 6 weeks of the administration. These results suggest that cinnamon extract has a regulatory role in blood glucose level and lipids and it may also exert a blood glucose-suppressing effect by improving insulin sensitivity or slowing absorption of carbohydrates in the small intestine. *Reference: Anti-diabetic effect of cinnamon extract on blood glucose in db/db mice. Journal of Ethnopharmacology. 104(1-2):119-123, 2006. Kim, S. H., et al. Department of Hygienic Chemistry, College of Pharmacy, Kyung Hee University, Seoul, Republic of Korea.*

According to previous studies, cinnamon may have a positive effect on the glycaemic control and the lipid profile in patients with diabetes mellitus type 2. The aim of this trial was to determine whether an aqueous cinnamon purified extract improves glycated haemoglobin A1c (HbA1c), fasting plasma glucose, total cholesterol, low-density lipoprotein (LDL), high-density lipoprotein (HDL) and triacylglycerol concentrations in patients with type 2 diabetes. A total of 79 patients with diagnosed diabetes mellitus type 2 not on insulin therapy but treated with oral antidiabetics or diet were randomly assigned to take either a cinnamon extract or a placebo capsule three times a day for 4 months in a double-blind study. The amount of aqueous cinnamon extract corresponded to 3 g of cinnamon powder per day. The mean absolute and percentage differences between the pre- and post-intervention fasting plasma glucose level of the cinnamon and placebo groups were significantly different. There was a significantly higher reduction in the cinnamon group (10.3%) than in the placebo group (3.4%). No significant intragroup or intergroup differences were observed regarding HbA1c, lipid profiles or differences between the pre- and post-intervention levels of these variables. The decrease in plasma glucose correlated significantly with the baseline concentrations, indicating that subjects with a higher initial plasma glucose level may benefit more from cinnamon intake. No adverse effects were observed. The cinnamon extract seems to have a moderate effect in reducing fasting plasma glucose concentrations in diabetic patients with poor glycaemic control. *Reference: Effects of a cinnamon extract on plasma glucose, HbA, and serum lipids in diabetes mellitus type 2. Eur J Clin Invest. 36(5):340-344, 2006. Mang, B., et al. Nutrition Physiology and Human Nutrition Unit, Institute of Food Science, University of Hannover, Hannover, Germany.*

The objective of this study was to determine the effects of a dried aqueous extract of cinnamon on antioxidant status of people with impaired fasting glucose that are overweight or obese. Twenty-two subjects, with impaired fasting blood glucose with BMI ranging from 25 to 45, were enrolled in a double-blind placebo-controlled trial. Subjects were given capsules containing either a placebo or 250 mg of an aqueous extract of cinnamon (Cinnulin PF) two times per day for 12 weeks. Plasma malondialdehyde (MDA) concentrations were assessed using high performance liquid chromatography and plasma antioxidant status was evaluated using ferric reducing antioxidant power (FRAP) assay. Erythrocyte Cu-Zn superoxide (Cu-Zn SOD) activity was measured after hemoglobin precipitation by monitoring the auto-oxidation of pyrogallol and erythrocyte glutathione peroxidase (GPx) activity by established methods. FRAP and plasma thiol (SH) groups increased, while plasma MDA levels decreased in subjects receiving the cinnamon extract. Effects were larger after 12 than 6 weeks. There was also a positive correlation ($r = 0.74$; $p = 0.014$) between MDA and plasma glucose. This study supports the hypothesis that the inclusion of water soluble cinnamon compounds in the diet could reduce risk factors associated with diabetes and cardiovascular disease. *Reference: Antioxidant effects of a cinnamon extract in people with impaired fasting glucose that are overweight or obese. J Am Coll Nutr. 28(1):16-21, 2009. Roussel, A. M., et al. INSERM, Grenoble, France.*

Coenzyme Q10

Antioxidant supplementations have the potential to alleviate the atherosclerotic damage caused by excessive production of reactive oxygen species (ROS). The present study evaluated the effects of prolonged antioxidant treatment on arterial elasticity, inflammatory and metabolic measures in patients with multiple cardiovascular risk factors. Study participants were randomly assigned to two groups. Group 1 received oral supplementation with 2 capsules per day of Mid Life Guard, SupHerb, Israel. In each capsule vitamin C (500 mg) vitamin E (200 iu), co-enzyme Q10 (60 mg) and selenium (100 mcg), Group 2 received matching placebo(SupHerb) for 6 months. Patients were evaluated for lipid profile, HbA1C, insulin, C-peptide, hs-CRP, endothelin, aldosterone, plasma renin activity and Homeostasis model assessment-insulin resistance (HOMA-IR). Arterial elasticity was evaluated using pulse wave contour analysis (HDI CR 2000, Eagan, Minnesota). Antioxidant-treated patients exhibited significant increases in large arterial elasticity index (LAEI) as well as small arterial elasticity index (SAEI). A significant decline HbA1C and a significant increase in HDL-cholesterol were also observed. In the placebo group, significant changes in LAEI, SAEI or metabolic measures were not observed. Antioxidant supplementation significantly increased large and small artery elasticity in patients with multiple cardiovascular risk factors. This beneficial vascular effect was associated with an improvement in glucose and lipid metabolism as well as decrease in blood pressure. *Reference: Nutr Metab (Lond). 2010; 7: 55. Published online 2010 July 6. doi: 10.1186/1743-7075-7-55. PMCID: PMC2911454. Effect of long-term treatment with antioxidants (vitamin C, vitamin E, coenzyme Q10 and selenium) on arterial compliance, humoral factors and inflammatory markers in patients with multiple cardiovascular risk factors. Marina Shargorodsky, Ortal Debby, Zipora Matas, and Reuven Zimlichman, Department of Endocrinology, Wolfson Medical Center, Holon, 58100, Israel. Brunner Institute for Cardiovascular Research, Wolfson Medical Center, Holon, 58100, Israel. Sackler School of Medicine, Tel Aviv University, Tel Aviv, Israel. Department of Biochemistry, Wolfson Medical Center, Holon, 58100, Israel. Department of Medicine, Wolfson Medical Center, Holon, 58100, Israel.*

This study investigated the level of platelet malondialdehyde (MDA) as a marker of oxidative stress and coenzyme Q10 (CoQ10) as an index of antioxidant capacity in patients with type 2 diabetes mellitus and their relation to glycemic control. The study group consisted of 28 patients with type 2 diabetes mellitus (10 men and 18 women) with mean age of 48 +/- 2 years. Ten healthy individuals, age and sex matched with the patients, were used as a control group. Laboratory investigations in the form of lipid profile, glycosylated hemoglobin, plasma MDA, platelet MDA and plasma CoQ10 were assessed for all patients and controls. The study revealed that plasma and platelet MDA, as a marker of oxidative stress, were significantly higher in diabetic patients than in controls. The level of CoQ10, as antioxidant capacity, was significantly lower in diabetic patients than in controls. There was a negative correlation between plasma CoQ10 concentrations and glycosylated hemoglobin. Type 2 diabetic patients are at increased risk of oxidative stress manifested by increased plasma MDA as well as platelet MDA and decreased CoQ10, and this oxidative stress increases with poor glycemic control. *Reference: Malondialdehyde and coenzyme Q10 in platelets and serum in type 2 diabetes mellitus: correlation with glycemic control. Blood Coagul Fibrinolysis. 20(4):248-251, 2009. El-Ghoroury, E. A., et al. Clinical and Chemical Pathology Department, National Research Center, Cairo, Egypt.*

A possible relationship between the pathogenesis of type 2 diabetes and coenzyme Q10 (CoQ10) deficiency has been proposed. The aim of this study was to assess the effect of CoQ10 on metabolic control in 23 type 2 diabetic patients in a randomized, placebo-controlled trial. Treatment with CoQ10 100 mg bid caused a more than 3-fold rise in serum CoQ10 concentration (p < 0.001). No correlation was observed between serum CoQ10 concentration and metabolic control. No significant changes in metabolic parameters were observed during CoQ10 supplementation. The treatment was well tolerated and did not interfere with glycemic control, therefore CoQ10 may be used as adjunctive therapy in patients with associated cardiovascular diseases. *Reference: The effect of coenzyme Q10 administration on metabolic control in patients with type 2 diabetes mellitus. Biofactors. 9(2-4):315-318, 1999. Eriksson, J. G., et al. National Public Health Institute, Department of Epidemiology and Health Promotion, Helsinki, Finland.*

A stimulus to mitochondrial respiratory activity is a crucial component of the signal transduction mechanism whereby increased plasma glucose evokes insulin secretion by beta-cells. Efficient function of the glycerol-3-phosphate shuttle is important in this regard, and the rate-limiting enzyme in this shuttle - the mitochondrial glycerol-3-phosphate dehydrogenase (G3PD) - is under expressed in the beta cells of human type II diabetics as well of rodents that are models for this disorder. Suboptimal tissue levels of coenzyme Q10 (CoQ) could be expected to further impair G3PD activity. Clinical reports from Japan suggest that supplemental CoQ may often improve beta-cell function and glycemic control in type II diabetics. It is proposed that correction of suboptimal CoQ status, by aiding the efficiency of G3PD and of respiratory chain function, will improve the glucose-stimulated insulin secretion of diabetic beta-cells. *Reference: Can correction of sub-optimal coenzyme Q status improve beta-cell function in type II diabetics? Medical Hypotheses. 52(5):397-400, 1999. McCarty, M. F. NutriGuard Research, Encinitas, CA, USA.*

The authors assessed whether dietary supplementation with coenzyme Q(10) improves endothelial function of the brachial artery in patients with Type II (non-insulin-dependent) diabetes mellitus and dyslipidaemia. A total of 40 patients with Type II diabetes and dyslipidaemia were randomized to receive 200 mg of coenzyme Q(10) or placebo orally for 12 weeks. Endothelium-dependent and independent function of the brachial artery was measured as flow-mediated dilatation and glyceryl-trinitrate-mediated dilatation, respectively. A computerized system was used to quantitate vessel diameter changes before and after intervention. Arterial function was compared with 18 non-diabetic subjects. Oxidative stress was assessed by measuring plasma F(2)-isoprostane concentrations, and plasma antioxidant status by oxygen radical absorbance capacity. The diabetic patients had impaired flow-mediated dilation [3.8 % (SEM 0.5) vs 6.4 % (SEM 1.0), p = 0.016], but preserved glyceryl-trinitrate-mediated dilation, of the brachial artery compared with non-diabetic subjects. Flow-mediated dilation of the brachial artery increased by 1.6 % (SEM 0.3) with coenzyme Q10 and decreased by -0.4 % (SEM 0.5) with placebo (p = 0.005); there were no group differences in the changes in pre-stimulatory arterial diameter, post-ischaemic hyperaemia or glyceryl-trinitrate-mediated dilation response. Coenzyme Q10 treatment resulted in a threefold increase in plasma coenzyme Q10 (p < 0.001) but did not alter plasma F(2)-isoprostanes, oxygen radical absorbance capacity, lipid concentrations, glycaemic control or blood pressure. Coenzyme Q10 supplementation improves endothelial function of conduit arteries of the peripheral circulation in dyslipidaemic patients with Type II diabetes. The mechanism could involve increased endothelial release and/or activity of nitric oxide due to improvement in vascular oxidative stress, an effect that might not be reflected by changes in plasma F(2)-isoprostane concentrations. *Reference: Coenzyme Q10 improves endothelial dysfunction of the brachial artery in Type II diabetes mellitus. Diabetologia. 45(3):420-426, 2002. Watts, G. F., et al. Department of Medicine, University of Western Australia, Royal Perth Hospital, Perth, Australia.*

Metformin

References:

- *Use of Metformin in Patients with Kidney and Cardiovascular Diseases. David Klachko, Adam Whaley-Connell. Cardiorenal Med. 2011 May; 1(2): 87–95. Published online 2011 April 14. doi: 10.1159/000327151.*
- *Cellular and molecular mechanisms of metformin: an overview. Benoit Viollet, Bruno Guigas, Nieves Sanz Garcia, Jocelyne Leclerc, Marc Foretz, Fabrizio Andreelli. Clin Sci (Lond) Author manuscript; available in PMC 2012 July 18. Published in final edited form as: Clin Sci (Lond). 2012 March; 122(6): 253–270. doi: 10.1042/CS20110386.*
- *Efficacy of metformin in patients with non-insulin-dependent diabetes mellitus. The Multicenter Metformin Study Group. DeFronzo, R. A., et al. N Engl J Med . 333(9): 541-549, 1995.*

Metformin has been shown to not only contribute to a better glycemic control but also to induce some weight loss (especially in the visceral depot) which may contribute to the improvement of the features of the metabolic syndrome. Metformin treatment may represent a relevant element of an integrated lifestyle modification-pharmacotherapy to prevent not only type 2 diabetes but also cardiovascular disease. *Reference: Potential contribution of metformin to the management of cardiovascular disease risk in patients with abdominal obesity, the metabolic syndrome and type 2 diabetes. Diabetes Metab. 29(4 Part 2):53-61, 2003. Despres, J.*

Type 2 diabetes is characterized by insulin resistance in association with clustering of atherothrombotic risk factors (dysglycaemia, hyperinsulinaemia, hypertension, raised triglyceride, low HDL cholesterol and increased levels of plasminogen activator inhibitor-1 (PAI-1) and clotting factor VII). There is a 3-5 fold increase in risk of myocardial infarction rising to 10-20 fold in the presence of microalbuminuria and overall around 70-75% of subjects with type 2 diabetes die of cardiovascular disease. However, classical risk factors which associate with insulin resistance do not account for all the increased burden of vascular disease in diabetic subjects. Metformin is a biguanide compound which is antihyperglycaemic, reduces insulin resistance and has cardioprotective effects on lipids, thrombosis and blood flow. Metformin has a weight neutral/weight lowering effect and reduces hypertriglyceridaemia, elevated levels of PAI-1, factor VII and C-reactive protein. In addition recent studies indicate that metformin has direct effects on fibrin structure/function and stabilises platelets, two important components of arterial thrombus. The United Kingdom Prospective Diabetes Study (UKPDS) reported that metformin was associated with a 32% reduction in any diabetes related endpoint (p<0.002), a 39% reduction in myocardial infarction (p<0.01) and a non-significant 29% fall in microvascular complications. The figures for macrovascular complications compare favourably for those described for other cardio protective agents such as ACE inhibitors and statins. These findings confirm metformin as first line therapy in the management of obese insulin resistant type 2 diabetes and in the prevention of the vascular complications of this common condition. *Reference: Beneficial effects of metformin on haemostasis and vascular function in man. Diabetes Metab. 29(4 Part 2):44-52, 2003. Grant, P.*

The objective of this study was to evaluate evidence from the medical literature that metformin is effective in preventing type 2 diabetes. Primary literature was accessed via a MEDLINE search (1966-December 2003) using the terms metformin, type 2 diabetes, and prevention. Two studies evaluated metformin's potential to prevent type 2 diabetes, finding that metformin maintained or reduced fasting blood glucose in non-diabetics. Recently, a large study by the Diabetes Prevention Program showed that metformin may reduce the incidence of diabetes. Researchers compared lifestyle changes, metformin therapy, and placebo groups. They found that both lifestyle changes (58%) and metformin therapy (31%) significantly reduced the occurrence of type 2 diabetes versus placebo. These studies provide evidence that metformin may reduce the occurrence of type 2 diabetes. Because long-term efficacy has not been determined, further studies are needed. *Reference: Metformin for prevention of type 2 diabetes. Ann Pharmacother. 2004. Raabe College of Pharmacy, Ohio Northern University, Ada, OH, USA. Hess, A. M., et al.*

Establishing and maintaining control of glycaemia is a key step in the reduction of diabetic microvascular complications. By contrast, macrovascular disease which is the most important complication and shortens the lives of many people with type 2 diabetes is not reduced by glycaemic control alone. The landmark UK Prospective Diabetes Study (UKPDS) showed that intensive glycaemic management with metformin significantly reduced the risk of a range of debilitating and/or life-threatening macrovascular complications, compared with other oral agents, diet and insulin who achieved similar overall glycaemic control. The benefits observed included diabetes-related mortality (reduced by 42%, compared with diet treatment, p=0.017), all-cause mortality (reduced by 36%, p=0.011), myocardial infarction (reduced by 39%, p=0.01), and any diabetes-related endpoint (reduced by 32%, p=0.002). Other clinical and experimental studies have shown metformin to be associated with improved outcomes and support the conclusions from the UKPDS. In addition, a well-designed retrospective analysis has shown significantly lower mortality rates in patients receiving metformin compared with patients treated with sulphonylurea monotherapy. Metformin provides a greater degree of cardiovascular protection than would be expected from its antihyperglycaemic actions alone and is the first drug of choice for the treatment of type 2 diabetes unless there are contraindications in the individual patient. *Reference: Improving survival with metformin: the evidence base today. Diabetes Metab. 29(4 Part 2):36-43, 2003. Scarpello, J. Department of Diabetes and Endocrinology, University Hospital of North Staffordshire NHS Trust, Stoke-on-Trent, UK.*

The timely series of state-of-the-art reviews contained within this supplement provide a valuable overview of the current state of diabetes care, and the pharmacological interventions we have available. Experts agree that one of the most important lessons to emerge recently concerns the magnitude of the malign influence on clinical outcomes of the cardiovascular risk factors associated with the dysmetabolic (insulin resistance) syndrome. Metformin is unique in being not only as effective as any other oral antidiabetic therapy in controlling blood glucose, but also having an unparalleled clinical database relating to improved clinical outcomes in pre-diabetic subjects, and patients with established type 2 diabetes. *Reference: Metformin: drug of choice for the prevention of type 2 diabetes and cardiovascular complications in high-risk subjects. Diabetes Metab. 29(4 Part 2):121-122, 2003. Standl, E. Munich Diabetes Research Institute, Germany.*

The metabolic effects and mechanism of action of metformin are still poorly understood, despite the fact that it has been used to treat patients with non-insulin-dependent diabetes mellitus (NIDDM) for more than 30 years. In 10 obese patients with NIDDM, the authors used a combination of isotope dilution, indirect calorimetry, bioimpedance, and tissue-balance techniques to assess the effects of metformin on systemic lactate, glucose, and free-fatty-acid turnover; lactate oxidation and the conversion of lactate to glucose; skeletal-muscle glucose and lactate metabolism; body composition; and energy expenditure before and after four months of treatment. Metformin treatment decreased the mean (+/- SD) glycosylated hemoglobin value from 13.2 +/- 2.2 percent to 10.5 +/- 1.6 percent (P < 0.001) and reduced fasting plasma glucose concentrations from 220 +/- 41 to 155 +/- 28 mg per deciliter (12.2 +/- 0.7 to 8.6 +/- 0.5 mmol per liter) (P < 0.001). Although resting energy expenditure did not change the patients lost 2.7 +/- 1.3 kg of weight (P < 0.001), 88 percent of which was adipose tissue. The mean (+/- SE) rate of plasma glucose turnover (hepatic glucose output and systemic glucose disposal) decreased from 2.8 +/- 0.2 to 2.0 +/- 0.2 mg per kilogram of body weight per minute (15.3 +/- 0.9 to 10.8 +/- 0.9 mumol per kilogram per minute) (P < 0.001), as a result of a decrease in hepatic glucose output; systemic glucose clearance did not change. The rate of conversion of lactate to glucose (gluconeogenesis) decreased by 37 percent (P < 0.001), whereas lactate oxidation increased by 25 percent (P < 0.001). There were no changes in the plasma lactate concentration, plasma lactate turnover, muscle lactate release, plasma free-fatty-acid turnover, or uptake of glucose by muscle. Metformin acts primarily by decreasing hepatic glucose output, largely by inhibiting gluconeogenesis. It also seems to induce weight loss, preferentially involving adipose tissue. *Reference: Metabolic effects of metformin in non-insulin-dependent diabetes mellitus. New England Journal of Medicine. 333(9):550-554, 1995. Stumvoll, M., et al.*

In patients with type 2 diabetes, intensive blood-glucose control with insulin or sulphonylurea therapy decreases progression of microvascular disease and may also reduce the risk of heart attacks. This study investigated whether intensive glucose control with metformin has any specific advantage or disadvantage. Of 4075 patients recruited to UKPDS in 15 centres, 1704 overweight (>120% ideal bodyweight) patients with newly diagnosed type 2 diabetes, mean age 53 years, had raised fasting plasma glucose (FPG; 6.1-15.0 mmol/L) without hyperglycemic symptoms after 3 months' initial diet. 753 were included in a randomized controlled trial, median duration 10.7 years, of conventional policy, primarily with diet alone (n=411) versus intensive blood-glucose control policy with metformin, aiming for FPG below 6 mmol/L (n=342). A secondary analysis compared the 342 patients allocated metformin with 951 overweight patients allocated intensive blood-glucose control with chlorpropamide (n=265), glibenclamide (n=277), or insulin (n=409). The primary outcome measures were aggregates of any diabetes-related clinical endpoint, diabetes-related death, and all-cause mortality. In a supplementary randomized controlled trial, 537 non-overweight and overweight patients, mean age 59 years, who were already on maximum sulphonylurea therapy but had raised FPG (6.1-15.0 mmol/L) were allocated continuing sulphonylurea therapy alone (n=269) or addition of metformin (n=268). Median glycated haemoglobin (HbA1c) was 7.4% in the metformin group compared with 8.0% in the conventional group. Patients allocated metformin, compared with the conventional group, had risk reductions of 32% for any diabetes-related endpoint, 42% for diabetes-related death, and 36% for all-cause mortality. Among patients allocated intensive blood-glucose control, metformin showed a greater effect than chlorpropamide, glibenclamide, or insulin for any diabetes-related endpoint, all-cause mortality, and stroke. Early addition of metformin in sulphonylurea-treated patients was associated with an increased risk of diabetes-related death (96% increased risk) compared with continued sulphonylurea alone. A combined analysis of the main and supplementary studies demonstrated fewer metformin-allocated patients having diabetes-related endpoints (risk reduction 19%). Epidemiological assessment of the possible association of death from diabetes-related causes with the concurrent therapy of diabetes in 4416 patients did not show an increased risk in diabetes-related death in patients treated with a combination of sulphonylurea and metformin (risk reduction 5%. Since intensive glucose control with metformin appears to decrease the risk of diabetes-related endpoints in overweight diabetic patients, and is associated with less weight gain and fewer hypoglycaemic attacks than are insulin and sulphonylureas, it may be the first-line pharmacological therapy of choice in these patients. **Reference:** *UK Prospective Diabetes Study (UKPDS) Group. Effect of intensive blood-glucose control with metformin on complications in overweight patients with type 2 diabetes (UKPDS 34). Lancet. 352(9131):854-865, 1998.*

EARACHES

Xylitol

Upper respiratory problems have been increasing since the early 1970s, owing to environmental factors that include poorly conceived drug therapy. Otitis media, asthma, sinusitis, and allergies can all be related to chronic faulty hygiene in the nasopharynx. A nasal spray, consisting of xylitol (a naturally occurring food substance) in saline, has been developed to aid the self-cleansing mechanism of the nasopharynx and to reduce local pathogens. The preventive value of the nasal spray is demonstrated in 3 case reports. **Reference:** *Alonzo, H., et al. Intranasal xylitol, recurrent otitis media, and asthma: report of three cases. Clinical Practice of Alternative Medicine. 2(2), 2001.*

Xylitol (8 – 10 grams per day taken a five equally divided doses) has been desmonstrated to inhibit Streptococcus pneumoniae and Haemophilus influenzae infections and to reduce the requirement for antibiotics in persons infected with these pathogens. Xylitol may help to prevent otitis media infections in children. **Reference:** *Cronin, J. R. Xylitol: a sweet for healthy teeth and more. Alternative & Complementary Therapies. 9(3):139-141, 2003.*

To obejctive of this study was to examine whether xylitol, which reduces the growth of Streptococcus pneumoniae, might have clinical importance in the prevention of acute otitis media. A double blind randomised trial with xylitol administered in chewing gum was instituted in Eleven day care nurseries in the city of Oulu. Most of the children had had problems with recurrent acute otitis media. Subjects were 306 day care children: 149 children in the sucrose group (76 boys; mean (SD) age 4.9 (1.5) years) and 157 in the xylitol group (80 boys; 5.0 (1.4) years). Either xylitol (8.4 g a day) or sucrose (control) chewing gum was administered for two months. The authors measured the occurrence of acute otitis media and antimicrobial treatment received during the intervention and nasopharyngeal carriage of S pneumoniae. During the two month monitoring period at least one event of acute otitis media was experienced by 31/149 (20.8%) children who received sucrose compared with 19/157 (12.1%) of those receiving chewing gum containing xylitol (difference 8.7%; 95% confidence interval 0.4% to 17.0%; P = 0.04). Significantly fewer antimicrobials were prescribed among those receiving xylitol: 29/157 (18.5%) children had at least one period of treatment versus 43/149 (28.9%) (difference 10.4%; 0.9% to 19.9%; P = 0.032). The carriage rate of S pneumoniae varied from 17.4% to 28.2% with no difference between the groups. Two children in the xylitol group experienced diarrhea, but no other adverse effects were noted among the xylitol users. Xylitol seems to have a preventive effect against acute otitis media. **References:** *Lagace, E. Xylitol for prevention of acute otitis media. J Fam Pract. 48(2):89,*

1999. -- Mitchell, A. A. Xylitol prophylaxis for acute otitis media: tout de suite? Pediatrics. 102(4 Part 1):974-975, 1998. -- Uhari, M., et al. Xylitol chewing gum in prevention of acute otitis media: double blind randomised trial. BMJ. 313(7066):1180-1184, 1996.

Xylitol, a commonly used sweetener, is effective in preventing dental caries. As it inhibits the growth of pneumococci, the authors evaluated whether xylitol could be effective in preventing acute otitis media (AOM). Altogether, 857 healthy children recruited from day care centers were randomized to one of five treatment groups to receive control syrup (n = 165), xylitol syrup (n = 159), control chewing gum (n = 178), xylitol gum (n = 179), or xylitol lozenge (n = 176). The daily dose of xylitol varied from 8.4 g (chewing gum) to 10 g (syrup). The design was a 3-month randomized, controlled trial, blinded within the chewing gum and syrup groups. The occurrence of AOM each time the child showed any symptoms of respiratory infection was the main outcome. Although at least one event of AOM was experienced by 68 (41%) of the 165 children who received control syrup, only 46 (29%) of the 159 children receiving xylitol syrup were affected, for a 30% decrease (95% confidence interval [CI]: 4.6%-55.4%). Likewise, the occurrence of otitis decreased by 40% compared with control subjects in the children who received xylitol chewing gum (CI: 10.0%-71.1%) and by 20% in the lozenge group (CI: -12.9%-51.4%). Thus, the occurrence of AOM during the follow-up period was significantly lower in those who received xylitol syrup or gum, and these children required antimicrobials less often than did controls. Xylitol was well tolerated. Xylitol sugar, when given in a syrup or chewing gum, was effective in preventing AOM and decreasing the need for antimicrobials. **Reference:** *Uhari, M., et al. A novel use of xylitol sugar in preventing acute otitis media. Pediatrics. 102(4 Part 1):879-884, 1998.*

Grapefruit Seed Extract
Reference: *Sachs, Allan, D.C., C.C.N. The Authoritative Guide to Grapefruit Seed Extract. Life Rhythm, Mendocino, California, USA, 1997:83.*

Zinc
Recurrent acute otitis media (rAOM) is frequently encountered in infants and children and the lack of any definitive treatment has led parents and physicians to try complementary and alternative therapies. The authors evaluated the efficacy of a propolis and zinc suspension in preventing AOM in 122 children aged 1-5 years with a documented history of rAOM, who were prospectively, blindly, randomized 1:1 to receive the suspension plus elimination of environmental risk factors or elimination of environmental risk factors only. AOM- and respiratory-related morbidity were assessed at study entry and every four weeks. In the 3-month treatment period AOM was diagnosed in 31 (50.8%) children given the propolis and zinc suspension and in 43 (70.5%) controls (p=0.04). The mean number of episodes of AOM per child/month was 0.23 -/+ 0.26 in the

propolis and zinc group and 0.34 -/+ 0.29 in controls (reduction 32.0%, p=0.03). The administration of a propolis and zinc suspension to children with a history of rAOM can significantly reduce the risk of new AOM episodes and AOM-related antibiotic courses, with no problem of safety or tolerability, and with a very good degree of parental satisfaction. No effect can be expected on respiratory infections other than AOM. **Reference:** *Marchisio, P., et al. Effectiveness of a propolis and zinc solution in preventing acute otitis media in children with a history of recurrent acute otitis media. Int J Immunopathol Pharmacol. 23(2):567-575, 2010. -- Department of Maternal and Pediatric Sciences, University of Milan, Italy.*

Milk and Soy Allergy

Cow's milk allergy (CMA) affects 2% to 3% of young children and presents with a wide range of immunoglobulin E (IgE-) and non-IgE-mediated clinical syndromes, which have a significant economic and lifestyle impact. Definitive diagnosis is based on a supervised oral food challenge (OFC), but convincing clinical history, skin prick testing, and measurement of cow's milk (CM)-specific IgE can aid in the diagnosis of IgE-mediated CMA and occasionally eliminate the need for OFCs. It is logical that a review of CMA would be linked to a review of soy allergy, as soy formula is often an alternative source of nutrition for infants who do not tolerate cow's milk. The close resemblance between the proteins from soy and other related plants like peanut, and the resulting cross-reactivity and lack of predictive values for clinical reactivity, often make the diagnosis of soy allergy far more challenging. This review examines the epidemiology, pathogenesis, clinical features, natural history and diagnosis of cow's milk and soy allergy. Cross-reactivity and management of milk allergy are also discussed. **Reference:** *Jacob D. Kattan, MD,a Renata R. Cocco, MD,b and Kirsi M. Järvinen, MD, PhDc.*

Whether ingested calcium is absorbed more efficiently from freely water-soluble calcium salts than from poorly soluble salts is unclear. It is also unknown whether calcium is absorbed better from dairy products than from calcium salts. Using a method by which the net absorption of calcium can be accurately measured after a single dose, the authors studied eight healthy fasting subjects after they took a 500-mg dose of calcium from each of five calcium salts with various degrees of water solubility and from milk. The order of administration of the agents given was randomly determined. The mean (+/- SEM) net calcium absorption, in decreasing order of the solubility of the salts, was 32 +/- 4 percent from calcium acetate, 32 +/- 4 percent from calcium lactate, 27 +/- 3 percent from calcium gluconate, 30 +/- 3 percent from calcium citrate, and 39 +/- 3 percent from calcium carbonate. The differences in absorption were not statistically significant according to analysis of variance. On the basis of in vitro solubility experiments in acid mediums, the authors hypothesize that acid dissolution in the gastrointestinal tract may be responsible for the similar absorption of calcium from salts with widely different water solubilities. Calcium absorption from whole milk (31 +/- 3 percent) was similar to absorption from calcium salts. Calcium absorption from carbonate, acetate, lactate, gluconate, and citrate salts of calcium, and from whole milk, is similar in fasting healthy young subjects. Further study will be required to determine whether the results would be different in older subjects, with a higher dose of calcium, or if the calcium was ingested with food. **Reference:** *Sibtain, M. Gastrointestinal absorption of calcium from milk & calcium salts. NEJM. 317(9):532, 1987.*

Vitamin A

Since the first characterization and description of vitamin A this is used in otolaryngologic therapy for different forms of hearing disorders, and its relation to the inner ear is subject of investigation. Animal experiments and clinical studies were done to clarify the significance of vitamin A for the function of hearing. Besides this there were a lot of observations describing correlations between vitamin A metabolism and hearing loss. Recent investigations showed that vitamin A is present in high concentrations in the inner ear and stored there. Morphological experiments revealed different and in some way contradictory results, but they showed that vitamin A seems to be essential for inner-ear morphogenesis. **Reference:** *Biesalski, H. K. [Vitamin A and the ear. Review of the literature.] Z Ernahrungswiss. 23(2):104-112, 1984.*

Morphological investigation of tongue, olfactory epithelia, trachea and inner ear in vitamin A deficiency are reported. The results support assumptions concerning the loss of sensory function as been at least a secondary effect of alterations of the neighbourhood of the sensory cells caused by vitamin A deficiency. Taste buds are hindered in function by a dense layer of squamous cells and olfaction is decreased by atrophy of the surrounding respiratory epithelium. Inner ear functionality seems to be affected by vitamin A status via a stabilizing effect on the endolymph-perilymph barrier. **Reference:** *Biesalski, H. K., et al. Vit. A deficiency and sensory function. Acta Vitaminol Enzymol. 7(Suppl.):45-54, 1985.*

With the sole exception of the hair cells of the inner ear, where information is lacking, all special somatic afferent receptor cells have been shown to be dependent upon vitamin A for normal function. In view of the paucity of information on the role of vitamin A in the inner ear, three experiments were performed to examine this relationship. Temporal bone histopathology was studied in rats deprived of vitamin A. In a second experiment, vitamin A-deficient rats were maintained with vitamin A acid and the histopathology was studied under the light microscope. In the third experiment, a microfluorometric estimate of the content of vitamin A in the guinea pig cochlea was performed. A fluorescent compound with the exact spectral characteristics of vitamin A was found in the guinea pig cochlea at a concentration of 21.2 micrograms/gm, which is ten times the vitamin A concentration found in most other tissues. **Reference:** *Chole, R. A. Experimental studies on the role of vitamin A in the inner ear. Otolaryngology. 86(4 Part 1):595-620, 1978.*

ESCHERICHIA COLI
(E. COLI)

Ginger & Honey

To evaluate the in vitro effects of ginger and honey on micro-organisms on carious teeth by employing antibiotic sensitivity test. Methods: Two hundred and fifty (250) extracted, carious teeth were aseptically collected into sterile peptone water. Bacterial species were isolated from the peptone water broth, characterized and identified according to standard methods described in the Manual of Clinical Microbiology. Aqueous ginger extract and honey were employed for sensitivity test. Suspensions of the bacterial isolates were made in sterile normal saline and adjusted to the 0.5 McFarland's standard. Each Mueller Hinton (MH) agar plate was uniformly seeded by means of sterile swab dipped in the suspension and streaked on the agar plate surface, and the plates left on the bench for excess fluid to be absorbed. Approximately 100 mL of the extracts were dropped into each well which filled them respectively to fullness. The setup was allowed to stabilize for 3 h before being incubated at 37 degrees (C) for 24 hours. The mean zones of inhibition were thereafter measured in mm, for all the individual isolates. Results: Streptococcus mutans (88.0%) and Lactobacillus acidophilus (L. acidophilus) (39.0%) were most prevalent as compared with other isolates. The diameter of the zone of inhibition ranged from (17.5 to 18.5) mm to (26.0 to 28.0) mm for ginger and (19.5 to 20.5) mm to (26.3 to 27.7) mm for honey, as compared with (17.3 to 18.7) mm to (22.5 to 23.5) mm for gentamycin, at the various concentrations used. Results indicate a considerable antibacterial activity of ginger and honey. The combined extracts were most effective against Staphylococcus aureus (30.0.0 plus/minus 1.5) mm but least effective against L. acidophilus (21.0 plus/minus 0.7) mm. Conclusions: For the prevention of the emergence of resistant microorganisms, use of combination of herbal preparations is more useful.Considering in vitro data obtained in this study, there is a significant synergistic effect of antimicrobial activity from the combination of ginger and honey, against isolates from carious teeth. *Reference: Omoya, F.O and Akharaiyi, F.C International Journal on Pharmaceutical and Biomedical Research (IJPBR), Vol. 2(1), 2011, 39-47, Mixture of honey and ginger extract for antibacterial assessment on some clinical isolates. OMOYA, F. O AND AKHARAIYI, F. C. Microbiology Department, Federal University of Technology, P.M.B 704, Akure, Ondo State, Nigeria.*

Ginger is one of the most commonly used fresh herbs and spices. Enterotoxigenic Escherichia coli heat-labile enterotoxin (LT)-induced diarrhea is the leading cause of infant death in developing countries. In this study, we demonstrated that ginger significantly blocked the binding of LT to cell-surface receptor G M1, resulting in the inhibition of fluid accumulation in the closed ileal loops of mice. Biological-activity-guided searching for active components showed that zingerone (vanillylacetone) was the likely active constituent responsible for the antidiarrheal efficacy of ginger. Further analysis of chemically synthesized zingerone derivatives revealed that compound 31 (2-[(4-methoxybenzyl)oxy]benzoic acid) significantly suppressed LT-induced diarrhea in mice via an excellent surface complementarity with the B subunits of LT. In conclusion, our findings provide evidence that ginger and its derivatives may be effective herbal supplements for the clinical treatment of enterotoxigenic Escherichia coli diarrhea. **Reference:** *J Agric Food Chem. 2007 Oct 17;55(21):8390-7. Epub 2007 Sep 20. Ginger and its bioactive component inhibit enterotoxigenic Escherichia coli heat-labile enterotoxin-induced diarrhea in mice. Chen JC, Huang LJ, Wu SL, Kuo SC, Ho TY, Hsiang CY. Graduate Institute of Chinese Pharmaceutical Sciences, Department of Biochemistry, Graduate Institute of Chinese Medical Science, Department of Microbiology, China Medical University, Taichung 40402, Taiwan.*

A *"medicinal grade"* honey called Revamil killed about 99% of antibiotic-resistant E. coli, Pseudomonas aeruginosa, Staphylococcus epidermidis, Enterococcus faecium, and Burkholderia cepacia, and methicillin-resistant Staphylococcus aureus (MRSA) after two hours contact and about 99.99% in 24 hours. **Reference:** *Kwakman PH, de Boer L, Ruyter-Spira CP, Creemers-Molenaar T, Helsper JP, Vandenbroucke-Grauls CM, Zaat SA, te Velde AA. Medical-grade honey enriched with antimicrobial peptides has enhanced activity against antibiotic-resistant pathogens. Eur J Clin Microbiol Infect Dis. 2011 Feb;30(2):251-7. Epub 2010 Oct 7.*

FIBROMYALGIA

Low energy

Correcting testosterone deficiency in hypogonadal men results in significant subjective and objective improvement in energy and vitality. *Reference: Alexander G. M., et al. Androgen-behavior correlations in hypogonadal men and eugonadal men, I: mood and response to auditory sexual stimuli. Horm Behav. 31:110-119, 1997.*

Scrotal transdermal patches improve energy in elderly men with suboptimal testosterone production. *Reference: Bals-Pratsch, M., et al. Transdermal testosterone substitution therapy for male hypogonadism. Lancet. 2:943-946, 1986.*

Fatigue

Hypogonadal men were given AndroGel for 180 days. Normal testosterone levels were attained on the first day of treatment and maintained for the duration of the study. Men receiving AndroGel reported improvement in fatigue. *Reference: Wang, C., et al. Transdermal testosterone gel improves sexual function, mood, and muscle strength and body composition parameters in hypogonadal men. Testosterone gel study group. J Clin Endocrinol Metab. 85(8):2839-2853, 2000.*

Depression

This study was designed to evaluate the safety and effectiveness of testosterone therapy for clinical symptoms of hypogonadism (low libido, low mood, low energy, loss of appetite/weight) in human immunodeficiency virus-positive men with CD4 cell counts less than 400 cells/mm3 and deficient or low normal serum testosterone levels. The trial consisted of 8 weeks of open treatment with 400 mg of intramuscular testosterone cypionate biweekly. Responders were maintained at this dosage for another 4 weeks and then were randomized in a double-blind, placebo-controlled, 6-week discontinuation trial. Of the 112 men who completed at least 8 weeks of treatment, 102 (91%) were rated as responders on a global assessment of sexual desire/function. Of the 34 study completers with major depressive disorder and/or dysthymia, 79% reported significant improvement in mood at week 8. Average weight change was a gain of 3.7 pounds, with 45% gaining more than 5 pounds. Eighty-four men entered and 77 completed the double-blind phase; of these, 78% of completers randomized to testosterone and 13% randomized to placebo maintained their response. Testosterone therapy was well tolerated and effective in ameliorating symptoms of clinical hypogonadism, and equally so for men with and without testosterone deficiency. For patients with major depression and/or dysthymia, improvement was equal to that achieved with standard antidepressants.

Reference: *Rabkin, J. G., et al. Testosterone therapy for human immunodeficiency virus-positive men with and without hypogonadism. J Clin Psychopharmacol. 19(1):19-27, 1999.*

Rheumatoid Arthritis

Rheumatoid arthritis (RA) is a multifactorial disease in which both environmental and genetic factors play a role. Data also suggest that neuroendocrine factors are involved. I briefly summarize observations that support this hypothesis. RA is characterized by striking age-sex disparities. The incidence of disease in women increases steadily from the age of menarche to its maximal incidence around menopause. The disease is uncommon in men under age 45, but its incidence increases rapidly in older men and approaches the incidence in women. These observations strongly suggest that androgens play a major suppressive role, and, in fact, testosterone levels are depressed in most men with RA. Mechanistically, many data indicate that testosterone suppresses both cellular and humoral immune responses. Dehydroepian-drosterone (DHEA), an adrenal product, is the major androgen in women. Its production is strikingly dependent upon age. Peak production is in the 2nd and 3rd decades, but levels decline precipitously thereafter. DHEA levels are low in both men and women with RA, and recent data show that levels of this hormone may be depressed before the onset of disease. The role of DHEA in immune diseases, however, is controversial. The menopausal peak of RA onset suggests estrogen and/or progesterone deficiency play a role in the disease, and many data indicate that estrogens suppress cellular immunity but stimulate humoral immunity, i.e., deficiency promotes cellular (Th1-type) immunity. Recent data also indicate that progesterone stimulates a switch for Th1 to Th2-type immune responses. RA often develops or flares in the postpartum period, particularly if the mother breastfeeds. This is again consistent with gonadal steroid deficiency playing a role in the onset of disease. Breastfeeding is associated with blunted hypothalamic-pituitary-adrenal function and elevated prolactin synthesis. Gonadal and adrenal steroid hormone deficiency, plus elevated prolactin, probably greatly facilitates the expression of Th1-type immunity, which is widely believed to be critical in the pathogenesis of RA. By contrast, RA typically remits during pregnancy, in parallel with the increasing levels of corticosteroids, estrogens, and progesterone. Pregnancy is characterized by a shift in immune function from Th1-type to Th2-type. Oral contraceptives, which generate a condition of pseudopregnancy, also decrease the risk of RA. These data argue that adrenal and gonadal steroid hormones suppress the development of RA. Several studies indicate that corticosteroid production is inappropriately low in patients with RA, and are reminiscent of observations in Lewis rat models of chronic erosive arthritis. A growing body of data indicates that RA develops as a consequence of a deficiency in both adrenal and gonadal steroid hormone production. **Reference:** *Wilder, R. L. Adrenal & gonadal steroid hormone deficiency in the etiopathogenesis of rheumatoid arthritis. Journ of Rheumatology. 23(suppl 44):10-12, 1996.*

Estradiol/Testosterone

References:
- *Sex hormones and pain in regularly menstruating women with fibromyalgia syndrome. Okifuji A, Turk DC. J Pain. 2006 Nov;7(11):851-9. PMID: 17074627 [PubMed - indexed for MEDLINE]*
- *Hypothalamic-pituitary-gonadal axis and cortisol in young women with primary fibromyalgia: the potential roles of depression, fatigue, and sleep disturbance in the occurrence of hypocortisolism. Gur A, Cevik R, Sarac AJ, Colpan L, Rheum Dis. 2004 Nov;63(11):1504-6.*
- *Cortisol and hypothalamic-pituitary-gonadal axis hormones in follicular-phase women with fibromyalgia and chronic fatigue syndrome and effect of depressive symptoms on these hormones. Gur A, Cevik R, Nas K, Colpan L, Sarac S. Arthritis Res Ther. 2004;6(3):R232-8. Epub 2004 Mar 15.*
- *Bone turnover and hormonal perturbations in patients with fibromyalgia. El Maghraoui A, Tellal S, Achemlal L, Nouijai A, Ghazi M, Mounach A, Bezza A, Derouiche el M. Clin Exp Rheumatol. 2006 Jul-Aug;24(4):428-31.*
- *Hyposecretion of adrenal androgens and the relation of serum adrenal steroids, serotonin and insulin-like growth factor-1 to clinical features in women with fibromyalgia. Dessein PH, Shipton EA, Joffe BI, Hadebe DP, Stanwix AE, Pain. 1999 Nov;83(2):313-9.*

Adrenal insufficiency

References:
- *[Addison's disease imitating fibromyalgia]. Fliciński J, Prajs K, Przepiera-Bedzak H. Ann Acad Med Stetin. 2010;56 Suppl 1 :70-2. Review. Polish. PMID: 21365946.*
- *Investigation of the hypothalamo-pituitary-adrenal axis (HPA) by 1 microg ACTH test and metyrapone test in patients with primary fibromyalgia syndrome. Calis M, Gökçe C, Ates F, Ulker S, Izgi HB, Demir H, Kirnap M, Sofuoglu S, Durak AC, Tutus A, Kelestimur F. J Endocrinol Invest. 2004 Jan;27(1):42-6. PMID:15053242.*
- *Fibromyalgia, chronic fatigue syndrome, and Addison disease. Baschetti R. Arch Intern Med. 1999 Nov 8;159(20):2481; author reply 2482-3. No abstract available. PMID:10665898*

Chlorella

The objective of this study was to find evidence of the potential of chlorella (Chlorella pyrenoidosa) dietary supplements to relieve signs and symptoms, improve quality of life, and normalize body functions in people with chronic illnesses, specifically fibromyalgia, hypertension, and ulcerative colitis in several double-blind, placebo-controlled, randomized clinical trials. Fifty-five subjects with fibromyalgia, 33 with hypertension, and 9 with ulcerative colitis were recruited. Subjects consumed 10 g of pure chlorella in tablet form and 100 mL of a liquid containing an extract of chlorella each day for 2 or 3 months. For fibromyalgia patients, assessments of pain and overall quality of life was measured. Daily dietary supplementation with chlorella may reduce high blood pressure, lower serum cholesterol levels, accelerate wound healing, and enhance immune functions. The potential of chlorella to relieve symptoms, improve quality of life, and normalize body functions in patients with fibromyalgia, hypertension, or ulcerative colitis suggests that larger, more comprehensive clinical trials of chlorella are warranted. **Reference:** *Merchant, R. E., et al. A review of recent clinical trials of the nutritional supplement Chlorella pyrenoidosa in the treatment of fibromyalgia, hypertension, & ulcerative colitis. Altern Ther Health Med. 7(3):79-91, 2001.*

Fibromyalgia syndrome is a common, chronic musculoskeletal disorder of unknown aetiology. While available therapy is often disappointing, most patients can be helped with a combination of medication, exercise and maintenance of a regular sleep schedule. The objective of the present study was to determine if adding nutritional supplements derived from the unicellular green alga, Chlorella pyrenoidosa, produced any improvements in the clinical and functional status in patients with moderately severe symptoms of fibromyalgia syndrome. Eligible patients had 2+ palpable tenderness at 11 or more of 18 defined tender points and had a tender point index (TPI) of at least 22. Each day for 2 months, participants consumed two commercially available Chlorella-based products, 10 g of 'Sun Chlorella' tablets and 100 mL of liquid 'Wakasa Gold'. Any amelioration of symptoms was validated and quantified using semi-objective and subjective outcome measures systematically administered at clinic visits on days 0, 30 and 60 of the diet therapy. Eighteen of the 20 patients enrolled completed the 2 month trial. The average TPI for the group which at onset was 32, decreased to a mean of 25 after 2 months. This decrease was statistically significant ($p = 0.01$), representing a 22% decrease in pain intensity. Blood samples taken on each occasion indicated no significant alterations in serum chemistries, formed elements, and circulating lymphocyte subsets. Compilations of the results of patient interviews and self-assessment questionnaires revealed that seven patients felt that the dietary supplement had improved their fibromyalgia symptoms, while six thought they had experienced no change, and five believed the symptoms had worsened over the time of the trial. The results of this pilot study suggest that dietary Chlorella supplementation may help relieve the symptoms of fibromyalgia in some patients and that a larger, more comprehensive double-blind, placebo-controlled clinical trial in these patients is warranted. **References:** *Merchant, R. E., et al. Nutritional supplementation with Chlorella pyrenoidosa for patients with fibromyalgia syndrome: a pilot study. Phytother Res. 14(3):167-173, 2000. -- Departments of Anatomy and Internal Medicine, Virginia Commonwealth Univ, Medical College of Virginia Richmond, VA, USA.*

Aloe vera

Fifty subjects with a physician diagnosis of fibromyalgia and/or chronic fatigue syndrome were interviewed using a structured interview form.

Each subject was interviewed initially, and again nine months later (follow-up). Subjects had, on their own, consumed nutritional supplements including freeze-dried aloe vera gel extract; a combination of freeze-dried aloe vera gel extract and additional plant-derived saccharides; freeze-dried fruits and vegetables in combination with the saccharides; and a formulation of dioscorea complex containing the saccharides and a vitamin/mineral complex. With medical treatments, approximately 25 percent of fibromyalgia patients improve, but the beneficial effects of medical treatment rarely persist more than a few months. All subjects in this study had received some form of medical treatment prior to taking the nutritional supplements, but none with enduring success. Nutritional supplements resulted in a remarkable reduction in initial symptom severity, with continued improvement in the period between initial assessment and the follow-up. **Reference:** *Dykman, K. D., et al. The effects of nutritional supplements on the symptoms of fibromyalgia and chronic fatigue syndrome. Integr Physiol Behav Sci. 33(1):61-71, 1998.*

Ginkgo biloba

An open, uncontrolled study was undertaken to measure the subjective effects of coenzyme Q10 combined with a Ginkgo biloba extract in volunteer subjects with clinically diagnosed fibromyalgia syndrome. Anecdotal reports from patients with fibromyalgia syndrome have claimed benefits from the use of these supplements. The aim of this study was to determine if these reports could be substantiated in a pilot clinical trial. Patient questioning had determined that poor quality of life was a major factor in the condition and a quality-of-life questionnaire was used to measure potential benefit. Subjects were given oral doses of 200 mg coenzyme Q10 and 200 mg Ginkgo biloba extract daily for 84 days. Quality of life was measured, using the well-validated Dartmouth Primary Care Cooperative Information Project/World Organization of Family Doctors (COOP/WONCA) questionnaire that measures seven different subjective responses, at 0-, 4-, 8-, and 12-week intervals. The subjects were asked for an overall self-rating at the end of the study. A progressive improvement in the quality-of-life scores was observed over the study period and at the end, the scores showed a significant difference from those at the start. This was matched by an improvement in self-rating with 64% claiming to be better and only 9% claiming to feel worse. Adverse effects were minor. A controlled study is planned. **Reference:** *Lister, R. E. An open, pilot study to evaluate the potential benefits of coenzyme Q10 combined with Ginkgo biloba extract in fibromyalgia syndrome. J Int Med Res. 30(2):195-199, 2002.*

Saint John's Wort

Atypical depression, somatoform disorder, neurasthenia and fibromyalgia seem to form a spectrum of disorders, who share a common biological basis, i.e. a reduced activity of the hypothalamus-pituitary-adrenocortical (HPA)-system. This is similar to the situation in Cushing's disease, where the central part of the hypothalamus-pituitary-adrenocortical-system is decreased by an increased feedback via increased intracerebral cortisol concentration. Cushing's disease is accompanied by features of atypical depression and of somatisation. Treatment with Hypericum seems to disinhibit the hypothalamus-pituitary-adrenocortical-system in healthy subjects and patients with a depression. Furthermore it decreases intracerebral corticosteroids, possibly by increasing the expression of p-glycoprotein at the blood brain barrier. Therefore hypericum might be especially effective in patients with a symptom cluster of atypical depressive features and somatisation. Clinical studies with patients with depression with atypical features like the seasonal affective disorder (SAD) and with patients with a depressive syndrome accompanied by somatic complaints or fatigue support this view. *Reference: Murck, H., et al. [Atypical depression and related illnesses - neurobiological principles for their treatment with Hypericum extract.] Wien Med Wochenschr. 152(15-16):398-403, 2002.*

Iodine

Recent reports of the World Health Organization show iodine deficiency to be a worldwide occurring health problem. As iodine status is based on median urinary iodine excretion, even in countries regarded as iodine sufficient, a considerable part of the population may be iodine deficient. Iodine is a key element in the synthesis of thyroid hormones and as a consequence, severe iodine deficiency results in hypothyroidism, goiter, and cretinism with the well known biochemical alterations. However, it is also known that iodine deficiency may give rise to clinical symptoms of hypothyroidism without abnormality of thyroid hormone values. This led us to the hypothesis that iodine deficiency may give rise to subtle impairment of thyroid function leading to clinical syndromes resembling hypothyroidism or diseases that have been associated with the occurrence of hypothyroidism. The authors describe several clinical conditions possibly linked to iodine deficiency, a connection that has not been made thus far. In this paper the authors focus on the relationship between iodine deficiency and obesity, attention deficit hyperactivity disorder (ADHD), psychiatric disorders including depression, fibromyalgia, and malignancies. *Reference: Verheeesen, R. H., et al. Iodine deficiency, more than cretinism and goiter. Med Hypotheses. 71(5):645-648, 2008.*

Magnesium

Primary fibromyalgia (FM) is a common clinical condition affecting mainly middle-aged women. Of the etiologies previously proposed, chronic hypoxia seems the one best supported by recent biochemical and histological findings. The authors postulate that FM symptoms are predominantly caused by enhanced gluconeogenesis with breakdown of muscle proteins, resulting from a deficiency of oxygen and other substances needed for ATP synthesis. The authors present data supporting a critical role for magnesium and malate in ATP production under aerobic and hypoxic conditions; and indirect evidence for magnesium and malate deficiency in FM. After treating 15 FM patients for an average of 8 weeks with an oral dosage form with dosages of 1200 -

335

2400 mg of malate and 300 - 600 mg of magnesium, the tender point index (TPI) scores (x +/-SE) were 19 6 +/- 2 1 prior to treatment and 8 +/- 1.1 and 6.5 +/- 0.74, respectively, after an average of 4 and 8 weeks on the magnesium malate combination (p<0.001). Subjective improvement of myalgia occurred within 48 hours of supplementation. In six FM patients, following 8 weeks of treatment, the mean TPI was 6.8 +/- 0.75. After 2 weeks on placebo tablets, the TPI values increased to a mean +/- SE of 21.5 +/- 1.4 (p<0-001). Again, subjective worsening of muscle pain occurs within 48 h of placebo administration. A double-blind placebo control trial is currently underway. *Reference: Abraham, G. E., et al. Mgmt fibromyalgia: rationale for the use of magnesium and malic acid. J Nutr Med. 3:49-59, 1992.*

Fibromyalgia patients were found to have low red blood cell levels of magnesium. This low magnesium status was linked to abnormal metabolism of vitamin B1. *Reference: Eisinger, J., et al. Selenium & magnesium status in fibromyalgia. Magn. Research. 7(3-4):285-288, 1994.*

Reduced erythrocyte magnesium levels have been reported in fibromyalgia patients. *Reference: Romano, T. J. Magnesium deficiency in systemic lupus erythematosus. Journ Nutr & Envir Med. 107-111, 1997.*

The authors examined the association between serum trace elements and clinical findings such as number of sensitive tender points, severity of fatigue and functional status in patients with fibromyalgia (FM). Thirty-two patients diagnosed as having FM according to the ACR 1990 criteria and 32 normal healthy controls (NHC) were included in this study. The demographic data, disease duration, number of tender points and accompanying symptoms (fatigue, sleep disorders, headache, paresthesia, irritable bowel syndrome, sicca symptoms, Raynaud's phenomena) of the patients were noted. Visual analog scale (10 cm) was implemented to estimate daily severity of pain and fatigue. Fibromyalgia impact questionnaire was used for functional assessment. Serum selenium (microg/dL) and serum zinc (microg/dL) levels were measured by atomic absorption spectrometer. Serum magnesium (mmol/L) level was measured by the original kits of Abbott Aeroset auto-analyzer. The mean age of patients in FM group and NHC were calculated as 42.9 (SD = 7.7) years and 41.3 (SD = 9.7) years, respectively. Serum levels of zinc (P = 0.001) and magnesium (P = 0.002) were significantly decreased in FM groups, whereas there was no considerable difference with selenium levels of both groups (P > 0.05). Association between serum zinc level and number of tender points (P = 0.008) and that between fatigue and magnesium level (P = 0.003) was found as meaningful. According to the results of this study, it was asserted that serum magnesium and zinc levels may play an important role in the pathophysiology of FM. *Reference: Sendur, O. F., et al. The relationship between serum trace element levels and clinical parameters in patients with fibromyalgia. Rheumatol Int. 28(11):1117-1121, 2008.*

Coenzyme Q10

Coenzyme Q10 (CoQ(10)) is an essential electron carrier in the mitochondrial respiratory chain and a strong antioxidant. Signs and symptoms associated with muscular alteration and mitochondrial dysfunction, including oxidative stress, have been observed in patients with fibromyalgia (FM). The aim was to study CoQ(10) levels in plasma and mononuclear cells, and oxidative stress in FM patients. The authors studied CoQ(10) level by HPLC in plasma and peripheral mononuclear cells obtained from patients with FM and healthy control subjects. Oxidative stress markers were analyzed in both plasma and mononuclear cells from FM patients. Higher level of oxidative stress markers in plasma was observed respect to control subjects. CoQ(10) level in plasma samples from FM patients was doubled compared to healthy controls and in blood mononuclear cells isolated from 37 FM patients was found to be about 40% lower. Higher levels of ROS production was observed in mononuclear cells from FM patients compared to control, and a significant decrease was induced by the presence of CoQ(10). The distribution of CoQ(10) in blood components was altered in FM patients. Also, the results confirm the oxidative stress background of this disease probably due to a defect on the distribution and metabolism of CoQ(10) in cells and tissues. The protection caused in mononuclear cells by CoQ(10) would indicate the benefit of its supplementation in FM patients. *Reference: Cordero, M. D., et al. Coenzyme Q10 distribution in blood is altered in patients with fibromyalgia. Clin Biochem. 2008.*

An open, uncontrolled study was undertaken to measure the subjective effects of coenzyme Q10 combined with a Ginkgo biloba extract in volunteer subjects with clinically diagnosed fibromyalgia syndrome. Anecdotal reports from patients with fibromyalgia syndrome have claimed benefits from the use of these supplements. The aim of this study was to determine if these reports could be substantiated in a pilot clinical trial. Patient questioning had determined that poor quality of life was a major factor in the condition and a quality-of-life questionnaire was used to measure potential benefit. Subjects were given oral doses of 200 mg coenzyme Q10 and 200 mg Ginkgo biloba extract daily for 84 days. Quality of life was measured, using the well-validated Dartmouth Primary Care Cooperative Information Project/World Organization of Family Doctors (COOP/WONCA) questionnaire that measures seven different subjective responses, at 0-, 4-, 8-, and 12-week intervals. The subjects were asked for an overall self-rating at the end of the study. A progressive improvement in the quality-of-life scores was observed over the study period and at the end, the scores showed a significant difference from those at the start. This was matched by an improvement in self-rating with 64% claiming to be better and only 9% claiming to feel worse. Adverse effects were minor. A controlled study is planned. *Reference: Lister, R. E. An open, pilot study to evaluate the potential benefits of coenzyme Q10 combined with Ginkgo biloba extract in fibromyalgia syndrome. J Int Med Res. 30(2):195-199, 2002.*

GOUT

Chrysin

That flavonoids inhibit xanthine oxidase from cow milk was confirmed by measuring oxygen consumption with an oxygen electrode. In contrast, flavonoids did not inhibit glucose oxidase, another oxygen consuming enzyme. Among the flavonoids tested, quercetin, kaempferol, myricetin, chrysin, quercitrin, and morin were potent inhibitors of xanthine oxidase; their inhibition rates (%) were 80, 70, 69, 62, 59, and 51 at 100 microM (except chrysin at 50 microM), respectively. The xanthine oxidase-inhibiting activities of the flavonoids were not always well correlated with the suppressive activities of the flavonoids on cytochrome c reduction by a xanthine-xanthine oxidase system. The inhibition of xanthine oxidase by quercetin was not affected by cupric ion. The partition rates of the flavonoids between n-butanol and a buffer solution seemed to account for some of the inhibition. *Reference: Lio, M., et al. Effects of flavonoids on xanthine oxidation as well as on cytochrome c reduction by milk xanthine oxidase. J Nutr Sci Vitaminol (Tokyo). 32(6):635-642, 1986.*

Various dietary flavonoids were evaluated in vitro for their inhibitory effect on xanthine oxidase, which has been implicated in oxidative injury to tissue by ischemia-reperfusion. Xanthine oxidase activity was determined by directly measuring uric acid formation by HPLC. The structure-activity relationship revealed that the planar flavones and flavonols with a 7-hydroxyl group such as chrysin, luteolin, kaempferol, quercetin, myricetin, and isorhamnetin inhibited xanthine oxidase activity at low concentrations (IC50 values from 0.40 to 5.02 microM) in a mixed-type mode, while the nonplanar flavonoids, isoflavones and anthocyanidins were less inhibitory. These results suggest that certain flavonoids might suppress in vivo the formation of active oxygen species and urate by xanthine oxidase. *References: Nagao, A., et al. Inhibition of xanthine oxidase by flavonoids. Biosci Biotechnol Biochem. 63(10):1787-1790, 1999. -- National Food Research Institute, Ministry of Agriculture, Forestry and Fisheries, Tsukuba, Ibaraki, Japan.*

A known and a new caffeic ester (1 and 2), new inhibitors of xanthine oxidase (XO), were isolated from leaves of Perilla frutescens var. acuta and their structures have been established as (Z,E)-2-(3,4-dihydroxy-phenyl)ethenyl ester (1) and (Z,E)-2-(3,5-dihydroxyphenyl)ethenyl ester (2) of 3-(3,4-dihydroxyphenyl)-2-propenoic acid, respectively, based on detailed spectral studies, including 2D COSY, long range COSY, difference NOE, etc. Both caffeic esters strongly inhibited XO in vitro and especially, the inhibition by 1 was as potent as that by allopurinol. The inhibition mode of 1 was also shown to be non-competitive. *References: Nakanishi, T., et al. Two new potent inhibitors of xanthine oxidase from leaves of Perilla frutescens Britton var. acuta Kudo. Chem Pharm*

Bull. 38(6):1772-1774, 1990. -- Faculty of Pharmaceutical Sciences, Setsunan University, Osaka, Japan.

Rhododendron caucasicum

Clinical studies at the hospital demonstrated that when as few as 2 to 3 doses of Rhododendron caucasicum were administered to gout patients, relief occurred shortly thereafter. According to the results of the clinical trials performed by Prof. Rossiski (170 volunteers with severe attacks of gout), the extract of Rhododendron caucasicum increased the discharge of uric acid. His study showed that a few hours after 5 to 6 doses, the pain and disagreeable symptoms associated with gout were relieved. In another clinical study, on humans, 150 mg of Rhododendron caucasicum extract were given to 320 gout patients. After administration of the test dose, the average discharge of uric acid increased by between 35% and 60% and in a few hours, the pain and disagreeable symptoms disappeared. They found that when the treatment was continued over several days, the symptoms of gout significantly decreased, and it helped to prevent future attacks of gout. *Reference: Samartzev, A. D., et al. Effect of Rhododendron caucasicum extract on gout and sodium release in urine. Russian clinical research, Dagestan Scientific Publisher, 112 pages, 1965.*

Skullcap

Baicalein, at 10 µM inhibited xanthine oxidase by 64% in vitro, while the standard gout medication allopurinol showed 43% inhibition at this concentration. *Reference: Chang, W., et al. Inhibitory effects of flavonoids on xanthine oxidase. Anticancer Res. 13:2165-2170, 1993.*

Cherry juice

This study involved 12 gout patients consuming 227 grams of cherries (or the equivalent quantity of cherry juice) for 3 days to 3 months. Cherries were found to prevent gout attacks. The types of cherries found to be effective included black, red sour and sweet yellow cherries. *Reference: Blau, L. W. Cherry diet control for gout and arthritis. TX Report on Biology & Medicine. 8(3):309-311, 1950.*

To assess the physiologic effects of cherry consumption, the authors measured plasma urate, antioxidant and inflammatory markers in 10 healthy women who consumed Bing sweet cherries. The women, age 22-40 years, consumed two servings (280 g) of cherries after an overnight fast. Blood and urine samples were taken before the cherry dose, and at 1.5, 3 and 5 h postdose. Plasma urate decreased 5 h postdose, mean +/- SEM = 183 +/- 15 micro mol/L compared with predose baseline of 214 +/- 13 micro mol/L ($P < 0.05$). Urinary urate increased postdose, with peak excretion of 350 +/- 33 micro mol/mmol creatinine 3 h postdose compared with 202 +/- 13 at baseline ($P < 0.01$). Plasma C-reactive protein (CRP) and nitric oxide (NO) concentrations had decreased marginally 3 h postdose ($P < 0.1$), whereas plasma albumin and tumor necrosis factor-alpha were unchanged. The vitamin C content of the cherries was solely as dehydroascorbic acid, but postdose increases in plasma ascorbic acid indicated that dehydroascorbic acid in fruits is bioavailable as vitamin C. The decrease in plasma urate after cherry consumption supports the reputed anti-gout efficacy of cherries. The trend toward decreased inflammatory indices (CRP and NO) adds to the in vitro evidence that compounds in cherries may inhibit inflammatory pathways. **Reference**: *Jacob, R. A., et al. Consumption of cherries lowers plasma urate in healthy women. Journal of Nutrition. 133(6):1826-1829, 2003.*

HEADACHES

Cayenne Pepper (Capsaicin)

Preliminary studies have shown that repeated nasal applications of capsaicin prevented the occurrence of cluster headache attacks. The present study was designed to verify the difference in efficacy of treatment with nasal capsaicin, depending on the side of application. Fifty-two patients affected by episodic form were divided into 2 groups, one receiving the treatment on the same side where the attacks occurred (ipsilateral side), the other on the controlateral side. Eighteen patients with a chronic form alternately received both ipsilateral and controlateral treatments. Seventy percent of the episodic patients, treated on the ipsilateral side, showed a marked amelioration whereas no improvement was noted in the patients treated on the contralateral side. The efficacy of ipsilateral treatment was emphasized by the results obtained in chronic patients. However, in these patients, the maximum period of amelioration lasted no more than 40 days. The difference between the effects of the two treatments (contralateral and ipsilateral) was statistically significant in both episodic and chronic sufferers. The efficacy of repeated nasal applications of capsaicin in cluster headache is congruent with previous reports on the therapeutic effect of capsaicin in other pain syndromes (post-herpetic neuralgia, diabetic neuropathy, trigeminal neuralgia) and supports the use of the drug to produce a selective analgesia. **Reference**: *Fusco B. M., et al. Preventative effect of repeated nasal applications of capsaicin in cluster headache. Pain. 59(3):321-325, 1994.*

This double-blind, placebo-controlled study found that 70% of cluster headache patients benefited when capsaicin was applied to the nostril on the same side of the head as the headache and when capsaicin was applied to the opposite nostril, patients did not improve. **Reference**: *Marks, D.R., et al. A double-blind placebo-controlled trial of intranasal capsaicin for cluster headache. Cephalalgia. 13 (2):114-116, 1993. -- Clinical Immunology Unit, Massachusetts General Hospital, Boston, USA.*

Recent studies support the role of extracranial perivascular afferents in a substantial percentage of migraineurs. Perivascular afferent fibres of the superficial temporal artery contain peptides, like calcitonin gene-related peptide (CGRP) and substance P (SP). CGRP and SP are considered relevant in the genesis of migraine pain. Capsaicin is an agonist of the transient receptor potential vanilloid type 1. It causes membrane depolarisation of sensory neurons, which release CGRP, SP and other pain peptides; excitation is followed by a refractory state, causing inactivation. Topical capsaicin has been found to be efficacious in several types of neuropathic pain. The authors attempted to verify whether topical periarterial capsaicin could ameliorate pain in absence of and during a migraine attack. On 23 migraineurs showing pain at pressure on scalp arteries, the authors administered topical capsaicin 0.1% or vaseline jelly on painful arteries in absence of migraine attack. In those having pain reduction > 50%, the authors made the same comparison during a migraine attack. Topical capsaicin caused > 50% reduction of arterial pain in absence of attack in 17/23 patients, as opposed to two with vaseline. During attacks of mild- to moderate-intensity, > 50% improvement was obtained in 11/17 with capsaicin and in one with vaseline. Although referring to a small number of patients, these data show that topical capsaicin may relieve arterial pain in absence of and during a migraine attack in a substantial number of patients experiencing scalp arterial tenderness. More active capsacinoids might be tried in the future and could provide a new method for treating migraine attacks. *Reference: Cianchetti, C. Capsaicin jelly against migraine pain. Int J Clin Pract. 64(4):457-459, 2010.*

Feverfew and Ginger

Treatment of migraine headaches is often delayed due to assessing the potential severity of an evolving headache or anticipating unwanted consequences from prescription medication. Studies have demonstrated improved pain-free response when prescription treatments are taken during the mild headache phase of a migraine. This study was designed to evaluate the efficacy of an OTC product, GelStat Migraine((R)), when taken in the early, mild pain phase of migraine. An open-label study enrolling 30 subjects, male and female, with a one-year history of migraine meeting IHS diagnostic criteria with or without aura, 2-8 migraines per month and 15 headache days per month. Inclusion required having migraines that consistently started at mild and worsened to moderate or severe, if untreated, in at least 75% of attacks. Subjects also had to be able to distinguish migraine from non-migraine headaches and reliably identify migraine early in the course of an attack. One headache was treated in the mild pain phase with GelStat Migraine((R)), a combination of feverfew and ginger. 29 evaluable subjects completed the study, all treating at mild pain. Two hours after treatment, 48% were pain-free with 34% reporting a headache of only mild severity. 29% reported a recurrence within 24 hours. Side effects were minimal and not serious. 59% of subjects were satisfied with Gelstat Migraine((R)) therapy and 41% preferred GelStat Migraine((R)) or felt it was equal to their pre-study medication. GelStat Migraine((R)) is effective as a first line abortive treatment for migraine when initiated early during the mild headache phase. *References: Cady, R. K., et al. Gelstat Migraine (sublingually administered feverfew and ginger compound) for acute treatment of migraine when administered during the mild pain phase. Med Sci Monit. 11(9):PPI65-PI69, 2005. -- Clinvest, Inc., Springfield and Headache Care Center, Springfield, Missouri, U.S.A.*

Migraine is considered as a neurological disorder with little convincing evidence of the involvement of some vascular phenomenon. Recent understanding of the mechanisms behind migraine pain generation and perception have considerably helped the development of modern migraine drugs. Most migraine drugs in use, i.e., ergotamine and dihydroergotamine, iprazochrome, pizotifen and diazepam; and non-steroidal anti-inflammatory drugs (i.e. aspirin, paracetamol, persantin, etc.) have side-effects and are prescribed with caution for a limited duration. Ginger is reported in Ayurvedic and Tibb systems of medicine to be useful in neurological disorders. It is proposed that administration of ginger may exert abortive and prophylactic effects in migraine headache without any side-effects. *Reference: Srivasta, K. C., et al. Ginger (Zingiber officinale) in migraine headache. J Ethnopharmacol. 29(3):267-273, 1992.*

The efficacy and tolerability of a CO(2)-extract of feverfew (MIG-99, 6.25 mg t.i.d.) for migraine prevention were investigated in a randomized, double-blind, placebo-controlled, multicentre, parallel-group study. Patients (N = 170 intention-to-treat; MIG-99, N = 89; placebo, N = 81) suffering from migraine according to International Headache Society criteria were treated for 16 weeks after a 4-week baseline period. The primary endpoint was the average number of migraine attacks per 28 days during the treatment months 2 and 3 compared with baseline. Safety parameters included adverse events, laboratory parameters, vital signs and physical examination. The migraine frequency decreased from 4.76 to 1.9 attacks per month in the MIG-99 group and by 1.3 attacks in the placebo group (P = 0.0456). Logistic regression of responder rates showed an odds ratio of 3.4 in favour of MIG-99 (P = 0.0049). Adverse events possibly related to study medication were 9/107 (8.4%) with MIG-99 and 11/108 (10.2%) with placebo (P = 0.654). MIG-99 is effective and shows a favourable benefit-risk ratio. *Reference: Diener, H. C., et al. Efficacy and safety of 6.25 mg t.i.d. feverfew CO2-extract (MIG-99) in migraine prevention - a randomized, double-blind, multicentre, placebo-controlled study. Cephalagia. 25(11):1031-1041, 2005.*

Seventeen patients who ate fresh leaves of feverfew daily as prophylaxis against migraine participated in a double blind placebo controlled trial of the herb: 8 patients received capsules containing freeze dried feverfew powder and 9 placebo. Those who received placebo had a significant increase in the frequency and severity of headache, nausea, and vomiting with the emergence of untoward effects during the early months of treatment. The group given capsules of feverfew showed no change in the frequency or severity of symptoms of migraine. This provides evidence that feverfew taken prophylactically prevents attacks of migraine, and confirmatory studies are now indicated, preferably with a formulation controlled for sesquiterpene lactone content, in migraine sufferers who have never treated themselves with this herb. *Reference: Johnson, E. S., et al. Efficacy of feverfew as prophylactic treatment of migraine. British Medical Journal. 291(6495):569-573, 1985.*

Feverfew has been used since antiquity to treat fevers and other inflammatory conditions. Feverfew extracts were found to inhibit ADP, thrombin, or collagen-induced aggregation of human platelets, but significantly, did not affect aggregation induced by arachidonic acid. Synthesis of thromboxane B2 from exogenous 14C-arachidonic acid was also not inhibited. Washed platelets prelabelled with 14C-AA responded normally to thrombin by releasing 14C-TXB2. This was completely blocked by feverfew. A purified platelet phospholipase A2 was inhibited by the material with an I50 of 0.1 antiplatelet units. The pharmacological properties of feverfew may thus be due to an inhibitor of cellular phospholipases, which prevents release of arachidonic acid in response to appropriate physiological stimuli. *Reference: Makheja, A. N., et al. A platelet phospholipase inhibitor from the medicinal herb feverfew (tanacetum parthenium). Prostaglandins, Leukotrienes & Med. 8(6):653-660, 1982.*

The use of feverfew (Tanacetum parthenium) for migraine prophylaxis was assessed in a randomised, double-blind, placebo-controlled crossover study. After a one-month single-blind placebo run-in, 72 volunteers were randomly allocated to receive either one capsule of dried feverfew leaves a day or matching placebo for four months and then transferred to the other treatment limb for a further four months. Frequency and severity of attacks were determined from diary cards which were issued every two months; efficacy of each treatment was also assessed by visual analogue scores. 60 patients completed the study and full information was available in 59. Treatment with feverfew was associated with a reduction in the mean number and severity of attacks in each two-month period, and in the degree of vomiting; duration of individual attacks was unaltered. Visual analogue scores also indicated a significant improvement with feverfew. There were no serious side-effects. *References: Murphy, J. J., et al. Randomized double-blind placebo-controlled trial of feverfew in migraine prevention. Lancet. 2(8604):189-192, 1988. -- Department of Medicine, University Hospital, Nottingham.*

To assess the effectivness of feverfew for the treatment of migraine, this clinical trial was conducted over a period of four months. 57 chronic migraine sufferers (43% of whom experienced more than ten attacks per month) were selected at random and divided into two groups. Both groups received feverfew (100 mg per day of dried leaves containing 0.2 mg pathenolide) in the preliminary phase that lasted for two months. In the second and third phases, which continued for an additional two months, a double-blind, placebo-controlled, crossover study was conducted. Results in phase 2 demonstrated that feverfew caused a significant reduction in pain and intensity of migraine compared with placebo. A significant reduction in typical migraine symptoms was observed (vomiting, nausea and sensitivity to noise and light). Transferring the feverfew group to placebo in phase 3 resulted in increased pain intensity and other symptoms. *Reference: Palevitch, E., et al. Phytotherapy Research. 11:508-511, 1997.*

Feverfew has been used in traditional medicine in the treatment of migraine for a long time. In 1985 researchers positive results of prophylactic use of this herb in migraine. Since 1994 through 1996 the authors studied in their Centre of Migraine Therapy the efficacy of feverfew in migraine treatment. The authors had 24 patients (women 19-61 years old) in their group. The drug was administered once daily (5 ml of the sap) for 30-60 days. The authors observed significant reduction of Migraine Index in 8 patients, less significant in additional 5. Feverfew may be beneficial in migraine prophylaxis as an additive drug. Further controlled studies need to be done, especially to establish the optimal dose of the drug. **Reference**: *Prusinski, A., et al. [Feverfew as a prophylactic treatment of migraine.] Neurol Neurochir Pol. 33(Supplement 5):89-95, 1999.*

Tanacetum parthenium (TP) is a member of the Asteracee family long used empirically as a herbal remedy for migraine. So far, however, clinical trials have failed to prove consistently the effectiveness of TP extracts in preventing migraine attacks, probably as a consequence of the uncertainty as regards the active principle. In this study, the biological effects of different TP extracts and purified parthenolide were tested in an animal model of migraine based on the quantification of neuronal activation induced by nitroglycerin. The extract enriched in parthenolide significantly reduced nitroglycerin-induced Fos expression in the nucleus trigeminalis caudalis. Purified parthenolide inhibited nitroglycerin-induced neuronal activation in additional brain nuclei and, significantly, the activity of nuclear factor-kappaB. These findings strongly suggest that parthenolide is the component responsible for the biological activity of TP as regards its antimigraine effect and provide important information for future controlled clinical trials. **Reference**: *Tassorelli, C., et al. Parthenolide is the component of tanacetum parthenium that inhibits nitroglycerin-induced Fos activation: studies in an animal model of migraine. Cephalagia. 25(8):612-621, 2005. -- Laboratory of Pathophysiology of Integrative Autonomic Systems, IRCCS Neurological Institute C. Mondino Foundation and University Centre for the Study of Adaptive Disorder and Headache, Pavia, Italy.*

Feverfew may be effective against migraines via prostaglandin-inhibiting effects. A more likely explanation is the ability of feverfew to interact with the protein kinase C pathway resulting in an inhibition of granule secretion from platelets (this would cause an anti-migraine effect). **Reference**: *Bone, K. Feverfew and migraine. Mediherb Newsletter. October 1987.*

HEMORRHOIDS

Psyllium

The aim of this study was to assess the role of micronized purified flavonidic fraction in the management of bleeding nonprolapsed hemorrhoids. Patients were randomly assigned to receive psyllium seed husk alone, rubber band ligation plus psyllium seed husk, or micronized purified flavonidic fraction plus ispaghula husk. Other colorectal diseases were excluded by colonoscopy. Blinded observers noted the time for bleeding to stop completely, recurrences, and treatment complications. A total of 162 patients were randomly assigned with no significant differences in the age and gender distributions among the groups. Hemorrhoidal bleeding was relieved most expediently in the micronized purified flavonidic fraction plus psyllium seed husk group (psyllium seed husk alone n = 66, mean (standard error of the mean) 10.6 (2.3) days; rubber band ligation plus psyllium seed husk n = 57, 5.6 (1.1) days; micronized purified flavonidic fraction plus psyllium seed husk n = 39, 3.9 (1.2) days; P = 0.03). However, there were no significant differences in the recurrences at six months of follow-up (psyllium seed husk alone n = 8 (12 percent); rubber band ligation plus psyllium seed husk n = 12 (21 percent); micronized purified flavonidic fraction plus psyllium seed husk n = 2 (5.1 percent); P = 0.075). No complications or side-effects were noted. Micronized purified flavonidic fraction used with fiber supplements rapidly and safely relieved bleeding from nonprolapsed hemorrhoids. **Reference**: *Ho. Y. H., et al. Micronized purified flavonidic fraction compared favorably with rubber band ligation and fiber alone in the management of bleeding hemorrhoids:random controlled trial. Dis Colon Rectum.43(1):66-69, 2000.*

The aim of this study is to assess prospectively the effect of fiber additions on internal bleeding hemorrhoids. Fifty patients with bleeding internal hemorrhoids are studied and randomized in two groups. Patients in the study group were treated with a commercially available preparation of Plantago Ovata and those in the control group were treated with a placebo. Endoscopy was performed on every patient before and after treatment to establish: a) the degree of hemorrhoidal prolapse, b) the number of congested hemorrhoidal cushions and c) contact bleeding hemorrhoids. During the 15 days of treatment, the average number of bleeding episodes was 4.8 +/- 3.8 for the study group versus 6.4 +/- 3 for the control group (n.s.). During the following 15 days, it decreased to 3.1 +/- 2.7 in the study group versus 5.5 +/- 3.2 (p < 0.05) in the control group and in the last 10 days of treatment a further reduction to 1.1 +/- 1.4 was found in the study group versus 5.5 +/- 2.9 (p < 0.001). The number of congested hemorrhoidal cushions diminished from 2.6 +/- 1 to 1.6 +/- 2.2 after fiber treatment (p < 0.01) and no differences were found in the control group. In the fiber group, hemorrhoids bled on contact in 5 out of 22 patients before treatment and in none after treatment; no differences were found in the control group. No modification of the degree of prolapse was observed after treatment. Addition of dietary fiber may improve internal bleeding hemorrhoids although with no immediate effect. Fiber addition should be ensured in patients who refuse invasive treatment, waiting for a more defined form of treatment, or with contraindications. *Reference: Perez-Miranda, M., et al. Effect of fiber supplements on internal bleeding hemorrhoids. Hepatogastroenterology. 43(12):1504-1507, 1996.*

Horse Chestnut

Horse chestnut's ability to alleviate hemorrhoids may involve its ability to inhibit elastase and hyaluronidase. *Reference: Mackay, D. Hemorrhoids and varicose veins: a review of treatment options. Alternative Medicine Review. 6(2):126-140, 2001.*

This double-blind, placebo-controlled trial, demonstrated that horse chestnut seed extract (HCSE) (40-mg aescin tablet three times daily for two months) given to patients with acute symptomatic hemorrhoids significantly improved symptoms, endoscopic evaluation, and bleeding after less than a week of treatment. Of 38 patients receiving aescin, 31 (82%) reported significant improvement in symptoms (pain, itching, burning, swelling), compared to only 11 of 34 (32%) in the placebo group. Endoscopic evaluation revealed significantly decreased bleeding in 26 patients taking aescin compared to 13 in the placebo group, as well as decreased swelling in 29 patients taking aescin compared to 12 in the placebo group. Average time to symptom improvement was six days for the aescin group. *Reference: Pirard, J., et al. Rev Med Liege. 31(10):343-345, 1976. -- Monograph: Aesculus hippocastanum (Horse chestnut). Alternative Medicine Review. 14(3):278-283, 2009.*

Buthcher's Broom

In this open trial, 75% of physicians rated butcher's broom's efficacy for the treatment of acute hemorrhoids as good or excellent. *Reference: Bennani, A., et al. Acute attack of hemorrhoids: efficacy of Cyclo 3 Forte [R] based on results in 124 cases. Phlebologie. 52:89-93, 1999.*

Several botanical extracts have been shown to improve microcirculation, capillary flow, and vascular tone, and to strengthen the connective tissue of the perivascular amorphous substrate.   Oral supplementation with Ruscus aculeatus (butcher's broom) may prevent time-consuming, painful, & expensive complications of hemorrhoids. *Reference:Chabanon, R. Experimentation du Proctolog dans les hemorroides et les fissures anales. Gaz Med De France. 83:3013, 1976. Mackay, D. Hemorrhoids & varicose veins: a review of treatment options. Alt Med Review. 6(2):126-140, 2001.*

Grape Seed (extract)

Grape seed extract (150 - 300 mg per day) alleviates/prevents hemorrhoids by inhibiting the collagenase enzyme that damages the blood vessels of the walls of the anus that occurs in hemorrhoids. **Reference**: *Clouatre, D. All about Grape seed Extract. Avery Publishing Group. Garden City, New York, USA. 1998:56-57.*

INFLUENZA ("THE FLU")

Elderberry extract

Sambucus nigra L. products - Sambucol - are based on a standardized black elderberry extract. They are natural remedies with antiviral properties, especially against different strains of influenza virus. Sambucol was shown to be effective in vitro against 10 strains of influenza virus. In a double-blind, placebo-controlled, randomized study, Sambucol reduced the duration of flu symptoms to 3-4 days. Convalescent phase serum showed a higher antibody level to influenza virus in the Sambucol group, than in the control group. The present study aimed to assess the effect of Sambucol products on the healthy immune system - namely, its effect on cytokine production. The production of inflammatory cytokines was tested using blood - derived monocytes from 12 healthy human donors. Adherent monocytes were separated from PBL and incubated with different Sambucol preparations i.e., Sambucol Elderberry Extract, Sambucol Black Elderberry Syrup, Sambucol Immune System and Sambucol for Kids. Production of inflammatory cytokines (IL-1 beta, TNF-alpha, IL-6, IL-8) was significantly increased, mostly by the Sambucol Black Elderberry Extract (2-45 fold), as compared to LPS, a known monocyte activator (3.6-10.7 fold). The most striking increase was noted in TNF-alpha production (44.9 fold). We conclude from this study that, in addition to its antiviral properties, Sambucol Elderberry Extract and its formulations activate the healthy immune system by increasing inflammatory cytokine production. Sambucol might therefore be beneficial to the immune system activation and in the inflammatory process in healthy individuals or in patients with various diseases. Sambucol could also have an immunoprotective or immunostimulatory effect when administered to cancer or AIDS patients, in conjunction with chemotherapeutic or other treatments. In view of the increasing popularity of botanical supplements, such studies and investigations in vitro, in vivo and in clinical trials need to be developed. *Reference:* *Eur Cytokine Netw. 2001 Apr-Jun;12(2):290-6. The effect of Sambucol, a black elderberry-based, natural product, on the production of human cytokines: I. Inflammatory cytokines. Barak V, Halperin T, Kalickman I. Immunology Laboratory for Tumor Diagnosis, Department of Oncology, Hadassah University Hosp, Jerusalem, Israel. PMID: 11399518.*

Background- Black elderberries (Sambucus nigra L.) are well known as supportive agents against common cold and influenza. It is further known that bacterial super-infection during an influenza virus (IV) infection can lead to severe pneumonia. We have analyzed a standardized elderberry extract (Rubini, BerryPharma AG) for its antimicrobial and antiviral activity using the microtitre broth micro-dilution assay against three Gram-positive bacteria and one Gram-negative bacteria responsible for infections of the upper respiratory tract, as well as cell culture experiments for two different strains of influenza virus. **Methods-** The antimicrobial activity of the elderberry extract was determined by bacterial growth experiments in liquid cultures using the extract at concentrations of 5%, 10%, 15% and 20%. The inhibitory effects were determined by plating the bacteria on agar plates. In addition, the inhibitory potential of the extract on the propagation of human pathogenic H5N1-type influenza A virus isolated from a patient and an influenza B virus strain was investigated using MTT and focus assays. **Results-** For the first time, it was shown that a standardized elderberry liquid extract possesses antimicrobial activity against both Gram-positive bacteria of Streptococcus pyogenes and group C and G Streptococci, and the Gram-negative bacterium Branhamella catarrhalis in liquid cultures. The liquid extract also displays an inhibitory effect on the propagation of human pathogenic influenza viruses. **Conclusion-** Rubini elderberry liquid extract is active against human pathogenic bacteria as well as influenza viruses. The activities shown suggest that additional and alternative approaches to combat infections might be provided by this natural product. Licorice root contains a compound called "glycyrrhizin" that has been found to have pretty potent antiviral effects against serious diseases (such as HIV and SARS) and a number of studies have found that licorice root extracts can fight off the flu, including strains of the avian flu virus. **CAUTION:** The compounds found in licorice root cause the body to eliminate potassium, for this reason a potassium supplement is recommended during its use. For many years it has been known that the polyphenols in green tea polyphenols actively suppress many strains of the influenza virus. EGCG, one of the main polyphenols in green tea, is mainly responsible for this suppression. ECGC binds to the haemagglutinin of the influenza virus, which blocks it from attaching to (and infecting) target receptor cells, and EGCG also alters the virus cell membrane, which further inhibits its ability to infect other cells. Another important component of green tea is the amino acid L-theanine, which has been shown to cause a specific type of lymphocyte ("gamma-delta T-cells") to proliferate and make interferon-gamma (a potent antimicrobial cytokine). *Reference: BMC Complement Altern Med. 2011; 11: 16. Published online 2011 February 25. doi: 10.1186/1472-6882-11-16. Inhibitory activity of a standardized elderberry liquid extract against clinically-relevant human respiratory bacterial pathogens and influenza A & B viruses. Christian Krawitz, Mobarak Abu Mraheil, Michael Stein, Can Imirzalioglu, Eugen Domann, Stephan Pleschka, Torsten Hain.*

Chimpanzees given Sambucol orally, as either a prophylactic or as a symptom-dependent treatment experienced fewer flu-like, upper respiratory ailments than chimpanzees administered a placebo. During the first fall and winter "flu season" of the study, five chimpanzees in an experimental group received 10 ml of Sambucol daily, while five chimpanzees constituting a control group received sugar syrup. When chimpanzees in the experimental group exhibited flu-like symptoms, they received an increased dose of Sambucol, 15 ml, twice daily. During the six months of the trial, the control group exhibited flu-like symptoms over a total of 39 days, whereas the experimental group had symptoms for a total of 12 days. During the second flu season, chimpanzees were strictly treated symptomatically with 15 ml of Sambucol twice daily. Symptoms lasted for fewer than 24 hours in all animals treated symptomatically. *Reference: Burge, B., et al. The effect of Sambucol on flu-like symptoms in chimpanzees: prophylactic and symptom-dependent treatment. International Zoo News. 46(1):16-19, 1999.*

An ionization technique in mass spectrometry called Direct Analysis in Real Time Mass Spectrometry (DART TOF-MS) coupled with a Direct Binding Assay was used to identify and characterize anti-viral components of an elderberry fruit (Sambucus nigra L.) extract without either derivatization or separation by standard chromatographic techniques. The elderberry extract inhibited Human Influenza A (H1N1) infection in vitro with an IC(50) value of 252+/-34 microg/mL. The Direct Binding Assay established that flavonoids from the elderberry extract bind to H1N1 virions and, when bound, block the ability of the viruses to infect host cells. Two compounds were identified, 5,7,3',4'-tetra-O-methylquercetin (1) and 5,7-dihydroxy-4-oxo-2-(3,4,5-trihydroxyphenyl) chroman-3-yl-3,4,5-trihydroxy-cyclohexanecarboxylate (2), as H1N1-bound chemical species. Compound 1 and dihydromyricetin (3), the corresponding 3-hydroxy-flavonone of 2, were synthesized and shown to inhibit H1N1 infection in vitro by binding to H1N1 virions, blocking host cell entry and/or recognition. Compound 1 gave an IC(50) of 0.13 microg/mL (0.36 microM) for H1N1 infection inhibition, while dihydromyricetin (3) achieved an IC(50) of 2.8 microg/mL (8.7 microM). The H1N1 inhibition activities of the elderberry flavonoids compare favorably to the known anti-influenza activities of Oseltamivir (Tamiflu; 0.32 microM) and Amantadine (27 microM). *Reference: Roschek, B. Jr., et al. Elderberry flavonoids bind to and prevent H1N1 infection in vitro. Phytochemistry. 70(10):1255-1261, 2009. HerbalScience Group LLC, Naples, FL, USA.*

Carbohydrate binding properties of a new plant lectin isolated from elderberry (Sambucus nigra L.) (SNA) bark were studied using the techniques of quantitative precipitation, hapten inhibition, and equilibrium dialysis. Purified SNA precipitates highly sialylated glycoproteins such as fetuin, orosomucoid, and ovine submaxillary mucin, but not their asialo derivatives. Hapten inhibition experiments showed that both D-Gal and D-GalNAc are weak inhibitors of SNA-glycophorin precipitation, but neither New5Ac nor Neu5Gc is an inhibitor. A series of oligosaccharides which contain the terminal Neu5Ac(alpha 2-6)Gal sequence showed an extremely high inhibitory potency (1,600-10,000 times more inhibitory than Gal). On the other hand, oligosaccharides with the Neu5Ac(alpha 2-3)Gal linkage were only 30-80 times more inhibitory than Gal, thus showing a marked preference for the 2,6-linked isomer. Hapten inhibition with Gal and its epimers suggested that the equatorial OH at C-3 and the axial OH at C-4 of the D-pyranose ring are strict requirements for binding. Conversion of the Neu5Ac residue to its 7-carbon analogue by selective periodate oxidation of its glyceryl side chain, followed by $NaBH_4$ reduction, completely destroyed the ability of fetuin and orosomucoid to precipitate with SNA. Moreover, the same treatment of Neu5Ac(alpha 2-3) lactitol also abolished its ability to inhibit the precipitation reaction, suggesting that the glyceryl side chain of NBu5Ac (especially the C-8 and/or C-9 portion) is an important determinant for SNA. The increased inhibitory potency of various glycosides with beta-linked nonpolar aglycons suggested the presence of a hydrophibic interacting region adjacent to the carbohydrate binding site. The results of equilibrium dialysis using [3H] Neu5Ac(alpha 2-6) lactitol as ligand showed the presence of two equivalent, noninteracting carbohydrate binding sites in this tetrameric glycoprotein lectin (Ka = 3.9 X 10(5) M-1). *Reference:* *Shibuya, N., et al. The elderberry (Sambucus nigra L.) bark lectin recognizes the Neu5Ac(alpha 2-6)Gal/GalNAc sequence. Journal of Biological Chemistry. 262(4):1596-1601, 1987] Full text of this study can be viewed at: www.jbc.org/cgi/reprint/262/4/1596.*

27 patients with recent onset of influenza were given either placebo or elderberry extract (two tablespoons (30 ml) a day for children; four tablespoons (60 ml) per day for adults). In subjects receiving elderberry, within 24 hours diminished influenza symptoms were observed in 20% of subjects afflicted with influenza. 93.3% experienced significant improvement in their symptoms after two days, compared to 25% of the placebo group. A total cure occurred in almost 90% of the elderberry group within two to three days vs. at least six days for the placebo group. A standardized elderberry extract, Sambucol (SAM), reduced hemagglutination and inhibited replication of human influenza viruses type A/Shangdong 9/93 (H3N2), A/Beijing 32/92 (H3N2), A/Texas 36/91 (H1N1), A/Singapore 6/86 (H1N1), type B/Panama 45/90, B/Yamagata 16/88, B/Ann Arbor 1/86, and of animal strains from Northern European swine and turkeys, A/Sw/Ger 2/81, A/Tur/Ger 3/91, and A/Sw/Ger 8533/91 in Madin-Darby canine kidney cells. A placebo-controlled, double blind study was carried out on a group of individuals living in an agricultural community (kibbutz) during an outbreak of influenza B/Panama in 1993. Fever, feeling of improvement, and complete cure were recorded during 6 days. Sera obtained in the acute and convalescent phases were tested for the presence of antibodies to influenza A, B, respiratory syncytial, and adenoviruses. Convalescent phase serologies showed higher mean and mean geometric hemagglutination inhibition (HI) titers to influenza B in the group treated with SAM than in the control group. A significant improvement of the symptoms, including fever, was seen in 93.3% of the cases in the SAM-treated group within 2 days, whereas in the control group 91.7% of the patients showed an improvement within 6 days (p < 0.001). A complete cure was achieved within 2 to 3 days in nearly 90% of the SAM-treated group and within at least 6 days in the placebo group (p < 0.001). No satisfactory medication to cure influenza type A and B is available. Considering the efficacy of the extract in vitro on all strains of influenza virus tested, the clinical results, its low cost, and absence of side-effects, this preparation could offer a possibility for safe treatment for influenza A and B. *Reference:* *Zakay-Rones, Z., et al. Inhibition of several strains of influenza virus in vitro and reduction of symptoms by an elderberry*

extract (Sambucus nigra) during an outbreak of influenza in Panama. Journal of Alternative & Compl Medicine. 1(4):361-369, 1995.

Elderberry has been used in folk medicine for centuries to treat influenza, colds and sinusitis, and has been reported to have antiviral activity against influenza and herpes simplex. The authors investigated the efficacy and safety of oral elderberry syrup for treating influenza A and B infections. Sixty patients (aged 18-54 years) suffering from influenza-like symptoms for 48 h or less were enrolled in this randomized, double-blind, placebo-controlled study during the influenza season of 1999-2000 in Norway. Patients received 15 ml of elderberry or placebo syrup four times a day for 5 days, and recorded their symptoms using a visual analogue scale. Symptoms were relieved on average 4 days earlier and use of rescue medication was significantly less in those receiving elderberry extract compared with placebo. Elderberry extract seems to offer an efficient, safe and cost-effective treatment for influenza. These findings need to be confirmed in a larger study. **Reference:** *Zakay-Rones, Z., et al. Randomized study of the efficacy and safety of oral elderberry extract in the treatment of influenza A and B virus infections. J Int Med Res. 32(2):132-140, 2004], [Department of Virology, Hebrew University-Hadassah Medical School, Jerusalem, Israel.*

Licorice Root

Glycyrrhizin is known to exert antiviral and anti-inflammatory effects. Here, the effects of an approved parenteral glycyrrhizin preparation (Stronger Neo-Minophafen C) were investigated on highly pathogenic influenza A H5N1 virus replication, H5N1-induced apoptosis, and H5N1-induced pro-inflammatory responses in lung epithelial (A549) cells. Therapeutic glycyrrhizin concentrations substantially inhibited H5N1-induced expression of the pro-inflammatory molecules CXCL10, interleukin 6, CCL2, and CCL5 (effective glycyrrhizin concentrations 25 to 50 μg/ml) but interfered with H5N1 replication and H5N1-induced apoptosis to a lesser extent (effective glycyrrhizin concentrations 100 μg/ml or higher). Glycyrrhizin also diminished monocyte migration towards supernatants of H5N1-infected A549 cells. The mechanism by which glycyrrhizin interferes with H5N1 replication and H5N1-induced pro-inflammatory gene expression includes inhibition of H5N1-induced formation of reactive oxygen species and (in turn) reduced activation of NFκB, JNK, and p38, redox-sensitive signalling events known to be relevant for influenza A virus replication. Therefore, glycyrrhizin may complement the arsenal of potential drugs for the treatment of H5N1 disease. **Reference:** *PLoS One. 2011; 6(5): e19705. Published online 2011 May 17. doi: 10.1371/journal.pone.0019705. PMCID: PMC3096629. Glycyrrhizin Exerts Antioxidative Effects in H5N1 Influenza A Virus-Infected Cells and Inhibits Virus Replication and Pro-Inflammatory Gene Expression. Martin Michaelis, Janina Geiler, Patrizia Naczk, Patchima Sithisarn, Anke Leutz, Hans Wilhelm Doerr, Jindrich Cinatl, Jr. Institut für Medizinische Virologie, Klinikum der J.W. Goethe-Universität, Frankfurt am Main, Germany.*

Glycyrrhizic acid (GA), a derivative of licorice, selectively inhibits the growth of lymphocytes latently infected with Kaposi's sarcoma-associated herpesvirus. The mechanism involves the deregulation of the multicistronic latency transcript, including the failure to generate the mature forms of viral mRNA encoding LANA. We show here that GA disrupts an RNA polymerase II (RNAPII) complex that accumulates at the CTCF-cohesin binding site within the first intron of the latency transcript. GA altered the enrichment of the RNAPII pausing complex, along with pausing factors SPT5 and NELF-A, at the intragenic CTCF-cohesin binding sites. GA blocked the interaction of cohesin subunit SMC3 with another cohesin subunit, RAD21, and reduced SPT5 interaction with RNAPII. Covalent coupling of GA to a solid support revealed that GA interacts with several cellular proteins, including SMC3 and SPT5, but not their respective interaction partners RAD21 and RNAPII. GA treatment also inhibited the transcription of some cellular genes, like c-myc, which contain a similar CTCF-cohesin binding site within the first intron. We also found that GA leads to a more general loss of sister chromatid cohesion for cellular chromosomes. These findings suggest that RNAPII pauses at intragenic CTCF-cohesin binding sites and that abrogation of this pausing by GA leads to loss of proper mRNA production and defects in sister chromatid cohesion, a process important for both viral and cellular chromosome stability. ***Reference:*** *J Virol. 2011 November; 85(21): 11159–11169. doi: 10.1128/JVI.00720-11. PMCID: PMC31 94953. Mechanism of Glycyrrhizic Acid Inhibition of Kaposi's Sarcoma-Associated Herpesvirus: Disruption of CTCF-Cohesin-Mediated RNA Polymerase II Pausing and Sister Chromatid Cohesion. Hyojeung Kang and Paul M. Lieberman. This article has been cited by other articles in PMC.*

Background- Hepatitis C virus is a major cause of chronic liver diseases which can lead to permanent liver damage, hepatocellular carcinoma and death. The presently available treatment with interferon plus ribavirin, has limited benefits due to adverse side effects such as anemia, depression, fatigue, and "flu-like" symptoms. Herbal plants have been used for centuries against different diseases including viral diseases and have become a major source of new compounds to treat bacterial and viral diseases. **Material-** The present study was design to study the antiviral effect of Glycyrrhizin (GL) against HCV. For this purpose, HCV infected liver cells were treated with GL at non toxic doses and HCV titer was measured by Quantitative real time RT-PCR. **Results and Discussion-** Our results demonstrated that GL inhibit HCV titer in a dose dependent manner and resulted in 50% reduction of HCV at a concentration of 14 ± 2 µg. Comparative studies were made with interferon alpha to investigate synergistic effects, if any, between antiviral compound and interferon alpha 2a. Our data showed that GL exhibited synergistic effect when combined with interferon. Moreover, these results were verified by transiently transfecting the liver cells with HCV 3a core plasmid. The results proved that GL dose dependently inhibit the expression of HCV 3a core gene both at mRNA and protein levels while the GAPDH remained constant.

Conclusion- Our results suggest that GL inhibit HCV full length viral particles and HCV core gene expression or function in a dose dependent manner and had synergistic effect with interferon. In future, GL along with interferon will be better option to treat HCV infection. **Reference:** *J Transl Med. 2011; 9: 112. Published online 2011 July 18. doi: 10.1186/1479-5876-9-112. PMCID: PMC3169469. Glycyrrhizin as antiviral agent against Hepatitis C Virus. Usman A Ashfaq, Muhammad S Masoud, Zafar Nawaz, and Sheikh Riazuddin. Division of Molecular Medicine, National Centre of Excellence in Molecular Biology, University of the Punjab, Lahore, Pakistan. Braman Family Breast Cancer Institute, University of Miami, USA. Allama Iqbal Medical College, University of Health sciences, Lahore.*

The antiviral effect of glycyrrhizin (GR), an active component of licorice roots, was investigated in mice infected with influenza virus A2 (H2N2). When mice that had been exposed to ten x 50% lethal doses of the virus were treated intraperitoneally with 10 mg of glycyrrhizin per kg of body weight 1 day before infection and 1 and 4 days post infection, all of the mice survived over the 21-day experimental period. At the end of this period, the mean survival time (in days) for control mice treated with saline was 10.5 days, and there were no survivors. The grade of pulmonary consolidations and the virus titers in the lung tissues of infected mice treated with GR were significantly lower than those in the lung tissues of infected mice treated with saline. GR did not show any effects on the viability or replication of influenza virus A2 in vitro. When splenic T cells from GR-treated mice were adoptively transferred to mice exposed to influenza virus, 100% of the recipients survived, compared to 0% survival for recipient mice inoculated with naive T cells or splenic B cells and macrophages from GR-treated mice. The antiviral activities of glycyrrhizin on influenza virus infection in mice were not demonstrated when it was administered to infected mice in combination with anti-gamma interferon (anti-IFN-gamma) monoclonal antibody. These results suggest that glycyrrhizin may protect mice exposed to a lethal amount of influenza virus through the stimulation of interferon-gamma production by T cells, because T cells have been shown to be producer cells of IFN-gamma stimulated with the compound. **Reference:** *Utsunomiya, T., et al. Glycyrrhizin, an active component of licorice roots, reduces morbidity and mortality of mice infected with lethal doses of influenza virus. Antimicrobial Agents Chemother. 41(3):551-556, 1997.*

The authors investigated the mechanism by which glycyrrhizin (GL), the main active component of licorice roots, protects cells from infection with influenza A virus (IAV). The authors found that GL treatment leads to a clear reduction in the number of IAV-infected human lung cells as well as a reduction in the CCID50 titer by 90%. The antiviral effect, however, was limited to on or two virus replication cycles. Analysis of different GL treatment protocols suggested that the antiviral effect of GL was limited to an early step in the virus replication cycle. A direct inhibitory action of GL on IAV particles could be excluded and GL did not interact with the virus receptor either. The antiviral effect of GL was abolished by treatment 1h after virus infection, whereas pre-treatment and treatment during and after virus adsorption led to a reduction in the cytopathic effect, reduced viral RNA within the cells and in the cell supernatants, and reduced viral hemagglutination titers. Detailed virus uptake analyses unambiguously demonstrated reduced virus uptake in various GL-treated cells. These observations lead to the conclusion, that the antiviral activity of GL is mediated by an interaction with the cell membrane which most likely results in reduced endocytotic activity and hence reduced virus uptake inside the cells. These insights might help in the design of structurally related compounds leading to potent anti-influenza therapeutics. *Reference: Wolkerstorfer, A., et al. Glycyrrhizin inhibits influenza A virus uptake into the cell. Antiviral Research. 2009. Onepharm Research & Development GmbH, Vienna, Austria.*

Green Tea

Background- Experimental studies have revealed that green tea catechins and theanine prevent influenza infection, while the clinical evidence has been inconclusive. This study was conducted to determine whether taking green tea catechins and theanine can clinically prevent influenza infection. **Methods-** Design, Setting, and Participants: A randomized, double-blind, placebo-controlled trial of 200 healthcare workers conducted for 5 months from November 9, 2009 to April 8, 2010 in three healthcare facilities for the elderly in Higashimurayama, Japan. Interventions: The catechin/theanine group received capsules including green tea catechins (378 mg/day) and theanine (210 mg/day). The control group received placebo. Main Outcome Measures: The primary outcome was the incidence of clinically defined influenza infection. Secondary outcomes were (1) laboratory-confirmed influenza with viral antigen measured by immunochromatographic assay and (2) the time for which the patient was free from clinically defined influenza infection, i.e., the period between the start of intervention and the first diagnosis of influenza infection, based on clinically defined influenza infection. **Results-** Eligible healthcare workers (n = 197) were enrolled and randomly assigned to an intervention; 98 were allocated to receive catechin/theanine capsules and 99 to placebo. The incidence of clinically defined influenza infection was significantly lower in the catechin/theanine group (4 participants; 4.1%) compared with the placebo group (13 participants; 13.1%) (adjusted OR, 0.25; 95% CI, 0.07 to 0.76, P = 0.022). The incidence of laboratory-confirmed influenza infection was also lower in the catechin/theanine group (1 participant; 1.0%) than in the placebo group (5 participants; 5.1%), but this difference was not significant (adjusted OR, 0.17; 95% CI, 0.01 to 1.10; P = 0.112). The time for which the patient was free from clinically defined influenza infection was significantly different between the two groups (adjusted HR, 0.27; 95% CI, 0.09 to 0.84; P = 0.023). **Conclusions-** Among healthcare workers for the elderly, taking green tea catechins and theanine may be effective prophylaxis for influenza infection. *Reference: C Complement Altern Med. 2011; 11: 15. Published online 2011 February 21. doi: 10.1186/1472-6882-11-15. PMCID:*

PMC3049752. Effects of Green Tea Catechins and Theanine on Preventing Influenza Infection among Healthcare Workers: A Randomized Controlled Trial. Keiji Matsumoto, Hiroshi Yamada, Norikata Takuma, Hitoshi Niino, and Yuko M Sagesaka. Department of Drug Evaluation & Informatics, Graduate School of Pharmaceutical Sciences, University of Shizuoka, 52-1 Yada, Suruga-ku, Shizuoka 422-8526, Japan.

The authors set their attention on the activity of the endonuclease of the A-type virus that depends on RNA polymerase and investigated whether green tea catechins inhibit this activity directly. Initially they performed endonuclease assays through the incubation of the influenza's PA subunit—of three principal subunits that comprise polymerase, PA is the one most closely associated with replication - using four different concentrations of EGCG. From this analysis they found that EGCG was the best inhibitor of the endonuclease activity of the PA N-terminal domain† at the highest dosage used (10 µM). The researchers report that this is the first demonstration of the inhibition of influenza A virus endonuclease by a green tea catechin. [Green, R. H. Inhibition of multiplication of influenza virus by extracts of tea. Proc Soc Exp Biol Med. 71(1):84, 1949], **Reference:** *Kuzuhara, T., et al. Green tea catechins inhibit the endonuclease activity of influenza A virus RNA polymerase. PLoS Currents Influenza. 2009 Oct 13:RRN1052.*

(-)Epigallocatechin gallate (EGCg) and theaflavin digallate (TF3) (1-10 microM) inhibited the infectivity of both influenza A virus and influenza B virus in Madin-Darby canine kidney (MDCK) cells in vitro. Study by electron microscope revealed that EGCg and TF3 (1 mM) agglutinated influenza viruses as well as did antibody, and that they prevented the viruses from adsorbing to MDCK cells. EGCg and TF3 more weakly inhibited adsorption of the viruses to MDCK cells. EGCg and TF3 (1-16 microM) also inhibited haemagglutination by influenza viruses. These findings suggest that tea polyphenols bind to the haemagglutinin of influenza virus, inhibit its adsorption to MDCK cells, and thus block its infectivity. **Reference:** *Nakayama, M., et al. Inhibition of the infectivity of influenza virus by tea polyphenols. Antiviral Res. 21:289-299, 1993.*

Polyphenolic compound catechins ((-)-epigallocatechin gallate (EGCG), (-)-epicatechin gallate (ECG) and (-)-epigallocatechin (EGC)) from green tea were evaluated for their ability to inhibit influenza virus replication in cell culture and for potentially direct virucidal effect. Among the test compounds, the EGCG and ECG were found to be potent inhibitors of influenza virus replication in MDCK cell culture and this effect was observed in all influenza virus subtypes tested, including A/H1N1, A/H3N2 and B virus. The 50% effective inhibition concentration (EC(50)) of EGCG, ECG, and EGC for influenza A virus were 22-28, 22-40 and 309-318muM, respectively. EGCG and ECG exhibited hemagglutination inhibition activity, EGCG being more effective. However, the sensitivity in hemagglutination inhibition was widely different among three different subtypes of influenza viruses tested.   Quantitative RT-PCR analysis revealed that, at high concentration, EGCG and ECG also suppressed viral RNA synthesis in MDCK cells whereas EGC failed to show similar effect.   Similarly, EGCG and ECG inhibited the neuraminidase activity more effectively than the EGC.   The results show that the 3-galloyl group of catechin skeleton plays an important role on the observed antiviral activity, whereas the 5'-OH at the trihydroxy benzyl moiety at 2-position plays a minor role.   The results, along with the HA type-specific effect, suggest that the antiviral effect of catechins on influenza virus is mediated not only by specific interaction with HA, but altering the physical properties of viral membrane. **Reference:** *Song, J. M., et al. Antiviral effect of catechins in green tea on influenza virus. Antiviral Res. 2005, Dept of Biotechnology, College of Engineering, Yonsei Univ, Seoul, South Korea.*

The objective of this study was to evaluate the effects of gargling tea catechin extracts on the prevention of influenza infection in elderly nursing home residents. This was a prospective study conducted for 3 months from January to March 2005. The setting was a nursing home in Japan. A total of 124 elderly residents of at least 65 years of age were enrolled in the study. 76 residents   (83 +/-8.2 years, mean +/-standard deviation; 24 men, 52 women) gargled with tea catechin extract (catechin group) and were compared with 48 age- and sex-matched residents who gargled without tea catechin extracts (control group). All the residents   were vaccinated with an influenza vaccine until early December 2004. The catechin group gargled with the tea catechin extract solution (200 mcg/mL catechins, 60% of catechins comprise epigallocatechin gallate). The control group gargled without the catechin extract solution. In both groups, gargling was performed three times daily for 3 months. The incidence of influenza infection during the study was compared between the two groups. A safety evaluation was conducted to observe adverse events during the study. The incidence of influenza infection was significantly lower in the catechin group (1.3%, one resident) than in the control group (10%, five residents) calculated by multivariate logistic regression analysis (p = 0.028; odds ratio, 15.711; 95% confidence interval, 1.883-399.658). No adverse events, such as respiratory tract irritation, an obstruction, or allergic bronchial spasm, were observed during the study.   This prospective study demonstrating the effect of catechin gargling on the prevention of influenza infection in the elderly is the first to be reported in the literature. Further randomized, controlled studies are needed to confirm the effects of catechin gargling on the prevention of influenza infection. **Reference:** *Yamada, H., et al. Gargling with tea catechin extracts for the prevention of influenza infection in elderly nursing home residents: a prospective clinical study. J Altern Complement Med. 12(7):669-672, 2006, Division of Drug Evaluation & Informatics, School of Pharmaceutical Sciences, University of Shizuoka, Shizuoka, Japan.*

LUPUS

Cordyceps Sinensis

The objective was to observe the effect of Cordyceps sinensis and artemisinin in preventing recurrence of lupus nephritis (LN). Sixty-one LN patients, who had no activities by corticosterone and cyclophosphamide (CTX) impacting therapy were randomly divided into two groups. The 31 cases in the treated group were given Cordyceps powder 2-4 g/d before meal and artemisinin 0.6 g/d after meal in three portions orally taken for 3 years. The 30 patients in the control group were treated with tripterygiitotorum and/or Baoshenkang tablet. The consecutive observation lasted for 5 years to monitor the clinical manifestations of lupus and laboratory indexes including blood creatinine, creatinine clearance rate (CCr) and antinuclear antibodies (ANA). The therapeutic effect showed markedly effective in 26 cases (83.9%), effective in 4 (12.9%) and ineffective in 1 (3.2%) in the treated group, while in the control group, the corresponding numbers were 15 (50.0%), 8 (26.7%) and 7 (23.3%), the difference between the two groups in markedly effective rate was significant (P < 0.01). In the treated group, C3 level was stabilized at above 1.21 +/- 0.20 g/L, which was over the normal range, CCr was unchanged as compared before and after treatment, which was significantly different from that in the control group. Moreover, the side-effects occurred in the treated group was less. Conclusion: Cordyceps and artemisinin could prevent the recurrence of LN and protect kidney function. *Reference: Zhongguo Zhong Xi Yi Jie He Za Zhi. 2002 Mar;22(3):169-71. [Study on effect of Cordyceps sinensis and artemisinin in preventing recurrence of lupus nephritis]. Department of Nephrology, Second People's Hospital of Guilin, Guangxi 541004.*

Systemic lupus erythematosus (SLE) is an important autoimmune disease with multiple organ system involvement. From preliminary studies, we have found that six Chinese herbs: Atractylodes ovata, Anqelica sinensis, Cordyceps sinensis, Liqustrum lucidum, Codonopsis pilosula and Homo sapiens can improve defective in vitro interleukin-2 (IL-2) production in patients with SLE. In order to investigate the in vivo effects of these herbs, the authors used NZB/NZW F1 mice, a typical lupus animal model used to test these herbs. It was found that C. pilosula, H. sapiens and C. sinensis could prolong the life span of female NZB/NZW F1 mice and inhibited anti-ds DNA production. Although A. sinensis could prolong the life span of experimental mice, it did not inhibit the production of anti-ds DNA antibody. These herbs may have great potential for the management of human SLE in the future. *Reference: Chen, J. R., et al. The effects of Chinese herbs on improving survival and inhibiting anti-ds DNA antibody production in lupus mice. American Journal of Chinese Medicine. 21(3-4):257-262, 1993. -- Department of Internal Medicine, School of Medicine, Kaohsiung Medical College, Taiwan.*

Graduate Institute and School of Traditional Chinese Medicine, Chang-Gung University, Center for Traditional Chinese Medicine, Chang-Gung Memorial Hospital, Taoyuan, Taiwan, China. Mycelia products from wild-form Cordyceps sinensis could be constantly produced in a large scale and would be a better source of this herbal medicine. The purpose was to investigate the immunological effects of an orally administered hot-water extract cultured mycelium of C. sinensis in lupus-prone (NZB/NZW) F1 hybrids. Forty female mice were divided into four groups and were given 2.4 mg/g/day oral doses of C. sinensis starting at three (group A), six (group B), or eight (group C) months of age, whereas the remaining group (group D) served as a control. Survival, proteinuria, and titers of anti-double-stranded DNA autoantibodies were evaluated. Treatment with C. sinensis resulted in increased survival, decreased proteinuria, and reduced titers of anti-double-stranded DNA antibody in groups A and B. Moreover, the mice in groups A and B showed significantly reduced percentages of CD4(+) T cells (*$P < 0.05$) and increased percentages of CD8(+) T cells in peripheral blood mononuclear cells (PBMC) after C. sinensis administration. At 6 months of age, the proliferation rate of BrdU-incorporated spleen cells was significantly decreased after 48 and 72 h of C. sinensis treatment (**$P < 0.01$) in group A of mice. Early medication with C. sinensis induced the redistribution of PBMC and attenuated the disease severity of lupus in (NZB/NZW) F1 mice. *Reference: Chen, J. L., et al. Immunological alterations in lupus-prone autoimmune (NZB/NZW) F1 mice by mycelia Chinese medicinal fungus Cordyceps sinensis-induced redistributions of peripheral mononuclear T lymphocytes. Clin Exp Med. 2009.*

The authors studied the effect of Cordyceps sinensis on inhibiting systemic lupus erythematosus (SLE) in MRL 1pr/1pr rats. The evalutions of lymphnoditis, proteinuria, kidney function and plasma antibody were adopted in MRL 1pr/1pr rats. Cordyceps sinensis could inhibit lymphadenectasis, induce the level of proteinuria and anti-ds-DNA antibody in plasma, and improve kidney function in SLE rats. Codyceps sinensis played an role on SLE rats. *Reference: Fu, T., et al. [Effect of Cordyceps sinensis on inhibiting systemic lupus erythematosus in MRL 1pr/1pr rats]. Zhong Yao Cai. 24(9):658-659, 2001.*

Pycnogenol

An increasing body of evidence indicates that Pycnogenol (PYC), a standardized extract of French maritime pine bark, has favorable pharmacological properties. Immunomodulation has been observed in both animal models as well as in patients with Lupus erythematosus. *Reference: Rohdewald, P. A review of the French maritime pine bark extract (Pycnogenol), a herbal medication with a diverse clinical pharmacology. Int J Clin Pharmacol. 40(4):158-168, 2002. Institute Pharmaceutical Chemistry, Westfalische Wilhelms-Universitat Munster, Germany.*

This pilot study investigated the effect of pycnogneol for the treatment of systemic lupus erythematosus (SLE). Eleven SLE patients received first-line pharmaceutical treatment for their SLE. Of these 11 patients, six also received pycnogenol and five also received a placebo. Pycnogenol was found to reduce the production of free radicals, reduce apoptosis, reduce p56lck specific activity and reduce the erythrocyte sedimentation rate. Pycnogenol is therefore useful as an adjunctive treatment for SLE. **Reference:** *Stefanescu, M., et al. Pycnogenol® efficacy in the treatment of systemic lupus erythematosus patients. Phytotherapy Research. 15(8):698-704, 2001.*

Fish Oil

The effect of dietary fish oil (Omega-3 fatty acids- eicosapentenoic acid [EPA] and docosahexaenoic acid [DHA]) on several mechanisms involved in immune, inflammatory and atherosclerotic vascular disease was determined in 12 subjects with systemic lupus erythematosus (SLE) and nephritis. These out-patients supplemented their usual diet for five weeks with daily doses of 6 g of fish oil, followed by a five-week washout period, then five weeks of 18 g of fish oil daily. The platelet EPA content rose six-fold with the lower and 15-fold with the higher dose of fish oil, and similar changes occurred to the platelet DHA content. The platelet arachidonic acid incorporation was reduced by 16 and 20%, respectively. These changes were associated with a reduction in collagen-induced platelet aggregation and an increase in red cell flexibility and a decrease in whole blood viscosity. Prostacyclin (PGI2) production was unaffected by the fish oil, but PGI3 formation correlated with its administration and dosage. Neutrophil leukotriene B4 release was reduced 78 and 42%, respectively, by the low and higher doses of fish oil. The higher fish oil dose induced a 38% decrease in triglyceride and a 39% reduction in VLDL cholesterol associated with a 28% rise in HDL, cholesterol. The fish oil had no effect on immune complex or anti-DNA antibody titer, albuminuria, intraplatelet serotonin or [14C]-serotonin release from platelets. In patients with lupus nephritis, dietary supplementation with fish oil affects the mechanisms involved in inflammatory and atherosclerotic vascular disease. **Reference:** *Clark, W. F., et al. Omega-3 fatty acid dietary supplementation in systemic lupus erythematosus. Kidney Int. 36(4):653-60, 1989.*

Systemic lupus erythematosus (SLE) is a chronic inflammatory condition characterised by arthritis, cutaneous rash, vasculitis, and involvement of central nervous system, renal and cardiopulmonary manifest-tations. Abnormalities in the cytokine network is believed to be involved in the pathobiology of this condition. The n-3 fatty acids such as eicosapentaenoic acid (EPA) and docosahexaenoic acid (DHA) can suppress T-cell proliferation and the production of interleukin-1, interleukin-2, and tumor necrosis factor by these cells both in vitro and in vivo. Oral supplementation of EPA and DHA induced prolonged remission of SLE in 10 consecutive patients without any side-effects. These results suggest that n-3 fatty acids, EPA and DHA, are useful in the management of SLE and possibly, other similar collagen vascular diseases. *Reference:* *Das, U. Beneficial effects of eicosapentaenoic acid and docosahexaenoic acids in the management of systemic lupus erythematosus and its relationship to the cytokine network. Prostaglandins, Leukotrienes, and Essential Fatty Acids. 51(3):207-213, 1994. Department of Medicine, Nizam's Institute of Medical Sciences, Punjagutta, Hyderabad, India.*

The objective of this study was to determine the effect of dietary supplementation with omega-3 fish oils with or without copper on disease activity in systemic lupus erythematosus (SLE). Fish oil supplementation has a beneficial effect on murine models of SLE, while exogenous copper can decrease the formation of lupus erythematosus cells in rats with a hydralazine-induced collagen disease. A double blind, double placebo controlled factorial trial was performed on 52 patients with SLE. Patients were randomly assigned to 4 treatment groups. Physiological doses of omega-3 fish oils and copper readily obtainable by dietary means were used. One group received 3 g MaxEPA and 3 mg copper, another 3 g MaxEPA and placebo copper, another 3 mg copper and placebo fish oil, and the fourth group received both placebo capsules. Serial measurements of disease activity using the revised Systemic Lupus Activity Measure (SLAM-R) and peripheral blood samples for routine hematological, biochemical, and immunological indices were taken at baseline, 6, 12, and 24 weeks. There was a significant decline in SLAM-R score from 6.12 to 4.69 ($p < 0.05$) in those subjects taking fish oil compared to placebo. No significant effect on SLAM-R was observed in subjects taking copper. Laboratory variables were unaffected by either intervention. In the management of SLE, dietary supplementation with fish oil may be beneficial in modifying symptomatic disease activity. *Reference: Duffy, E. M., et al. The clinical effect of dietary supplementation with omega-3 fish oils and/or copper in systemic lupus erythematosus. J Rheumatol. 31(8):1551-1556, 2004. Northern Ireland Center for Food and Health (NICHE), School of Biomedical Sciences, University of Ulster, Ulster, Northern Ireland.*

Dietary supplementation of fish oil as the exclusive source of lipid suppresses autoimmune lupus in MRL-lpr mice. This marine oil diet decreases the lymphoid hyperplasia regulated by the lpr gene, prevents an increase in macrophage surface Ia expression, reduces the formation of circulating retroviral gp70 immune complexes, delays the onset of renal disease, and prolongs survival. The authors show that a fatty acid component uniquely present in fish oil but not in vegetable oil decreases the quantity of dienoic prostaglandin E, thromboxane B, and prostacyclin normally synthesized by multiple tissues, including kidney, lung, and macrophages, and promotes the synthesis of small amounts of trienoic prostaglandin in autoimmune mice. This change in endogenous cyclooxygenase metabolite synthesis directly suppresses immunologic and/or inflammatory mediators of murine lupus. *Reference: Kelley, V. E., et al. A fish oil diet rich in eicosapentaenoic acid reduces cyclooxygenase metabolites, and suppresses lupus in MRL-lpr mice. Journal of Immun-ology. 134(3):1914-1919, 1985.*

The effect of dietary modifications has been extensively studied in lupus animal models. Calorie, protein, and especially fat restriction, caused a significant reduction in immune-complex deposition in the kidney, reduced proteinuria and prolongation of the mice's life span. The addition of polyunsaturated fatty acids (PUFAs), such as fish oil or linseed oil, was also related to decreased mice morbidity and mortality in animal models of lupus and of antiphospholipid syndrome. PUFAs such as eicosapetaenoic acid (EPA) and docosahexaenoic acid (DHA) competitively inhibit arachidonic acid with a resultant decrease in inflammatory eicosanoids and cytokines. Human studies support the effect of a PUFAs-enriched diet, both scrologically and clinically. ***Reference:*** *Leiba, A., et al. Diet and lupus. Lupus. 10(3):246-248, 2001. Research Unit of Autoimmune Diseases, Department of Medicine B Chaim Sheba Medical Center, Tel Hashomer, Israel.*

A menhaden oil diet, rich in eicosapentaenoic acid, protected female NZB X NZW/F1 mice from autoimmune nephritis. Only 15% of mice treated with the diet from weaning had died with severe renal disease at 19 months, versus 98% of controls on a beef tallow diet. The menhaden oil also protected these mice from renal disease when instituted at 4 and 5 months of age and, under these conditions, levels of anti-native DNA antibodies were similar in both dietary groups. These data suggest that the menhaden oil diet may act primarily to reduce inflammation via the ability of eicosapentaenoic acid to alter the production of prostaglandins and leukotrienes. ***Reference:*** *Prickett, J. D., et al. Effects of dietary enrichment with eicosa-pentaenoic acid upon autoimmune nephritis in female NZBxNZW/F1 mice. Arth Rheumat. 26(2):133-139, 1983.*

Dietary marine lipids markedly reduce the severity of glomerulonephritis and its associated mortality in inbred strains of mice developing autoimmune disease, a model for human systemic lupus erythematosus. The authors report the influence of varying the dose of menhaden oil and the timing of its administration on the mortality of female (NZB x NZW) F1 mice. After ingesting 25 wt% menhaden oil (MO) for periods of 1.5 weeks to 12 months, there was a stable content of tissue n-3 fatty acids, with total n-3 fatty acids of 28% and 35% in spleen and liver, respectively. The extent of protection from mortality was dependent on the dose of MO with marked protection at doses of 11 to 25%, marginal protection at 5.5% and no protection at 2.5% MO. Delay in the institution of MO until ages 5 or 7 months still resulted in large reductions of mortality. Institution of a MO diet from 6 weeks until ages 5 to 7 months followed by a change to beef tallow resulted in little protection. Serum levels of 4 cyclooxygenase products were reduced ranging from 26 to 76% in mice fed MO diets, compared to mice fed beef tallow, based on radioimmunoassay. The degree of reduction of mortality on different doses of MO was correlated best with tissue levels of C22:5, and levels of

C20:5 and C22:6 were similar at high and low doses of MO, suggesting that levels of 22:5 may be related to the protective effects of marine lipids on autoimmune disease. **Reference:** Robinson, D. R. *The protective effect of dietary fish oil on murine lupus. Prostaglandins. 30(1):51-75, 1985.*

A prospective, double blind, cross over study assessing the effects of a low fat, high marine oil diet in 27 patients with active systemic lupus erythematosus has been performed. The patients were given 20 g daily of MaxEPA (eicosapentaenoic acid) or 20 g of olive oil (placebo) in matching capsules added to a standardised isoenergetic low fat diet. When individual outcome measures of the 17 patients who completed the full 34 week study were considered 14 who were receiving MaxEPA achieved useful or ideal status, whereas 13 receiving placebo were rated as worse or no change. The difference between the two types of capsule was statistically significant. No major side effects were noted, and it is suggested that dietary modification with additional marine oil may be a useful way of modifying disease activity in systemic lupus erythematosus. **Reference:** Walton, A. J., et al. *Dietary fish oil and the severity of symptoms in patients with systemic lupus erythema-tosus. Annals of the Rheumatic Diseases. 50(7):463-466, 1991. Bloomsbury Rheumatology Unit, University College, London, UK.*

To determine the clinical effect of dietary supplementation with low dose omega-3-polyunsaturated fatty acids on disease activity and endothelial function in patients with systemic lupus erythematosus. A 24 week randomised double-blind placebo-controlled parallel trial of the effect of 3g of omega-3-polyunsaturated fatty acids on 60 patients with SLE was performed. Serial measurements of disease activity using the revised Systemic Lupus Activity Measure (SLAM-R) and British Isles Lupus Assessment Group index of disease activity for SLE (BILAG), endothelial function using flow mediated dilation of the brachial artery (FMD), oxidative stress using platelet 8-isoprostanes and analysis of platelet membrane fatty acids were taken at baseline, 12 and 24 weeks. In the fish oil group there was a significant improvement at 24 weeks in SLAM-R (from 9.4+/-3.0 to 6.3+/-2.5, $p<0.001$); in BILAG (from 13.6+/-6.0 to 6.7+/-3.8, $p<0.001$); in FMD (from 3.0% (-0.5-8.2) to 8.9% (1.3-16.9), $p<0.001$) and in platelet 8-isoprostanes (from 177pg/mg protein (23 - 387) to 90 pg/mg protein (32 - 182), $p = 0.007$). Low dose dietary supplementation with omega-3 fish oils in SLE not only has a therapeutic effect on disease activity but also improves endothelial function and reduces oxidative stress and may therefore confer cardiovascular benefits. **Reference:** Wright, S. A., et al. *A randomised placebo-controlled interventional trial of omega-3-polyunsaturated fatty acids on endothelial function and disease activity in systemic lupus erythematosus. Ann Rheum Dis. 2007. Musgrave Park Hospital, United Kingdom.*

LYME DISEASE

Silver

Borrelia burgdorferi & b hermsti, organisms associated with the causing the symptoms of Lyme Disease, were tested at the Department of Heath and Human Services, Rocky Mountain Laboratories, & Fox Chase Cancer Center, respectively in 1995. Colloidal silver in concentrations of 15 PPM And 150 PPM demonstrated that no live spirochetes of either borrellia burgdorferi (B310 or b hermsti (HS-1) survived after 24 hours of exposure. Ref. (11, 4-D) **Reference:** *Department of Health & Human Services (NIH) and cancer center laboratory test results, regarding Lyme disease.*

The Fox chase Cancer Center, Philadelphia, Pennsylvania, demonstrated growth inhibition of borrelia burgdorferi using colloidal silver in concentrations as low as two to ten PPM. Much more rapid effects demonstrated in higher concentrations e.g. fifteen to seventy-five PPM.

Cat's Claw

A tick-borne, multisystemic disease, Lyme borreliosis caused by the spirochete Borrelia burgdorferi has grown into a major public health problem during the last 10 years. The primary treatment for chronic Lyme disease is administration of various antibiotics. However, relapse often occurs when antibiotic treatment is discontinued. One possible explanation for this is that B. burgdorferi become resistant to antibiotic treatment, by converting from their vegetative spirochete form into different round bodies and/or into biofilm like colonies. There is an urgent need to find novel therapeutic agents that can eliminate all these different morphologies of B. burgdorferi. In this study, two herbal extracts, Samento and Banderol, as well as doxycycline (one of the primary antibiotics for Lyme disease treatment) were tested for their in vitro effectiveness on several of the different morphological forms of B. burgdorferi (spirochetes, round bodies, and biofilm like colonies) using fluorescent, darkfield microscopic, and BacLight viability staining methods. Our results demonstrated that both herbal agents, but not doxycycline, had very significant effects on all forms of B. burgdorferi, especially when used in combination, suggesting that herbal agents could provide an effective therapeutic approach for Lyme disease patients. **Reference:** *In Vitro Effectiveness of Samento and Banderol Herbal Extracts on the Different Morphological Forms of Borrelia Burgdorferi, by Akshita Datar, Navroop Kaur, Seema Patel, David F. Luecke, and Eva Sapi, PhD, Lyme Disease Research Group, University of New Haven.*

"Lyme Disease: Nutraceutical Breakthrough Using TOA-Free Cat's Claw"

Article: featured in the October 2003 Allergy Research Group Newsletter Focus.

Study Shows Pentacyclic Alkaloid Chemotype Uncaria tomentosa to be Effective In Treating Chronic Lyme Disease (Lyme Borreliosis)
INVESTIGATORS: William Lee Cowden, M.D. Hamid Moayad, D.O. Joan Vandergriff, N.D. Luis Romero, M.D., Ph.D. Svetlana Ivanova, M.D., Ph.D.

Control Group: A few patients experienced slight improvement, and the rest remained with no positive change in their clinical condition at the end of study. Experimental Group: 100% of patients experienced marked clinical improvement; 85% were seronegative for Lyme disease at the end of study. A 6-month pilot study was recently conducted with 28 patients suffering from Advanced Chronic Lyme disease. All the patients tested positive for Lyme disease utilizing the Western Blot blood test for Borrelia burgdorferi (Bb), the bacteria that causes Lyme disease. The control group was treated with conventional antibiotic treatment, and at the end of the study, from 14 patients in this group, 3 slightly improved, 3 got worse, and the rest remained with no change in their clinical condition. The experimental group was treated with Pentacyclic Alkaloid Chemotype Uncaria tomentosa. At the end of the study, 85% of the patients in this group tested negative for Bb, and all the patients experienced a dramatic improvement in their clinical condition. Pentacyclic Alkaloid Chemotype Uncaria tomentosa, also known as TOA-Free Cat's Claw, is a rare chemo - type of a medicinal plant commonly known as Cat's Claw, botanical name Uncaria tomentosa. Unlike traditional Cat's Claw products, this chemotype does not contain a group of chemical antagonists called tetracyclic oxindole alkaloids (TOAs) that act upon the central nervous system and can greatly inhibit the positive effect of the pentacyclic oxindole alkaloids (POAs). The Pentacyclic Alkaloid Chemotype Uncaria tomentosa that was utilized in the study contains a standardized amount of POAs that primarily affect the immune cells responsible for non-specific and cellular immunity, and demonstrate powerful immune system modulating properties. According to re search conducted in Austria, traditional Cat's Claw products may contain as much as 80% TOAs, and as little as 1% TOAs can cause a 30% reduction in immune system modulating properties that POAs provide. The latest research on Bb shows that it exists in at least three different forms: the spirochete, the spheroplast (also known as L-form), and the cyst. During the course of infection, Bb can shift among these three forms, converting from the spirochete form to the others when presented with an unfavorable environment (antibiotics, changes in pH of body fluids in chronic inflammation, etc.), and reverting back to the spirochete form to grow and reproduce upon being released from naturally aging and dying infected cells. It is during the growth period after re-conversion to the spirochete form, as well as in adult spirochete form, that Bb is most vulnerable and susceptible to antibiotics and natural elimination by the body's immune system. The severity of Lyme presentation is directly related to the spirochete load: low load results in mild or even asymptomatic infections. With increased spirochete load from subsequent re p e a t e d infections and/or reactivated dormant infections, the severity of the disease increases. Higher loads also impair key cells of the immune system and modify the immune response, thus making the immune system unable to fight the pathogen. The negative effects on the immune system increase the longer the spirochetes are present. To prevail in the effort to fight Lyme disease, it is necessary to not only restore the immune system to normal functioning, but to boost it as well. Even a normal functioning immune system is unable to attack and eliminate Bb in all its forms. The results of research on TOA - f re e Chemotype Cat's Claw demonstrate its powerful immune system modulating and stimulating properties, along with pronounced anti-inflammatory, antioxidant, and anti-infectious effects. The diverse spectrum of the biological activities of TOA - free Chemotype Cat's Claw is due to its biologically active compounds. The pentacyclic oxindole alkaloids (POAs) contained in this Chemotype are generally accepted as the principal immunomodulating and immunostimulating agents. POAs are actively involved in the repair of many elements and functional mechanisms of both the innate and acquire d immunity damaged by Bb and other coinfections, assisting in restoration of structural and functional integrity of the immune system, enhancing its ability to eliminate the pathogens in a natural way. In addition, this Chemotype contains quinovic acid glycosides – compounds with strong natural antibiotic properties (the latest generations of conventional synthetic antibiotics, "Quinolones," are based on quinovic acid glycosides), which further enhance the medicinal effect of TOA - free Chemotype Cat's Claw in fighting the infection. Considering the life-span of intracellular forms of Bb equivalent to the life-span of the cells invaded by these forms, they are constantly released into the surrounding environment upon natural cell death and destruction. The release of intracellular forms of Bb is gradual over time due to the various life-spans of various invaded cells. Since about 90% of these forms reside in various cells (including all blood cells) which have a life-span of 2-3 weeks to 6-8 months, it may be assumed that within a 6-8 month period, a significant majority of all intracellular forms of Bb will be released into the environment where they can be successfully attacked by a properly functioning immune system and a natural powerful antibiotic. Taking into account all the above, it can be assumed that continuous use of TOA-free Chemotype Cat's Claw over a period of time consistent with the lifespan of several generations of various infected cells (8-12 months), would more likely result in gradual killing and eliminating of Bb and co-existing infectious pathogens, with subsequent reduction of infectious load in the body and restoration of the person's health. It is believed that years can pass before symptoms appear in a patient who has been infected with Bb. In 1998, a study conducted in Switzerland demonstrated that only 12.5% of the patients that tested positive for Bb developed clinical symptoms confirming that the infection is often asymptomatic. A report fro m Germany outlines the case of a 12 year old boy that developed Lyme

Arthritis 5 years after being bit by a tick. The case indicates that the latency period between tick bite and onset of L y m e Arthritis may be as long as 5 years. All asymptomatic carriers of B b a re at risk of developing Lyme disease at some point. Stress, an increasing health concern for physicians worldwide, may have been the trigger that activated Lyme disease in a patient in Sweden, a 26 year-old woman with latent Lyme borreliosis that was concurrently activated with a herpes simplex virus type 1 infection. Immune suppression by stress may have caused activation of both infections.

Grapefruit Seed Extract (GSE)

In 2007, the journal "Infection" published a study looking at the effects of GSE on this gram-negative bacterium. B. burgdorferi has two forms, a motile form and a cystic form. This study looked at the effects of GSE on treating both forms in a laboratory setting. High concentrations of GSE completely destroyed both forms of the bacteria. *Reference: Brorson O, Brorson SH. Grapefruit seed extract is a powerful in vitro agent against motile and cystic forms of Borrelia burgdorferi sensu lato. Infection. 2007 Jun;35(3):206-8. No abstract available. PMID: 17565468 [PubMed - in process].*

MARFAN SYNDROME

Copper

Copper deficiency is a recognized but often overlooked cause of anemia and neutropenia. The authors began checking serum copper levels on patients referred for evaluation for unexplained anemia and neutropenia or myelodysplasia. Eight patients were identified as copper deficient (serum copper less than 70 microg/dL). The anemia was normochromic and normocytic in seven patients. Neutropenia was present in seven patients. Seven patients had been referred for evaluation of myelodysplasia. Three were seen for consideration for allogenic stem cell transplant. Five patients had concomitant peripheral neurological symptoms. Seven patients were treated with oral copper gluconate. All treated patients demonstrated a hematological response; seven had a complete remission. The improvement in anemia and neutropenia was rapid with normalization of blood counts within three to four weeks. In one patient, normalization of the underlying marrow dysplasia was demonstrated by bone marrow histology eight months after copper replacement. The cause of copper deficiency was felt to be gastrointestinal malabsorption in five of our patients. The authors conclude that copper deficiency should be considered in all patients with unexplained anemia and neutropenia or myelodysplasia. *Reference: Huff, J. D., et al. Copper deficiency causes reversible myelodysplasia. Am J Hematol. 82(7):625-630, 2007. - Section on Hematology and Oncology, Department of Internal Medicine, Wake Forest University School of Medicine, Winston-Salem, NC, USA.*

In the July 2005 issue of the Mayo Clinic Proceedings, Kumar et al described a woman with anemia, leukopenia, and lower limb weakness suspected of having myelodysplastic syndrome. Oral therapy with copper (8 mg/d) was initiated. Within several months, the patient's peripheral blood cell counts had normalized; within 6 months, her weakness had resolved. A diet low in copper may have been contributory. *Reference: Klevay, L. M. "Myelodysplasia," myeloneuropathy, and copper deficiency. Mayo Clin Proc. 81(1):132, 2006.*

The authors describe a patient with a suspected myelodysplastic syndrome that developed in association with a neurologic disorder resembling subacute combined degeneration but without vitamin B12 deficiency. Ultimately, the hematologic manifestations and the neurologic syndrome were linked to severe copper deficiency. Prompt and complete reversal of the hematologic abnormalities occurred with copper replacement (8 mg per day). Serum copper determination should be included in the work-up of patients with anemia and leukopenia of unclear etiology who have associated myeloneuropathy. The hematologic picture can resemble sideroblastic anemia or myelodysplastic syndrome. Hyperzincemia can be an accompanying abnormality even without exogenous zinc ingestion. The reason for the copper deficiency may not be evident. *Reference: Kumar, N., et al. "Myelodysplasia," myeloneuropathy, and copper deficiency. Mayo Clin Proc. 80(7):943-946, 2005. -- Department of Neurology, Mayo Clinic College of Medicine, Rochester, MN, USA.*

Aortic aneurysms are a key feature of Marfan syndrome. There are many studies linking copper deficiencies in humans and animals (turkeys, chickens, ostriches, waterfowl, rats, mice, pigs, cows and guinea pigs) to aortic aneurysms. Research has found that some animals develop aortic aneurysms because they have a genetic predisposition (not an incurable disorder) to be low in copper. Aneurysms in these animals are often reduced when they are fed a diet with sufficient copper. Interestingly, it has been noted that the symptoms of Mafan syndrome were similar to those of copper deficiency in chicks. Unfortunately, I couldn't find any studies of anyone ever actually testing people with Marfan syndrome for copper deficiencies. It would be a highly logical area to research. *Reference: Roes, E. M., et al. Effects of oral N-acetylcysteine on plasma homocysteine and whole blood glutathione levels in healthy, non-pregnant women. Clin Chem Lab Med. 40(5):496-498, 2002.*

N-acetylcysteine (NAC)

Elevated plasma homocysteine is a known risk factor for atherosclerotic vascular disease, but the strength of the relationship and the interaction of plasma homocysteine with other risk factors are unclear. The objective was to establish the magnitude of the vascular disease risk associated with an increased plasma homocysteine level and to examine interaction effects between elevated plasma homocysteine level and conventional risk factors. This was a case-control study. A total of 750 cases of atherosclerotic vascular disease (cardiac, cerebral, and peripheral) and 800 controls of both sexes younger than 60 years were studied. Plasma total homocysteine was measured while subjects were fasting and after a standardized methionine-loading test, which involves the administration of 100 mg of methionine per kilogram and stresses the metabolic pathway responsible for the irreversible degradation of homocysteine. Plasma cobalamin, pyridoxal 5'-phosphate, red blood cell folate, serum cholesterol, smoking, and blood pressure were also measured. The relative risk for vascular disease in the top fifth compared with the bottom four fifths of the control fasting total homocysteine distribution was 2.2 (95% confidence interval, 1.6-2.9). Methionine loading identified an additional 27% of at-risk cases. A dose-response effect was noted between total homocysteine level and risk. The risk was similar to and independent of that of other risk factors, but interaction effects were noted between homocysteine and these risk factors; for both sexes combined, an increased fasting homocysteine level showed a more than multiplicative effect on risk in smokers and in hypertensive subjects. Red blood cell folate, cobalamin, and pyridoxal phosphate, all of which modulate homocysteine metabolism, were inversely related to total homocysteine levels. Compared with nonusers of vitamin supplements, the small number of subjects taking such vitamins appeared to have a substantially lower risk of vascular disease, a proportion of which was attributable to lower plasma homocysteine levels. An increased plasma total homocysteine level confers an independent risk of vascular disease similar to that of smoking or hyperlipidemia. It powerfully increases the risk associated with smoking and hypertension. It is time to undertake randomized controlled trials of the effect of vitamins that reduce plasma homocysteine levels on vascular disease risk. *Reference: Graham, I. M., et al. Plasma homocysteine as risk factor for vascular disease. Journal of the American Medical Association. 277(22):1775-1781, 1997. Department of Cardiology, Adelaide Hospital, Trinity College, Dublin, Ireland.*

The objective of this study was to estimate the relations between established cardiovascular risk factors and total homocysteine (tHcy) in plasma. Health examination survey by the Norwegian Health Screening Service in 1992 and 1993. The setting was a general community, Hordaland County of Western Norway. A total of 7591 men and 8585 women, 40 to 67 years of age, with no history of hypertension, diabetes, coronary heart disease, or cerebrovascular disease were included. Plasma tHcy level was measured. The level of plasma tHcy was higher in men than in women and increased with age. In subjects 40 to 42 years old, geometric means were 10.8 mumol/L for 5918 men and 9.1 mumol/L for 6348 women. At age 65 to 67 years, the corresponding tHcy values were 12.3 mumol/L (1386 men) and 11.0 mumol/L (1932 women). Plasma tHcy level increased markedly with the daily number of cigarettes smoked in all age groups. Its relation to smoking was particularly strong in women. The combined effect of age, sex, and smoking was striking. Heavy-smoking men aged 65 to 67 years had a mean tHcy level 4.8 mumol/L higher than never-smoking women aged 40 to 42 years. Plasma tHcy level also was positively related to total cholesterol level, blood pressure, and heart rate and inversely related to physical activity. The relations were not substantially changed by multivariate adjustment, including intake of vitamin supplements, fruits, and vegetables. Elevated plasma tHcy level was associated with major components of the cardiovascular risk profile, ie, male sex, old age, smoking, high blood pressure, elevated cholesterol level, and lack of exercise. These findings should influence future studies on the etiology and pathogenesis of cardiovascular disease. *Reference: Nygard, O., et al. Total plasma homocysteine and cardiovascular risk profile. Journal of the American Medical Association. 274(19):1526-1533, 1995. Section for Medical Informatics and Statistics, University of Bergen, Norway.*

Oral N-acetylcysteine supplementation in nine young healthy females induced a quick and highly significant decrease in plasma homocysteine levels and an increase in whole blood concentration of the antioxidant glutathione. N-acetylcysteine impresses as an efficient drug in lowering homocysteine concentration and might be beneficial for individuals with hyperhomocysteinemia who are at increased risk of cardiovascular disease. *Reference: Stampfer, M. J., et al. Can lowering homocysteine levels reduce cardiovascular risk? New England Journal of Medicine. 332(5):328-329, 1995. -- Department of Obstetrics and Gynecology, University Medical Centre, Nijmegen, The Netherlands.*

A decrease of plasma homocysteine (Hcy) may represent a therapeutic promise for reducing the impact of atherosclerosis. N -Acetyl-cysteine (NAC) is a thiol-containing compound interfering with endogenous thiols, cysteine (Cys) and Hcy, by forming with them mixed disulphides with a possibly more efficient renal clearance. The aim of this work was to assess the effect of NAC intravenous infusion on plasma levels of different forms of Hcy and particularly to verify the effect on Hcy renal excretion. The authors collected basal blood samples at 0.5, 1, 2, 5, 8 and 24 h after the beginning of NAC infusion (50 mg kg(-1)body wt.) and also 24-h urine samples of the day of NAC infusion and of the day before and of the day after the infusion in ten healthy subjects (mean age 73+/-15). Urinary and plasma thiols (Hcy, Cys and NAC) were assayed by HPLC. Both total plasma Hcy (approx. 69%vs basal values) and Cys (approx. 40%vs basal values) fell progressively, reaching a minimum 5 h after infusion start; total free (i.e. not bound to proteins) Hcy (2.2+/-1.8 down from 4.4+/-4.2 nmol ml(-1)) and Cys (70.4+/-39.8 down from 113. 3+/-61.2 nmol ml(-1)) decreased as well. Reduced (thiolic-free form) Hcy and Cys decreased during infusion, though not as pronounced as for the other forms. Percentage-wise, out of the total plasma levels, Hcy and Cys total free form and reduced form tended to increase over infusion as well as their difference (i.e. the plasma mixed disulphide moiety), thus supporting the idea that excess NAC displaces thiols from their plasma binding sites forming mixed disulphides. Urinary total Cys and Hcy excretion significantly increased at the end of the day of NAC infusion (tenfold for Cys and fivefold for Hcy) and reduced appreciably on the following day. Also urinary excretion of the free form of Cys and Hcy increased at the end of the day of NAC infusion, although in a lower amount with respect of total amounts, meaning a reduction of percentage Cys and Hcy excreted as the free form; for none of the patients had proteinuria, the 'free' form of urine thiols has to be identified in the 'reduced' form, the difference between the total and free form reflecting the 'mixed disulphide' moiety. NAC intravenous administration induces an efficient and rapid reduction of plasma thiols, particularly of Hcy. These data support the hypothesis that NAC displaces thiols from their binding protein sites and forms, in excess of plasma NAC, mixed disulphides (NAC-Hcy) with an high renal clearance. This effect may represent the start of an alternative approach in the treatment of hyperhomocysteinemic conditions. *Reference: Ventura, P., et al. N -Acetyl-cysteine reduces homocysteine plasma levels after single intravenous administration by increasing thiols urinary excretion. Pharmacol Res. 40(4):345-350, 1999. Department of Internal Medicine, Chair of Geriatrics and Gerontology, University of Modena and Reggio Emilia, Modena, Italy.*

Acute administration of N-acetylcysteine (NAC) may induce alterations in plasma and urinary levels of homocysteine (Hcy) and cysteine (Cys). The authors studied the effects of continuous oral NAC therapy on different Hcy and Cys plasma and urinary forms in 40 healthy subjects assigned to three groups (groups A: n = 13, no therapy; group B: n = 14, NAC 600 mg/day, and group C: n = 14, NAC 1,800 mg/day) for 1 month (T(1)). After a 1-month washout period without therapy (T(2)), all subjects were treated with oral NAC (1,800 mg/day) for 2 months and (T(3) and T(4)) reassessed monthly for plasma and urinary thiols. The treated subjects showed a significant decrease in plasma total Hcy and a slight increase in total Cys levels; the alterations of different forms of plasma thiols suggested an NAC-induced increase in disulfide forms and an increase in urinary Hcy and Cys excretion as disulfide forms. The effects appeared to be dose dependent, being more marked in subjects treated with higher dosages. This approach may be important, as an association or alternative therapy in hyperhomocysteinemic conditions of poor responses to vitamins. *Reference:* *Ventura, P., et al. Urinary and plasma homocysteine and cysteine levels during prolonged oral N-acetylcysteine therapy. Pharmacology. 68(2):105-114, 2003. Currently, one of the most effective means for keeping homocysteine levels low is supplementation with NAC, (N-acetylcysteine). This is supplementation that can easily be justified by measuring plasma homocysteine levels if verification is needed. Department of Internal Medicine, Chair of Internal Medicine II, Modena, Italy.*

Magnesium

Dietary magnesium improves endothelial dependent relaxation of balloon injured arteries in rats. *Reference:* *Atherosclerosis. 1998 Aug;139(2):237-42. Fonseca FA, Paiva TB, Silva EG, Ihara SS, Kasinski N, Martinez TL.*

The purpose of the present study was to examine the importance of magnesium in endothelial function after arterial balloon injury. Male Wistar rats were fed normal, high or low concentrations of magnesium. Three weeks later the animals underwent endothelial injury of the thoracic aorta by a balloon catheter or a sham operation. Biochemical, histological and endothelial function analysis were performed 15 days after the surgical treatment. The animals fed a low magnesium diet presented the lowest level of serum magnesium and the highest ionized blood calcium levels. Histomorphometric analysis revealed no differences among groups neither regarding the magnitude of intimal thickening nor the recovery of endothelial coverage. However, when vasoreactivity responses were compared in the balloon-injured group, those animals fed high magnesium diet had the better endothelium-dependent vascular relaxation. In conclusion, a higher magnesium level in the diet was beneficial to vessels that underwent endothelial injury by balloon catheter. *Reference:* *Department of Medicine, Disciplina de Cardiologia, Universidade Federal de São Paulo, Escola Paulista de Medicina, SP, Brazil. ffonseca@mandic.com.br.*

MULTIPLE SCLEROSIS (MS)

Dental Amalgam

It was claimed by the Scientific Committee on Emerging and Newly Identified Health Risks (SCENIHR)) in a report to the EU-Commission that "....no risks of adverse systemic effects exist and the current use of dental amalgam does not pose a risk of systemic disease..." SCENIHR disregarded the toxicology of mercury and did not include most important scientific studies in their review. But the real scientific data show that: (a) Dental amalgam is by far the main source of human total mercury body burden. This is proven by autopsy studies which found 2-12 times more mercury in body tissues of individuals with dental amalgam. Autopsy studies are the most valuable and most important studies for examining the amalgam-caused mercury body burden. (b) These autopsy studies have shown consistently that many individuals with amalgam have toxic levels of mercury in their brains or kidneys. (c) There is no correlation between mercury levels in blood or urine, and the levels in body tissues or the severity of clinical symptoms. SCENIHR only relied on levels in urine or blood. (d) The half-life of mercury in the brain can last from several years to decades, thus mercury accumulates over time of amalgam exposure in body tissues to toxic levels. However, SCENIHR state that the half-life of mercury in the body is only "20-90 days". (e) Mercury vapor is about ten times more toxic than lead on human neurons and with synergistic toxicity to other metals. (f) Most studies cited by SCENIHR which conclude that amalgam fillings are safe have severe methodical flaws. *Reference: J Occup Med Toxicol. 2011; 6: 2. Published online 2011 January 13. doi: 10.1186/1745-6673-6-2. Is dental amalgam safe for humans? The opinion of the scientific committee of the European Commission. Joachim Mutter. This article has been cited by other articles in PMC.*

Air Pollution

Exposure to ambient air pollution is a serious and common public health concern associated with growing morbidity and mortality worldwide. In the last decades, the adverse effects of air pollution on the pulmonary and cardiovascular systems have been well established in a series of major epidemiological and observational studies. In the recent past, air pollution has also been associated with diseases of the central nervous system (CNS), including stroke, Alzheimer's disease, Parkinson's disease, and neurodevelopmental disorders. It has been demonstrated that various components of air pollution, such as nano sized particles, can easily translocate to the CNS where they can activate innate immune responses. Furthermore, systemic inflammation arising from the pulmonary or cardiovascular system can affect CNS health. Despite intense studies on the health effects of ambient air pollution, the underlying molecular mechanisms of susceptibility and disease remain largely elusive. However, emerging evidence suggests that air pollution-induced neuroinflammation, oxidative stress, microglial activation, cerebrovascular dysfunction, and alterations in the blood-brain barrier contribute to CNS pathology. A better understanding of the mediators and mechanisms will enable the development of new strategies to protect individuals at risk and to reduce detrimental effects of air pollution on the nervous system and mental health. *Reference: J Toxicol. 2012; 2012: 782462. Published online 2012 February 19. doi: 10.1155/2012/782462. PMCID: PMC3317189. The Adverse Effects of Air Pollution on the Nervous System. Sermin Genc, Zeynep Zadeoglulari, Stefan H. Fuss, and Kursad Genc.*

UV Radiation

French farmers and their families constitute an informative population to study multiple sclerosis (MS) prevalence and related epidemiology. We carried out an ecological study to evaluate the association of MS prevalence and ultraviolet (UV) radiation, a candidate climatologic risk factor. **Methods:** Mean annual and winter (December–March) UVB irradiation values were systematically compared to MS prevalence rates in corresponding regions of France. UVB data were obtained from the solar radiation database (SoDa) service and prevalence rates from previously published data on 2,667 MS cases registered with the national farmer health insurance system, Mutualité Sociale Agricole (MSA). Pearson correlation was used to examine the relationship of annual and winter UVB values with MS prevalence. Male and female prevalence were also analyzed separately. Linear regression was used to test for interaction of annual and winter UVB with sex in predicting MS prevalence. **Results:** There was a strong association between MS prevalence and annual mean UVB irradiation ($r = -0.80$, $p < 0.001$) and average winter UVB ($r = -0.87$, $p < 0.001$). Both female ($r = -0.76$, $p < 0.001$) and male ($r = -0.46$, $p = 0.032$) prevalence rates were correlated with annual UVB. Regression modeling showed that the effect of UVB on prevalence rates differed by sex; the interaction effect was significant for both annual UVB ($p = 0.003$) and winter UVB ($p = 0.002$). **Conclusions:** The findings suggest that regional UVB radiation is predictive of corresponding MS prevalence rates and supports the hypothesis that sunlight exposure influences MS risk. The evidence also supports a potential role for gender-specific effects of UVB exposure. *Reference: Neurology. 2011 February 1; 76(5): 425–431. doi: 10.1212/WNL. 0b013e31820a0a9f. PMCID: PMC3034408. Association of UV radiation with multiple sclerosis prevalence and sex ratio in France. S.-M. Orton, PhD, L. Wald, PhD, C. Confavreux, MD, S. Vukusic, PhD, J.P. Krohn, MSc, S.V. Ramagopalan, PhD, B.M. Herrera, PhD, A.D. Sadovnick, PhD, and G.C. Ebers, MD, FMedSci. From the Wellcome Trust Centre for Human Genetics and Department of Clinical Neurology (S.-M.O., J.P.K., S.V.R., B.M.H., G.C.E.), University of Oxford, Oxford, UK; Centre Energétique et Procédés (L.W.), MINES ParisTech, Sophia Antipolis cedex; Service de Neurologie A and EDMUS Coordinating Center (C.C., S.V.), Hôpital Neurologique Pierre Wertheimer, Hospices Civils de Lyon, Bron, France; INSERM U842 (C.C., S.V.), Lyon,*

France; Université Lyon 1 (C.C., S.V.), Lyon, France; and Department of Medical Genetics and Faculty of Medicine (A.D.S.), Division of Neurology, University of British Columbia, Vancouver, Canada.

Epidemiological, clinical and laboratory studies have implicated solar ultraviolet (UV) radiation in various skin diseases including premature aging of the skin and melanoma and nonmelanoma skin cancers. Chronic UV radiation exposure-induced skin diseases or skin disorders are caused by the excessive induction of inflammation, oxidative stress and DNA damage, etc.. The use of chemopreventive agents, such as plant polyphenols, to inhibit these events in UV-exposed skin is gaining attention. Chemoprevention refers to the use of agents that can inhibit, reverse, or retard the process of these harmful events in the UV-exposed skin. A wide variety of polyphenols or phytochemicals, most of which are dietary supplements, have been reported to possess substantial skin photoprotective effects. This review article summarizes the photoprotective effects of some selected polyphenols, such as green tea polyphenols, grape seed proanthocyanidins, resveratrol, silymarin and genistein, on UV-induced skin inflammation, oxidative stress, and DNA damage, etc., with a focus on mechanisms underlying the photoprotective effects of these polyphenols. The laboratory studies conducted in animal models, suggest that these polyphenols have the ability to protect the skin from the adverse effects of UV radiation, including the risk of skin cancers. It is suggested that polyphenols may favorably supplement sunscreens protection, and may be useful for skin diseases associated with solar UV radiation-induced inflammation, oxidative stress and DNA damage. **Reference:** *Arch Dermatol Res. 2010 March; 302(2): 71. Published online 2009 November 7. doi: 10.1007/s00403-009-1001-3. Skin photoprotection by natural polyphenols: Anti-inflammatory, anti-oxidant and DNA repair mechanisms. Joi A. Nichols and Santosh K. Katiyar.*

Animal Fat & Cow's Milk

Multiple sclerosis is a complex and multifactorial neurological disease, and nutrition is one of the environmental factors possibly involved in its pathogenesis. At present, the role of nutrition is unclear, and MS therapy is not associated to a particular diet. MS clinical trials based on specific diets or dietary supplements are very few and in some cases controversial. To understand how diet can influence the course of MS and improve the wellness of MS patients, it is necessary to identify the dietary molecules, their targets and the molecular mechanisms involved in the control of the disease. The aim of this paper is to provide a molecular basis for the nutritional intervention in MS by evaluating at molecular level the effect of dietary molecules on the inflammatory and autoimmune processes involved in the disease. *Nutrients to Avoid in MS*:   **Animal Fat** -- In principle, MS patients should avoid the intake of food containing molecules that are potentially harmful over time and should prefer healthy food containing those molecules that can improve their well-being by lowering, for example, the extent of inflammation. Among the dietary factors that have been considered most frequently for their deleterious influence on MS are saturated fatty acids of animal origin (found in whole milk, butter, cheese, meat, sausages ...). In 1950 Swank suggested that the consumption of saturated animal fat is directly related to the frequency of MS. In 2003, Swank and Goodwin reported that restriction of saturated fat induces remission of the disease and produces beneficial effects in MS patients. These effects have been ascribed to the fact that saturated fat forms aggregates that may be not capable of entering the smallest capillaries. Obstructions of the capillaries may contribute to MS and other diseases. In addition saturated fats decrease membrane fluidity, lead to the synthesis of cholesterol, activate the CD14/TLR4 receptor complex and favor the formation of TNF-α. As shown in hypercaloric diets rich in saturated lipids and lipogenesis favor several human diseases. Metabolic patterns and diseases correlated with lipogenesis. It is becoming clear now that the influence of fat on cells is more direct: is controlled at transcriptional level, and influences gene expression, cell metabolism, and cell growth, and differentiation. **Cow Milk** -- MFGM Proteins, and Molecular Mimicry in MS. MS is believed to be an autoimmune disease. Environmental (either microbial or dietary) factors can be associated with autoimmunity and myelin breakdown by molecular mimicry, that is, the amino acid homology between the autoantigen and microbial or dietary peptides. According to this hypothesis, molecular mimicry may disrupt immunological self-tolerance to CNS myelin antigens in genetically susceptible individuals.The best example of potential molecular mimicry between myelin autoantigens and dietary proteins is given by cow's milk. The hypothesis of a link between milk consumption and MS has been taken into consideration since the mid of 1970s. Later, epidemiological studies gave support to this hypothesis. The milk proteins that could be detrimental in MS are the proteins of the milk fat globule membrane (MFGM proteins). The MFGM proteins account for only 1-2% of the total protein fraction, and for this reason they are not relevant for their nutritional value. The protein which is most frequently suspected of the association with MS is butyrophilin (BTN), the most representative MFGM protein. BTN belongs to the Ig superfamily and is very similar to MOG, the myelin oligodendrocyte glycoprotein, one of the candidate autoantigen in MS. BTN inhibits the MOG-induced experimental autoimmune encephalomyelitis (EAE), but also induces inflammatory responses in the CNS, when injected alone into animals, and stimulates in vitro MOG-specific T cell responses. Antibody cross-reactivity between MOG and BTN has been observed in MS. Antibodies against BTN and other MFGM proteins have been detected also in two other diseases: autism and coronary heart disease (CHD).The MFGM proteins might have detrimental effects on health also because they are associated to milk saturated fat, another possibly deleterious dietary component. On these grounds, we have introduced the concept that the consumption of the MFGM proteins by MS patients should be discouraged. Different is the opinion of Spitsberg (2005) who reviewed the intake of MFGM proteins and milk fat and recommended them for their potential nutraceutical value. However, reports on the relationship between human health and cow milk do not substantiate such an assertion, at present. *Reference: Autoimmune Dis. 2010; 2010: 249842. Published online 2011 February 24. doi: 10.4061/2010/249842. PMCID: PMC3065662. May Diet and Dietary Supplements Improve the Wellness of Multiple Sclerosis Patients? A Molecular Approach. Paolo Riccio, Rocco Rossano, and Grazia Maria Liuzzi. Dipartimento di Biologia D.B.A.F., Università degli Studi della Basilicata, 85100 Potenza, Italy. Istituto Nazionale di Biostrutture e Biosistemi (INBB), 00100 Roma, Italy. Dipartimento di Biochimica e Biologia Molecolare "Ernesto Quagliariello", 70126, Bari, Italy.*

N-Acetylcysteine (NAC)

Following the initial acute stage of spinal cord injury, a cascade of cellular and inflammatory responses will lead to progressive secondary damage of the nerve tissue surrounding the primary injury site. The degeneration is manifested by loss of neurons and glial cells, demyelination and cyst formation. Injury to the mammalian spinal cord results in nearly complete failure of the severed axons to regenerate. We have previously demonstrated that the antioxidants N-acetylcysteine (NAC) and acetyl-L-carnitine (ALC) can attenuate retrograde neuronal degeneration after peripheral nerve and ventral root injury. The present study evaluates the effects of NAC and ALC on neuronal survival, axonal sprouting and glial cell reactions after spinal cord injury in adult rats. Tibial motoneurons in the spinal cord were pre-labeled with fluorescent tracer Fast Blue one week before lumbar L5 hemisection. Continuous intrathecal infusion of NAC (2.4 mg/day) or ALC (0.9 mg/day) was initiated immediately after spinal injury using Alzet 2002 osmotic minipumps. Neuroprotective effects of treatment were assessed by counting surviving motoneurons and by using quantitative immunohistochemistry and Western blotting for neuronal and glial cell markers 4 weeks after hemisection. Spinal cord injury induced significant loss of tibial motoneurons in L4–L6 segments. Neuronal degeneration was associated with decreased immunostaining for microtubular-associated protein-2 (MAP2) in dendritic branches, synaptophysin in presynaptic boutons and neurofilaments in nerve fibers. Immunostaining for the astroglial marker GFAP and microglial marker OX42 was increased. Treatment with NAC and ALC rescued approximately half of the motoneurons destined to die. In addition, antioxidants restored MAP2 and synaptophysin immunoreactivity. However, the perineuronal synaptophysin labeling was not recovered. Although both treatments promoted axonal sprouting, there was no effect on reactive astrocytes. In contrast, the microglial reaction was significantly attenuated. The results indicate a therapeutic potential for NAC and ALC in the early treatment of traumatic spinal cord injury. *Reference: Published online 2012 July 17. doi: 10.1371/journal.pone.0041086. Neuroprotective Effects of N-Acetyl-Cysteine and Acetyl-L-Carnitine after Spinal Cord Injury in Adult Rats. Amar Karalija, Liudmila N. Novikova, Paul J. Kingham, Mikael Wiberg, and Lev N. Novikov.*

Acetyl-L-Carnitine (ALC)

The effects of long-term treatment (11 months) with acetyl-L-carnitine (75 mg/kg daily) on the morphology of brain and optic nerve was studied in 16 senescent (22-month-old) Wistar rats (nine untreated, seven treated). Five young rats (aged 3 months) were used for comparison. Senescence was found to cause a structural disorganization of cerebral cortex, hippocampus and cerebellar cortex, and a decrease in the volume densities of the pyramidal neurons of layers 2 and 5 of the prefrontal cortex. An impaired myelination of the pyramidal tract and of the optic nerve was also observed. Besides improving the structural organization of the cerebral areas under study, treatment with acetyl-L-carnitine increased the volume densities of pyramidal neurons of the prefrontal cortex layers under observation. Myelination of the pyramidal tract and optic nerve was found to be less impaired after acetyl-L-carnitine administration. *Reference: Drugs Exp Clin Res. 14(9):593-601, 1988. Effect of long-term treatment with acetyl-L-carnitine on structural changes of ageing rat brain. Ramacci, M. T., et al. Biological Research Laboratories, Sigma Tau S.p.A., Pomezia, Rome, Italy.*

Treatment with acetyl l-carnitine (ALCAR) has been shown to improve fatigue in patients with chronic fatigue syndrome, but there have been no trials on the effect of ALCAR for treating fatigue in multiple sclerosis (MS). To compare the efficacy of ALCAR with that of amantadine, one of the drugs most widely used to treat MS-related fatigue, 36 MS patients presenting fatigue were enrolled in a randomised, double-blind, crossover study. Patients were treated for 3 months with either amantadine (100 mg twice daily) or ALCAR (1 g twice daily). After a 3-month washout period, they crossed over to the alternative treatment for 3 months. Patients were rated at baseline and every 3 months according to the Fatigue Severity Scale (FSS), the primary endpoint of the study. Secondary outcome variables were: Fatigue Impact Scale (FIS), Beck Depression Inventory (BDI) and Social Experience Checklist (SEC). Six patients withdrew from the study because of adverse reactions (five on amantadine and one on ALCAR). Statistical analysis showed significant effects of ALCAR compared with amantadine for the Fatigue Severity Scale (p=0.039). There were no significant effects for any of the secondary outcome variables. The results of this study show that ALCAR is better tolerated and more effective than amantadine for the treatment of MS-related fatigue. *Reference: J Neurol Sci. 218(1-2):103-108, 2004. Comparison of the effects of acetyl l-carnitine and amantadine for the treatment of fatigue in multiple sclerosis: results of a pilot, randomised, double-blind, crossover trial. Tomassini, V., et al. Department of Neurological Sciences, University of Rome, Rome, Italy.*

Recent studies suggest that NO and its reactive derivative peroxynitrite are implicated in the pathogenesis of multiple sclerosis (MS). Patients dying with MS demonstrate increased astrocytic inducible nitric oxide synthase activity, as well as increased levels of iNOS mRNA. Peroxynitrite is a strong oxidant capable of damaging target tissues, particularly the brain, which is known to be endowed with poor antioxidant buffering capacity.   Inducible nitric oxide synthase is upregulated in the central nervous system (CNS) of animals with experimental allergic encephalomyelitis (EAE) and in patients with MS.   The authors have recently demonstrated in patients with active MS a significant increase of NOS activity associated with increased nitration of proteins in the cerebrospinal fluid (CSF).   Acetylcarnitine is proposed as a therapeutic agent for several neurodegenerative disorders.   MS patients were treated for 6 months with acetylcarnitine and compared with untreated MS subjects or with patients noninflammatory neurological conditions, taken as controls.   Western blot analysis showed in MS patients increased nitrosative stress associated with a significant decrease of reduced glutathione (GSH).   Increased levels of oxidized glutathione (GSSG) and nitrosothiols were also observed.   Interestingly, treatment of MS patients with acetylcarnitine resulted in decreased CSF levels of NO reactive metabolites and protein nitration, as well as increased content of GSH and GSH/GSSG ratio.   These data sustain the hypothesis that nitrosative stress is a major consequence of NO produced in MS-affected CNS and implicate a possible important role for acetylcarnitine in protecting brain against nitrosative stress, which may underlie the pathogenesis of MS. **Reference:** *Neurochem Res.   28(9):1321-1328, 2003. Disruption of thiol homeostasis and nitrosative stress in the cerebrospinal fluid of patients with active multiple sclerosis: evidence for a protective role of acetylcarnitine. Calabrese, V., et al. Department of Chemistry, Section of Biochemistry and Molecular Biology. Faculty of Medicine, University of Catania, Catania, Italy.*

L-carnitine fumarate

Fumarates improve multiple sclerosis (MS) and psoriasis, two diseases in which both IL-12 and IL-23 promote pathogenic T helper (Th) cell differentiation. However, both diseases show opposing responses to most established therapies. First, we show in humans that fumarate treatment induces IL-4–producing Th2 cells in vivo and generates type II dendritic cells (DCs) that produce IL-10 instead of IL-12 and IL-23. In mice, fumarates also generate type II DCs that induce IL-4–producing Th2 cells in vitro and in vivo and protect mice from experimental autoimmune encephalomyelitis. Type II DCs result from fumarate-induced glutathione (GSH) depletion, followed by increased hemoxygenase-1 (HO-1) expression and impaired STAT1 phosphorylation. Induced HO-1 is cleaved, whereupon the N-terminal fragment of HO-1 translocates into the nucleus and interacts with AP-1 and NF-κB sites of the IL-23p19 promoter. This interaction prevents IL-23p19 transcription without affecting IL-12p35, whereas STAT1 inactivation prevents IL-12p35 transcription without affecting IL-23p19. As a consequence, GSH depletion by small molecules such as fumarates induces type II DCs in mice and in humans that ameliorate inflammatory autoimmune diseases. This therapeutic approach improves Th1- and Th17-mediated autoimmune diseases such as psoriasis and MS by interfering with IL-12 and IL-23 production. *Reference: J Exp Med. 2011 October 24; 208(11): 2291–2303. doi: 10.1084/jem.20100977. Fumarates improve psoriasis and multiple sclerosis by inducing type II dendritic cells. Kamran Ghoreschi, Jürgen Brück, Christina Kellerer, Caishu Deng, Haiyan Peng, Oliver Rothfuss, Rehana Z. Hussain, Anne R. Gocke, Annedore Respa, Ivana Glocova, Nadejda Valtcheva, Eva Alexander, Susanne Feil, Robert Feil, Klaus Schulze-Osthoff, Rudolf A. Rupec, Amy E. Lovett-Racke, Ralf Dringen, Michael K. Racke, and Martin Röcken.*

Vitamin D

Background - Multiple sclerosis is the most common chronic inflammatory disease of the central nervous system in young adults. Despite the fact that numerous lines of evidence link both the risk of disease development and the disease course to the serum level of 25-hydroxyvitamin D it still remains elusive whether multiple sclerosis patients benefit from boosting the serum level of 25-hydroxyvitamin D, mainly because interventional clinical trials that directly address the therapeutic effects of vitamin D in multiple sclerosis are sparse. We here present the protocol of an interventional clinical phase II study to test the hypothesis, that high-dose vitamin D supplementation of multiple sclerosis patients is safe and superior to low-dose supplementation with respect to beneficial therapeutic effects. **Methods/Design-** The EVIDIMS trial is a German multi-center, stratified, randomized, controlled and double-blind clinical phase II pilot study. Eighty patients with the diagnosis of definite multiple sclerosis or clinically isolated syndrome who are on a stable immunomodulatory treatment with interferon-β1b will be randomized to additionally receive either high-dose (average daily dose 10.200 IU) or low-dose (average daily dose 200 IU) cholecalciferol for a total period of 18 months. The primary outcome measure is the number of new lesions detected on T2-weighted cranial MRI at 3 tesla. Secondary endpoints include additional magnetic resonance imaging and optical coherence tomography parameters for neuroinflammation and -degeneration, clinical parameters for disease activity, as well as cognition, fatigue, depression, and quality of life. Safety and tolerability of high-dose vitamin D supplementation are further outcome parameters. **Discussion** - In light of the discrepancy between existing epidemiological and preclinical data on the one hand and available clinical data on the other the study design presented here has the potential to substantially contribute to the evaluation of the efficacy of vitamin D supplementation in MS and CIS patients. The randomized, controlled, double-blinded study design and the implementation of independent evaluation of outcome parameters fulfill the criteria for a high-quality clinical phase II trial in MS [34]. Some aspects of the study design however may deserve a closer discussion: Why was an active treatment regimen instead of a placebo treatment chosen for the control arm, i.e. low-dose vitamin D? In fact, this question was heavily debated. Although we do not know whether this represents rather a causal factor or a consequence, serum levels of 25-hydroxyvitamin D are often quite low in

MS patients. Thus, we expect that low serum levels or even vitamin D deficiency will be detected in a substantial number of screened study candidates. From an ethical point of view and bearing in mind the importance of vitamin D for bone metabolism it would be difficult not to supplement these patients with vitamin D. On the other hand, the daily dose provided in the control arm may not be immunologically active itself as this would prevent the detection of any difference between both groups. Thus, the daily dose recommended by the German Nutrition Society for this group of age which corresponds to 5 µg or 200 IU and which most probably has no immunomodulatory potential represents a compromise between ethical concerns and efficacy aspects. Another important question relates to the dose used in the high-dose arm. In fact, we do not know, at which minimum doses or serum levels vitamin D starts to have immunomodulatory effects. To prevent failure of the trial because of an insufficient treatment dose, we choose the maximum dose for which sufficient safety data are available, which currently corresponds to 10.000 IU per day. It might well be that already smaller doses would be sufficient, but on the other hand it is rather unlikely, that if this dose does not demonstrate any treatment effect, even higher daily doses would do. A further question might be why an add-on regimen to an established immunomodulatory treatment with interferon-β was chosen? In fact, from a methodological point of view, a monotherapeutic design would be preferable. However, since disease-modifying drugs are established and approved for the treatment of MS it would again be unethical to withhold these treatment options in favor of an experimental approach. The restriction to interferon-β as immunomodulatory treatment is explained by the need for maximum homogeneity in the trial cohort on the one hand and the reported synergistic effects of interferon-β and the vitamin D system on the other . Finally, one might suspect that in view of the rather small sample size of 80 participants the study might be underpowered to detect a significant difference between both groups. However, the study will be able to detect a difference in mean new T2-hyperintense lesions per year of 1.5 with a power of more than 0.8. In the pivotal interferon-β1b trial, verum treatment resulted in a reduction of 2.0 lesions per year as compared to a placebo arm. Thus, if high-dose supplementation with vitamin D is indeed effective, a reduction of 1.5 lesions per year would not be unrealistic. In **conclusion**, vitamin D has the potential for a safe, orally available and cheap treatment option in MS and the EVIDIMS trial may help to close the existing gap between available promising preclinical and the lacking clinical data on the immunomodulatory efficacy of vitamin D in MS. *Reference: Trials. 2012; 13: 15. Published online 2012 February 8. doi: 10.1186/1745-6215-13-15. Efficacy of Vitamin D Supplementation in Multiple Sclerosis (EVIDIMS Trial): study protocol for a randomized controlled trial. Jan Dörr, Stephanie Ohlraun, Horst Skarabis, and Friedemann Paul.*

Low vitamin D status has been associated with multiple sclerosis (MS) prevalence and risk, but the therapeutic potential of vitamin D in established MS has not been explored. The aim was to assess the tolerability of high-dose oral vitamin D and its impact on biochemical, immunologic, and clinical outcomes in patients with MS prospectively. An open-label randomized prospective controlled 52-week trial matched patients with MS for demographic and disease characteristics, with randomization to treatment or control groups. Treatment patients received escalating vitamin D doses up to 40,000 IU/day over 28 weeks to raise serum 25-hydroxyvitamin D [25(OH)D] rapidly and assess tolerability, followed by 10,000 IU/day (12 weeks), and further down titrated to 0 IU/day. Calcium (1,200 mg/day) was given throughout the trial. Primary endpoints were mean change in serum calcium at each vitamin D dose and a comparison of serum calcium between groups. Secondary endpoints included 25(OH)D and other biochemical measures, immunologic biomarkers, relapse events, and Expanded Disability Status Scale (EDSS) score. Forty-nine patients (25 treatment, 24 control) were enrolled [mean age 40.5 years, EDSS 1.34, and 25(OH)D 78 nmol/L]. All calcium-related measures within and between groups were normal. Despite a mean peak 25(OH)D of 413nmol/L, no significant adverse events occurred. Although there may have been confounding variables in clinical outcomes, treatment group patients appeared to have fewer relapse events and a persistent reduction in T-cell proliferation compared to controls. High-dose vitamin D (approximately 10,000 IU/day) in multiple sclerosis is safe, with evidence of immunomodulatory effects. This trial provides Class II evidence that high-dose vitamin D use for 52 weeks in patients with multiple sclerosis does not significantly increase serum calcium levels when compared to patients not on high-dose supplementation. The trial, however, lacked statistical precision and the design requirements to adequately assess changes in clinical disease measures (relapses and Expanded Disability Status Scale scores), providing only Class level IV evidence for these outcomes. *Reference: A phase I/II dose-escalation trial of vitamin D3 and calcium in multiple sclerosis. Neurology. 2010. Burton, J. M., et al.*

Experimental autoimmune encephalomyelitis (EAE) is an autoimmune disease believed to be a model for the human disease multiple sclerosis (MS). Induced by immunizing B10.PL mice with myelin basic protein (MBP). EAE was completely prevented by the administration of 1,25-dihydroxyvitamin D3 (1,25- (OH)2D3). 1,25-(OH)2D3 could also prevent the progression of EAE when administered at the appearance of the first disability symptoms. Withdrawal of 1,25-(OH)2D3 resulted in a resumption of the progression of EAE. Thus, the block by 1,25-(OH)2D3 is reversible. A deficiency of vitamin D resulted in an increased susceptibility to EAE. Thus, 1,25-(OH)2D3 or its analogs are potentially important for treatment of MS. *Reference: 1,25-dihydroxyvitamin D3 reversibly blocks the progression of relapsing encephalomyelitis, a model of multiple sclerosis. Proceedings of the National Academy of Sciences of the United States of America (USA). 93(15):7861-7864, 1996. Cantorna, M. T., et al.*

Multiple sclerosis (MS) is a demyelinating disease of the central nervous system that runs a chronic course and disables young people. The disease is more prevalent in the geographic areas that are farthest from the equator. No form of treatment is known to be effective in preventing MS or its disabling complications. A number of epidemiological studies have shown a protective effect of exposure to sunlight during early life and a recent longitudinal study confirmed that vitamin D supplementation reduced life-time prevalence of MS in women. Very little is known regarding the role of vitamin D on the developing brain but experimental data suggest that cerebral white matter is vitamin D responsive and oligodendrocytes in the brain and spinal cord and express vitamin D receptors. It is possible that differentiation and axonal adhesion of oligodendrocytes are influenced by vitamin D level during brain development and a relative lack of vitamin D may increase oligodendroglial apoptosis. The age effect of migration on susceptibility to develop MS could be explained by a role of vitamin D on brain development. In areas of high MS prevalence, dietary supplementation of vitamin D in early life may reduce the incidence of MS. In addition, like folic acid, vitamin D supplementation should also be routinely recommended in pregnancy. Prevention of MS by modifying an important environmental factor (sunlight exposure and vitamin D level) offers a practical and cost-effective way to reduce the burden of the disease in the future generations. **Reference:** *Why we should offer routine vitamin D supplementation in pregnancy and childhood to prevent multiple sclerosis. Med Hypotheses. 64(3):608-618, 2005. Chaudhuri, A., et al. Department of Neurology, Institute of Neurological Sciences, 1345 Govan Road, Glasgow, UK.*

The authors administered calcium (1,100 mg per day), magnesium (680 mg per day), and 20 grams of cod liver oil (which contains vitamin D) to 16 young MS patients for periods of one to two years. The number of multiple sclerosis exacerbations observed during the program was less than ½ the predicted number. **Reference:** *Multiple sclerosis: decreased relapse rate through dietary supplementation with calcium, magnesium and vitamin D. Medical Hypotheses 21:193-200, 1986. Goldberg, P., et al.*

Inheriting genetic risk factors for multiple sclerosis (MS) is not sufficient to cause this demyelinating disease of the central nervous system; exposure to environmental risk factors is also required. MS may be preventable if these unidentified environmental factors can be avoided. MS prevalence increases with decreasing solar radiation, suggesting that sunlight may be protective in MS. Since the vitamin D endocrine system is exquisitely responsive to sunlight, and MS prevalence is highest where environmental supplies of vitamin D are lowest, the authors proposed that the hormone, 1, 25-dihydroxycholecalciferol (1,25-(OH)2D3), may protect genetically-susceptible individuals from developing MS. Evidence consistent with this hypothesis comes not only from geographic studies, but also genetic and biological studies. Over-representation of the vitamin D receptor gene b allele was found in Japanese MS patients, suggesting it may confer MS susceptibility. Fish oil is an excellent vitamin D source, and diets rich in fish may lower MS prevalence or severity. Vitamin D deficiency afflicts most MS patients, as demonstrated by their low bone mass and high fracture rates. However, the clearest evidence that vitamin D may be a natural inhibitor of MS comes from experiments with experimental autoimmune encephalomyelitis (EAE), a model of MS. Treatment of mice with 1,25-(OH)2D3 completely inhibited EAE induction and progression. The hormone stimulated the synthesis of two anti-encephalitogenic cytokines, interleukin 4 and transforming growth factor beta-1, and influenced inflammatory cell trafficking or apoptosis. If vitamin D is a natural inhibitor of MS, providing supplemental vitamin D to individuals who are at risk for MS would be advisable. *Reference: Vitamin D: a natural inhibitor of multiple sclerosis. Proc Nutr Soc. 59(4):531-535, 2000. Hayes, C. E.*

Availability of vitamin D, decreases with increasing latitude in patterns closely correlated with increasing MS rates. Individuals with a high exposure to sunlight have a significantly lower risk of MS, independent of country of origin, age, sex, race, and socioeconomic status. This lowered risk may be attributable to sunshine stimulating vitamin D production. *Reference: Vitamin D and multiple sclerosis. Proc Soc Exper Biol Med. 216:21-27, 1997. Hayes, C. E., et al.*

Multiple sclerosis (MS) patients were randomized, in a double blind design, and placed into either a vitamin D supplemented group or a placebo control group. As expected, serum 25-hydroxyvitamin D levels increased significantly following 6 month vitamin D supplementation (17+/-6 ng/ml at baseline to 28+/-8 ng/ml at 6 months). Vitamin D supplementation also significantly increased serum transforming growth factor (TGF)-beta1 levels from 230+/-21 pg/ml at baseline to 295+/-40 pg/ml 6 months later. Placebo treatment had no effect on serum TGF-beta1 levels. Tumor necrosis factor (TNF)-alpha, interferon (IFN)-gamma, and interleukin (IL)-13 were not different following vitamin D supplementation. IL-2 mRNA levels decreased following vitamin D supplementation but the differences did not reach significance. Vitamin D supplementation of MS patients for 6 months was associated with increased vitamin D status and serum TGF-beta1. *Reference: Cytokine profile in patients with multiple sclerosis following vitamin D supplementation. J Neuroimmunol. 134(1-2):128-132, 2003. Mahon, B. D., et al. Graduate Program in Nutrition, Pennsylvania State University, University Park, PA, USA.*

Recent studies and commentaries link vitamin D with several autoimmune diseases, including multiple sclerosis (MS). Adequate vitamin D intake reduces inflammatory cytokines through control of gene expression, thus inadequate vitamin D intake is suggested as a mechanism that could contribute to inflammation and, consequently, development of MS. Poor vitamin D status has been associated with increased risk for development of MS, and patients with MS may suffer consequences of vitamin D deficiency, such as bone loss. Animal studies and very limited human data suggest possible benefit from vitamin D supplementation in patients with MS. Based on the current state of research, a key principle for practicing dietetics professionals is to include vitamin D status in nutritional assessment. For those at risk for poor vitamin D status, intake can be enhanced by food-based advice and, when indicated, vitamin D supplementation. *Reference: Vitamin D and autoimmune disease - implications for practice from the multiple sclerosis literature. J Am Diet Assoc. 106(3):418-424, 2006. Mark, B. L., et al.*

The active metabolite of vitamin D, 1alpha,25-dihydroxyvitamin D(3), suppresses autoimmune disease in several animal models including experimental autoimmune encephalomyelitis (EAE), a model of multiple sclerosis. The molecular mechanism of this immunosuppression is at present unknown. While 1alpha,25-dihydroxyvitamin D(3) is believed to function through a single vitamin D receptor, there are reports of other vitamin D receptors as well as a "nongenomic" mode of action. The authors have prepared the EAE model possessing the vitamin D receptor null mutation and determined if 1alpha,25-dihydroxyvitamin D(3) can suppress this disease in the absence of a functional vitamin D receptor. Vitamin D receptor null mice develop EAE although the incidence rate is one-half that of wild-type controls. The administration of 1alpha,25-dihydroxyvitamin D(3) had no significant effect on the incidence of EAE in the vitamin D receptor null mice, while it completely blocked EAE in the wild-type mice. 1alpha,25-dihydroxyvitamin D(3) functions to suppress EAE through the well-known VDR and not through an undiscovered receptor or through a "nongenomic" mechanism. *Reference: The vitamin D receptor is necessary for 1alpha,25-dihydroxyvitamin D(3) to suppress experimental autoimmune encephalomyelitis in mice. Arch Biochem Biophys. 408(2):200-204, 2002. Meehan, T. F., et al. Department of Biochemistry, College of Agricultural and Life Sciences, University of Wisconsin-Madison, Madison, WI, USA.*

The authors sought to determine if vitamin D status, a risk factor for multiple sclerosis, is associated with the rate of subsequent clinical relapses in pediatric-onset multiple sclerosis. This is a retrospective study of patients with pediatric-onset multiple sclerosis or clinically isolated syndrome who were consecutively recruited into a prospective cohort at their clinical visit at the pediatric multiple sclerosis center of University of California, San Francisco or State University of New York at Stony Brook. Of 171 eligible patients, 134 (78%) with multiple sclerosis/clinically isolated syndrome were included in the cohort; a further 24 were excluded from this analysis due to lack of available serum (n = 7) or lack of follow-up (n = 17). Serum 25-hydroxyvitamin D(3) levels were measured and were adjusted to reflect a deseasonalized value. The adjusted serum 25-hydroxyvitamin D(3) level was the primary predictor in a multivariate negative binomial regression model in which the main outcome measure was the number of subsequent relapses. Among the 110 subjects, the mean unadjusted 25-hydroxyvitamin D(3) level was 22 +/- 9 ng/ml. After adjustment for age, gender, race, ethnicity, disease duration, disease-modifying therapy, and length of follow-up, every 10 ng/ml increase in the adjusted 25-hydroxyvitamin D(3) level was associated with a 34% decrease in the rate of subsequent relapses (incidence rate ratio, 0.66; 95% confidence interval, 0.46-0.95; p = 0.024).   Lower serum 25-hydroxyvitamin D(3) levels are associated with a substantially increased subsequent relapse rate in pediatric-onset multiple sclerosis or clinically isolated syndrome, providing rationale for a randomized controlled trial of vitamin D supplementation. *Reference: Vitamin D status is associated with relapse rate in pediatric-onset multiple sclerosis. Ann Neurol. 67(5):618-624, 2010. Mowry, E. M., et al. MS Center, Department of Neurology, University of California, San Francisco, CA, USA.*

A protective effect of vitamin D on risk of multiple sclerosis (MS) has been proposed, but no prospective studies have addressed this hypothesis. Dietary vitamin D intake was examined directly in relation to risk of MS in two large cohorts of women: the Nurses' Health Study (NHS; 92,253 women followed from 1980 to 2000) and Nurses' Health Study II (NHS II; 95,310 women followed from 1991 to 2001).   Diet was assessed at baseline and updated every 4 years thereafter. During the follow-up, 173 cases of MS with onset of symptoms after baseline were confirmed. The pooled age-adjusted relative risk (RR) comparing women in the highest quintile of total vitamin D intake at baseline with those in the lowest was 0.67 (95% CI = 0.40 to 1.12; p for trend = 0.03). Intake of vitamin D from supplements was also inversely associated with risk of MS; the RR comparing women with intake of 400 IU/day with women with no supplemental vitamin D intake was 0.59 (95% CI = 0.38 to 0.91; p for trend = 0.006). No association was found between vitamin D from food and MS incidence. These results support a protective effect of vitamin D intake on risk of developing MS. *Reference: Vitamin D intake and incidence of multiple sclerosis. Neurology. 62(1):60-65, 2004. Department of Nutrition, Harvard School of Public Health, Boston, MA, USA. Munger, K. L., et al.*

Most multiple sclerosis patients have vitamin D deficiency, which leads to low bone mass and high risk of fracture, compounded by the osteopenic effects of the glucocorticoids widely used in MS therapy. *Reference: High prevalence of vitamin D deficiency and reduced bone mass in multiple sclerosis. Neurology. 44:1687-1692, 1994. Nieves, J., et al.*

Vitamin D is a principal regulator of calcium homeostasis.   However, recent evidence has indicated that vitamin D can have numerous other physiological functions including inhibition of proliferation of a number of malignant cells including breast and prostate cancer cells and protection against certain immune mediated disorders including multiple sclerosis (MS). The geographic incidence of MS indicates an increase in MS with a decrease in sunlight exposure. Since vitamin D is produced in the skin by solar or UV irradiation and high serum levels of 25-hydroxyvitamin D (25(OH)D) have been reported to correlate with a reduced risk of MS, a protective role of vitamin D is suggested. Mechanisms whereby the active form of vitamin D, 1,25-dihydroxyvitamin D(3) (1,25(OH)(2)D(3)) may act to mediate this protective effect are reviewed. Due to its immunosuppressive actions, it has been suggested that 1,25(OH)(2)D(3) may prevent the induction of MS. *Reference: Vitamin D and multiple sclerosis. J Cell Biochem. 105(2):338-443, 2008. Raghuwanshi, A., et al. Department of Biochemistry and Molecular Biology, UMDNJ-New Jersey Medical School, Newark, New Jersey USA.*

MS is a chronic, immune-mediated inflammatory and neuro-degenerative disease of the central nervous system (CNS), with an etiology that is not yet fully understood. The prevalence of MS is highest where environmental supplies of vitamin D are lowest. It is well recognized that the active hormonal form of vitamin D, 1,25-dihydroxyvitamin D (1,25-(OH)(2)D), is a natural immunoregulator with anti-inflammatory action. The mechanism by which vitamin D nutrition is thought to influence MS involves paracrine or autocrine metabolism of 25OHD by cells expressing the enzyme 1alpha-OHase in peripheral tissues involved in immune and neural function. Administration of the active metabolite 1,25-(OH)(2)D in mice and rats with experimental allergic encephalomyelitis (EAE, an animal model of MS) not only prevented, but also reduced disease activity. 1,25-(OH)(2)D alters dendritic cell and T-cell function and regulates macrophages in EAE. Interestingly, 1,25-(OH)(2)D is thought to be operating on CNS constituent cells as well. Vitamin D deficiency is caused by insufficient sunlight exposure or low dietary vitamin D(3) intake. Subtle defects in vitamin D metabolism, including genetic polymorphisms related to vitamin D, might possibly be involved as well. Optimal 25OHD serum concentrations, throughout the year, may be beneficial for patients with MS, both to obtain immune-mediated suppression of disease activity, and also to decrease disease-related complications, including increased bone resorption, fractures, and muscle weakness. *Reference: Multiple sclerosis and vitamin D: an update. Eur J Clin Nutr. 58(8):1095-1109, 2004. Van Amerongen, B. M., et al.*

A new theory for the etiology of multiple sclerosis (MS) has been developed which is compatible with epidemiologic, biochemical and genetic evidence. A predisposition for the disease is held to result from the development of abnormal myelin during puberty. Vitamin D and calcium are proposed as being essential for normal myelination. Curtailed supplies of these substances (from inadequate sunlight and phytate rich diets) correlate with geographic regions of high risk of MS. Conversely the prevalence of MS is lower where vitamin D is abundant, as in sunny climates, high altitudes, and littorals with dietaries rich in fish oils. *Reference: Multiple sclerosis: vitamin D and calcium as environmental determinants of prevalence (a viewpoint). I.: Sunlight, dietary factors and epidemiology. Int J Environ Stud. 6(1):19-27, 1971.*

Vitamin B12

Serum vitamin B12 levels and unsaturated vitamin B12 binding capacities were measured in 24 patients with multiple sclerosis (MS), 73 patients with other neurological disorders and 21 healthy subjects. There was no decrease in the vitamin B12 levels, however, a significant decrease in the unsaturated vitamin B12 binding capacities was observed in patients with MS when compared with other groups. A massive dose of methyl vitamin B12 (60 mg every day for six months) was administered to six patients with chronic progressive MS, a disease which usually had a morbid prognosis and widespread demyelination in the central nervous system. Although the motor disability did not improve clinically, the abnormalities in both the visual and brainstem auditory evoked potentials improved more frequently during the therapy than in the pre-treatment period. The authors concluded that a massive dose methyl vitamin B12 therapy may be useful as an adjunct to immunosuppressive treatment for chronic progressive MS. *Reference: Vitamin B12 metabolism and massive-dose methyl vitamin B12 therapy in Japanese patients with multiple sclerosis. Int Med. 33(2):82-86, 1994. Kira, J., et al.*

Patients with multiple sclerosis (MS) may have low serum vitamin B12 and folate levels and high levels of homocysteine. The authors aimed to evaluate serum vitamin B12, folate, homocysteine, mean corpuscular volume (MCV), hemoglobin (Hb), and hematocrit (Hct) levels in patients with MS. The authors examined the relationship between these parameters and age, sex, disease type, age at onset, disease duration, Expanded Disability Status Score, immunoglobulin G (IgG) index, oligoclonal band presence, visual evoked potentials (VEP) and posterior tibial somatosensory evoked potentials (SEP). These parameters were evaluated in 35 patients during an acute attack and compared to data collected from 30 healthy individuals (control subjects). Serum vitamin B12, folate, homocysteine, Hb, and Hct levels and MCV were low in a proportion of patients with MS (20%, 14.3%, 20%, 6.7%, 3.3% and 10% respectively), whereas only vitamin B12 and folate levels were low in only 3.3% of the control subjects. Homocysteine levels were high in 20% of patients with MS but were within normal limits in the control group. Elevated Hct levels were significantly correlated (p<0.05) with prolonged posterior tibial SEP P1 and P2 latencies compared to the control subjects. Patients with MS who had prolonged VEP and posterior tibial SEP P1 and P2 latencies also had lower vitamin B12 levels compared to patients with normal latencies. The authors found a significant relationship between MS and vitamin B12 deficiency, and also demonstrated a relationship between vitamin B12 deficiency, VEP and posterior tibial SEP in MS. *Reference: Serum vitamin B12, folate, and homocysteine levels and their association with clinical and electrophysiological parameters in multiple sclerosis. J*

Clin Neurosci. 2009. Kocer, B., et al. Department of Neurology, Ankara Numune Teaching and Research Hospital, Ankara, Turkey.

Multiple Sclerosis (MS) and vitamin B12 deficiency share common inflammatory and neurodegenerative pathophysiological characteristics. Due to similarities in the clinical presentations and MRI findings, the differential diagnosis between vitamin B12 deficiency and MS may be difficult. Additionally, low or decreased levels of vitamin B12 have been demonstrated in MS patients. Moreover, recent studies suggest that vitamin B12, in addition to its known role as a co-factor in myelin formation, has important immunomodulatory and neurotrophic effects. These observations raise the questions of possible causal relationship between the two disorders, and suggest further studies of the need to close monitoring of vitamin B12 levels as well as the potential requirement for supplementation of vitamin B12 alone or in combination with the immunotherapies for MS patients. **Reference:** *Vitamin B12, demyelination, remyelination and repair in multiple sclerosis. J Neurol Sci. 2005. Miller, A., et al. Division of Neuroimmunology and Multiple Sclerosis Center, Carmel Medical Center, Haifa, Israel.*

Vitamin B12 and folate concentrations were measured in serum and cerebrospinal fluid (CSF) in 293 neurological patients. Serum and CSF vitamin B12 concentrations showed a positive correlation. In individual patients CSF B12 concentrations varied considerably for a given serum concentration. The median serum vitamin B12 concentration of the Alzheimer's disease patients group was significantly lower compared with that of a control group. Lower median CSF vitamin B12 concentrations were found in groups of patients with multiple sclerosis and Alzheimer's disease. Five patients with heterogeneous clinical pictures had unexplained low serum and CSF B12 concentrations without macrocytosis. **Reference:** *Vitamin B12 and folate concentrations in serum and cerebrospinal fluid of neurological patients with special reference to multiple sclerosis and dementia. J Neurol Neurosurg Psychiatry. 53(11):951-954, 1990. Nijst, T. Q., et al.*

The authors describe 10 patients with a previously unreported, to our knowledge, association of multiple sclerosis and unusual vitamin B12 deficiency. The clinical features and the age at presentation were typical of multiple sclerosis, with eight cases occurring before age 40 years, which is a rare age for vitamin B12 deficiency. Nine patients had hematologic abnormalities, but only two were anemic. All six patients examined had low erythrocyte cobalamin levels. Only two patients had pernicious anemia; in the remaining patients the vitamin B12 deficiency was unexplained. A vitamin B12 binding and/or transport is suspected. The nature of the association of multiple sclerosis and vitamin B12 deficiency is unclear but is likely to be more than coincidental. Further studies of vitamin B12 metabolism, binding, and transport in multiple sclerosis are indicated, as these cases may offer a clue to the understanding of a still mysterious neurologic disorder. *Reference: Multiple sclerosis associated with vitamin B12 deficiency. Arch Neurol. 48(8):808-811, 1991. Reynolds, E. H., et al. Department of Neurology, King's College Hospital, London, England.*

Multiple sclerosis (MS) is occasionally associated with vitamin B12 deficiency. Recent studies have shown an increased risk of macrocytosis, low serum and/or CSF vitamin B12 levels, raised plasma homocysteine and raised unsaturated R-binder capacity in MS. The aetiology of the vitamin B12 deficiency in MS is often uncertain and a disorder of vitamin B12 binding or transport is suspected. The nature of the association of vitamin B12 deficiency and MS is unclear but is likely to be more than coincidental. There is a remarkable similarity in the epidemiology of MS and pernicious anaemia. Vitamin B12 deficiency should always be looked for in MS. The deficiency may aggravate MS or impair recovery. There is evidence that vitamin B12 is important for myelin synthesis and integrity. *Reference: Multiple sclerosis and vitamin B12 metabolism. J Neuroimmunol. 40(2-3):225-230, 1992. Reynolds, E. H. Multiple sclerosis patients generally have lower than normal CSF vitamin B12 levels.*

The authors have previously described 10 patients with multiple sclerosis (MS) and unusual vitamin B12 deficiency. They studied vitamin B12 metabolism in 29 consecutive cases of MS, 17 neurological controls, and 31 normal subjects. Patients with MS had significantly lower serum vitamin B 12 levels and significantly higher unsaturated R-binder capacities than neurological and normal controls, and they were significantly macrocytic compared with normal controls. Nine patients with MS had serum vitamin B12 levels less than 147 pmol/L and, in the absence of anemia, this subgroup was significantly macrocytic and had significantly lower red blood cell folate levels than neurological and normal controls. Nine patients with MS had raised plasma unsaturated R-binder capacities, including three patients with very high values. There is a significant association between MS and disturbed vitamin B12 metabolism. Vitamin B12 deficiency should always be looked for in patients with MS. The cause of the vitamin B12 disorder and the nature of the overlap with MS deserve further investigation. Coexisting vitamin B12 deficiency might aggravate MS or impair recovery from MS. *Reference: Vitamin B12 metabolism and multiple sclerosis. Arch Neurol. 49(6):649-652, 1992. Reynolds, E. H., et al.*

Attention has been focused recently on the association between vitamin B12 metabolism and the pathogenesis of multiple sclerosis (MS). Several recent reports have documented vitamin B12 deficiency in patients with MS. The etiology of this deficiency in MS is unknown. The majority of these patients do not have pernicious anemia and serum levels of the vitamin are unrelated to the course or chronicity of the disease. Vitamin B12 does not reverse the associated macrocytic anemia nor are the neurological deficits of MS improved following supplementation with vitamin B12. It has been suggested that vitamin B12 deficiency may render the patient more vulnerable to the putative viral and/or immunologic mechanisms widely suspected in MS. Serum vitamin B12 levels in MS patients are related to the age of onset of the disease. Specifically, in 45 MS patients vitamin B12 levels were significantly lower in those who experienced the onset of first neurological symptoms prior to age 18 years (N = 10) compared to patients in whom the disease first manifested after age 18 (N = 35). In contrast, serum folate levels were unrelated to age of onset of the disease. As vitamin B12 levels were statistically unrelated to chronicity of illness, these findings suggest a specific association between the timing of onset of first neurological symptoms of MS and vitamin B12 metabolism. In addition, since vitamin B12 is required for the formation of myelin and for immune mechanisms, the authors propose that its deficiency in MS is of critical pathogenetic significance. *Reference: Vitamin B12 and its relationship to age of onset of multiple sclerosis. Int J Neuroscience. 71(1-4):93-99, 1993. Sandyk, R., et al.*

Vitamin B3 (Nicotinic Acid)

Acute attacks of multiple sclerosis (MS) are most commonly treated with glucocorticoids, which can provide life-saving albeit only temporary symptomatic relief. The mechanism of action (MOA) is now known to involve induction of indoleamine 2,3-dioxygenase (IDO) and interleukin-10 (IL-10), where IL-10 requires subsequent heme oxygenase-1 (HMOX-1) induction. Ectopic expression studies reveal that even small changes in expression of IDO, HMOX-1, or mitochondrial superoxide dismutase (SOD2) can prevent demyelination in experimental autoimmune encephalomyelitis (EAE) animal models of MS. An alternative to glucocorticoids is needed for a long-term treatment of MS. A distinctly short list of endogenous activators of both membrane G-protein-coupled receptors and nuclear peroxisome proliferating antigen receptors (PPARs) demonstrably ameliorate EAE pathogenesis by MOAs resembling that of glucocorticoids. These dual activators and potential MS therapeutics include endocannabinoids and the prostaglandin 15-deoxy-Δ12,14-PGJ2. Nicotinamide profoundly ameliorates and prevents autoimmune-mediated demyelination in EAE via maintaining levels of nicotinamide adenine dinucleotide (NAD), without activating PPAR nor any G-protein-coupled receptor. By comparison, nicotinic acid provides even greater levels of NAD than nicotinamide in many tissues, while additionally activating the PPARγ-dependent pathway already shown to provide relief in animal models of MS after activation of GPR109a/HM74a. Thus nicotinic acid is uniquely suited for providing therapeutic relief in MS. However nicotinic acid is unexamined in MS research. Nicotinic acid penetrates the blood brain barrier, cures pellagric dementia, has been used for over 50 years clinically without toxicity, and raises HDL concentrations to a greater degree than any pharmaceutical, thus providing unparalleled benefits against lipodystrophy. Summary analysis reveals that the expected therapeutic benefits of high-dose nicotinic acid administration far outweigh any known adverse risks in consideration for the treatment of multiple sclerosis. *Reference: PPAR Res. 2009; 2009: 853707. Published online 2009 May 17. doi: 10.1155/2009/853707. PMCID: PMC2683338. Nicotinic Acid-Mediated Activation of Both Membrane and Nuclear Receptors towards Therapeutic Glucocorticoid Mimetics for Treating Multiple Sclerosis. W. Todd Penberthy. Department of Molecular Genetics, Biochemistry, and Microbiology, University of Cincinnati, 231 Albert Sabin Way P.O. Box 670524, 2938 CVC Mail Loc-0524, Cincinnati, Ohio 45237, USA.*

Magnesium

The effects of magnesium glycerophosphate oral therapy on spasticity was studied in a 35-year-old woman with severe spastic paraplegia resulting from multiple sclerosis (MS). The authors found a significant improvement in the spasticity after only 1 week from the onset of the treatment on the modified Ashworth scale, an improvement in the range of motion and in the measures of angles at resting position in lower limbs. No side-effects were reported and there was no weakness in the arms during the treatment. *Reference: Multiple sclerosis, an autoimmune inflammatory disease: prospects for its integrative management. Alternative Medicine Review. 6(6):540-566, 2001. Kidd, P. M. The effect of magnesium oral therapy on spasticity in a patient with multiple sclerosis. Eur J Neurol. 7(6):741-744, 2000. Rossier, P., et al. Rivermead Rehabilitation Centre, Abingdon Road, Oxford, UK.*

There are few reports of Mg in MS and none dealing with Mg content in erythrocytes. Mg concentration was determined in serum and in erythrocytes with the help of a BIOTROL Magnesium Calmagite colorimetric method (average sensitivity: 0.194 A per mmol/l) and a Hitachi autoanalyzer in 24 MS patients (7 men and 17 women, age 29-60; 37 years on average with the duration of the disease: 3-19; 11 years on average, at clinical disability stages according to the Kurtzke scale: 1-7; 3.2 on average, in remission stage. A statistically significant decrease (p < 0.001) of Mg concentration in erythrocytes and no changes in plasma of MS patients were found. The results obtained suggest the presence of changes in membrane of erythrocytes which could be connected with their shorter life and with affection of their function. *Reference: Magnesium concentration in plasma and erythrocytes in MS. Acta Neurol Scand. 92(1):109-111, 1995. Stelmasiak, Z., et al. Department of Clinical Analytics, School of Medicine, Lublin, Poland.*

Magnesium concentrations were studied in the brains of four multiple sclerosis patients and 5 control subjects. The magnesium contents were studied from 26 sites of central nervous system tissues, and visceral organs such as liver, spleen, kidney, heart and lung. The average magnesium content in the CNS tissues, as well as visceral organs except for spleen, of MS patients showed a significantly lower value than that seen in control cases. The most marked reduction of magnesium content was observed in CNS white matter including demyelinated plaques of MS samples. Whether or not these significantly lower magnesium contents found in CNS and visceral organs of MS patients may play an essential role in the demyelinating process remain unclear, requiring further studies on MS pathogenesis from the point of metal metabolism. *Reference: Magnesium concentration in brains from multiple sclerosis patients. Acta Neurology Scandinavia. 81(3):197-200, 1990. Yasui, M., et al.*

Zinc & Calcium

The proposed aetiologies of multiple sclerosis (MS) have included immunological mechanisms, genetic factors, virus infection and direct or indirect action of minerals and/or metals. The processes of these aetiologies have implicated magnesium. Magnesium and zinc have been shown to be decreased in central nervous system (CNS) tissues of MS patients, especially tissues such as white matter where pathological changes have been observed. The calcium content of white matter has also been found to be decreased in MS patients. The interactions of minerals and/or metals such as calcium, magnesium, aluminium and zinc have also been evaluated in CNS tissues of experimental animal models. These data suggest that these elements are regulated by pooling of minerals and/or metals in bones. Biological actions of magnesium may affect the maintenance and function of nerve cells as well as the proliferation and synthesis of lymphocytes. A magnesium deficit may induce dysfunction of nerve cells or lymphocytes directly and/or indirectly, and thus magnesium depletion may be implicated in the aetiology of MS. The action of zinc helps to prevent virus infection, and zinc deficiency in CNS tissues of MS patients may also be relevant to its aetiology. Magnesium interacts with other minerals and/or metals such as calcium, zinc and aluminium in biological systems, affecting the immune system and influencing the content of these elements in CNS tissues. Because of these interactions, a magnesium deficit could also be a risk factor in the aetiology of MS. *Reference: Experimental and clinical studies on dysregulation of magnesium metabolism and the aetiopathogenesis of multiple sclerosis. Magnesium Research. 5(4):295-302, 1992 Yasui, M., et al. Division of Neurological Diseases, Wakayama Med College, Japan.*

Enzymes

Clinical trials that test the efficacy of Phlogenzym (consisting of the hydrolytic enzymes bromelain and trypsin and the anti-oxidant rutosid) as a treatment for T cell-mediated autoimmune diseases including multiple sclerosis (MS), type 1 diabetes and rheumatoid arthritis are presently ongoing. The authors tested the effects of Phlogenzym treatment in the murine model for MS, experimental allergic encephalomyelitis (EAE), a disease induced in SJL mice by immunization with proteolipid protein (PLP) peptide 139-151. Oral administration of Phlogenzym resulted in complete protection from EAE. In Phlogenzym-treated mice, the dose response curve of the PLP:139-151-specific T cell response was shifted to the right, that is, the primed T cells required higher peptide concentrations to become activated. Additionally, the T cell response to this peptide was shifted towards the T helper 2 cytokine profile. Both effects are consistent with an increased T cell activation threshold. The accessory molecules CD4, CD44, and B7-1 (all of which are involved in T cell co-stimulation) were cleaved by Phlogenzym, while CD3 and MHC class II molecules (which are involved in the recognition of antigens by T cells) and LFA-1 were unaffected. These data show the efficacy of oral Phlogenzym treatment in an animal model of T cell-mediated autoimmune disease and suggest that the protective effect might be the result of an increase in the activation threshold of the autoreactive T lymphocytes brought about by the cleavage of accessory molecules involved in the interaction of T cells and antigen presenting cells. *Reference: Prevention of murine EAE by oral hydrolytic enzyme treatment. J Autoimmun. 12(3):191-198, 1999. Targoni, O. S., et al. Institute of Pathology, School of Medicine, Case Western Reserve University, Cleveland, Ohio, USA.*

Curcumin, Quercetin, Green Tea

Our understanding of the pathophysiological and biochemical basis of a number of neurological disorders has increased enormously over the last three decades. Parallel with this growth of knowledge has been a clearer understanding of the mechanism by which a number of naturally occurring plant extracts, as well as whole plants, can affect these mechanisms so as to offer protection against injury and promote healing of neurological tissues. Curcumin, quercetin, green tea catechins, balcalein, and luteolin have been extensively studied, and they demonstrate important effects on cell signaling that go far beyond their antioxidant effects. Of particular interest is the effect of these compounds on immunoexcitotoxicity, which, the authors suggest, is a common mechanism in a number of neurological disorders. By suppressing or affecting microglial activation states as well as the excitotoxic cascade and inflammatory mediators, these compounds dramatically affect the pathophysiology of central nervous system disorders and promote the release and generation of neurotrophic factors essential for central nervous system healing. We discuss the various aspects of these processes and suggest future directions for study. *Reference: Surg Neurol Int. 2012; 3: 19. Published online 2012 February 15. doi: 10.4103/2152-7806.92935. PMCID: PMC3307240. Natural plant products and extracts that reduce immunoexcitotoxicity-associated neurodegeneration and promote repair within the central nervous system. Russell L. Blaylock and Joseph Maroon. Theoretical Neurosciences, Department of Biology, Belhaven University, Jackson, MS 39157, USA.*

Nutrition

Multiple sclerosis is a complex and multifactorial neurological disease, and nutrition is one of the environmental factors possibly involved in its pathogenesis. At present, the role of nutrition is unclear, and MS therapy is not associated to a particular diet. MS clinical trials based on specific diets or dietary supplements are very few and in some cases controversial. To understand how diet can influence the course of MS and improve the wellness of MS patients, it is necessary to identify the dietary molecules, their targets and the molecular mechanisms involved in the control of the disease. The aim of this paper is to provide a molecular basis for the nutritional intervention in MS by evaluating at molecular level the effect of dietary molecules on the inflammatory and autoimmune processes involved in the disease. The rationale for the use of natural antioxidants in MS is based on the finding that oxidative stress and in particular the generation of reactive oxygen species (ROS), is one of the most important components involved in inflammation and neuronal damage. On these grounds, the administration of appropriate doses of antioxidants, such as the dietary polyphenols and carotenoids, could be very useful to restore the right balance between ROS generation and their destruction. Polyphenols include flavonoids and nonflavonoids molecules. Flavonoids, the most abundant polyphenols in plants, are more than 8000 different compounds which have in common the structure of diphenylpropanes (C6-C3-C6) with two benzene rings separated by a linear three-carbon chain forming an oxygenated heterocycle. Flavonoids can be divided into various classes: flavanols (catechin, epigallocatechin), flavones (luteolin, apigenin), flavanones (naringenin, hesperidin), flavonols (quercetin, myricetin), isoflavones (daidzein, genistein) and anthocyanidins (cyanidin, malvidin). Nonflavonoids are hydroxycinnamic or phenolic acids (caffeic acid, ferulic acid, including curcumin, a diferuloylmethane), lignans (secoisolariciresinol), stilbenes (resveratrol). They have only one or two phenolic rings. Alternatively, polyphenols can be divided into four different classes: (1) those containing the pyrocatechol unit (1,2 benzene diol) (hydroxytyrosol, caffeic acid, curcumin); (2) those containing the resorcinol unit (1,3 benzene diol) (resveratrol, genistein); (3) those containing both the pyrocathecol and resorcinol units (quercetin, catechins, anthocyanidins); (4) those containing the pyrogallol unit (1,2,3 benzene triol) (Epigallocathechin). This classification might are useful because different chemical groups might have different effects. For example, it has been reported that catechols have anti-inflammatory activity in stimulated microglia and neutrophils and thereby be useful for the treatment of neurodegenerative diseases. The most important polyphenols are quercetin (QRC), resveratrol (RSV), curcumin (CRC); hydroxytyrosol, catechins, daidzein, genistein. Among the carotenoids the most important is lycopene. They often have a complementary activity as antioxidants and radical scavengers. Quercetin is found in onion, apple, citrus, and wine. QRC occurs mainly as glycoside, with a sugar group bound to one of the hydroxyl groups of the flavonol. QRC has anti-inflammatory, immunomodulating and antiviral properties, reduces the proliferation of peripheral blood mononuclear cells (PBMCs) and decreases the production of IL-1β, TNF-α and MMP-9. These effects are additive to those of IFN-β. QRC passes the BBB, inhibits myelin phagocytosis by blocking the ROS released from the macrophages and inhibits the expression of inflammatory cytokines through inhibition of NF-κB. Furthermore, QRC inhibits angiogenesis, reduces the neutrophil dependent inflammation, and has neuroprotective effects. QRC inhibits or ameliorates the Experimental Allergic Encephalomyelitis (EAE) induced in SJL/J mice by mouse spinal cord homogenate. Apparently, QRC is not toxic, but its oxidation product, quercetin quinone (QQ), which is very reactive towards protein thiols and glutathione, could have a toxic effect. Resveratrol is found in red wine, chocolate, peanuts, berries, and black grapes. RSV is glucuronated in the liver and absorbed in this form mainly in the duodenum. Metabolic modification of RSV is inhibited by QRC. Only a few unmodified RSV molecules are absorbed. RSV has a neuroprotective effect and ameliorates MOG-EAE in C57BL/6 mice. RSV has anticarcinogenic, anti-inflammatory, and estrogenic activities and allows cardiovascular protection, free-radical scavenging, inhibition/induction of apoptosis, and inhibition of platelet aggregation. Depending on its concentration, RSV mediates cell death of a variety of cells by necrosis or apoptosis downregulating targets such as NF-κB, AP-1, cyclins, STAT 3, and others, and upregulating cytochrome c, caspases, cathepsin D, p53, JNK, and others. RSV acts as a nonsteroidal anti-inflammatory molecule and inhibits the production of TNF-α, IL-1α, IL-1β, IL-6, IL-8, IL-18, MMP-9, VEGF, COX-2, 5-lipoxygenase, and ROS. Moreover, RSV activates the sirtuins, a family of histone deacetylases, particularly SIRT2, and PPAR-α/γ. Curcumin (CRC) is the yellow pigment present in curry powder. Among its many biological properties, the most important in the present context are its anti-inflammatory properties and in particular the downregulation of NF-κB and AP-1. Catechins are polyphenols found in green tea. They have anti-inflammatory and anticarcinogenic activity, inhibit the activity of MMP-2, MMP-9 and MMP-12 and the intestinal absorption of lipids. Lycopene is a carotenoid that is found in tomato, water-melon, and pink grapefruit. As an antioxidant, it is two times better than beta-carotene and 100 times better than vitamin E and protects against cancer. Hydroxytyrosol is the main antioxidant found in olive oil and a very efficient scavenger of free radicals. Soy flavonoids as genistein downregulate proimatory cytokines and ameliorate MOG-EAE symptoms in C57BL/6 mice. Thiol-containing compounds such as alpha-lipoic acid (ALA), glutathione and N-acetylcysteine (NAC) might be effective as oral supplements in the complementary treatment of MS. ALA has immunomodulating effects, stimulates the production of cAMP, inhibits the synthesis of IFN-gamma and adhesion molecules, is effective in the treatment of EAE, affects T cell migration into CNS and stabilizes blood-brain barrier integrity. Studies in patients with multiple sclerosis with oral supplements of lipoic acid are underway to assess the right dosage of this thiol compound. NAC pass through the BBB and, like glucorticoids and interferons, is able to protect it against inflammation. ALA, NAC, and glutathione could be useful to reduce the possible toxic effect of quercetin quinones described above. Other useful compounds with antioxidant activity and a possible role as dietary supplements are: melatonin, vitamin. E, selenium, vitamin C.

Reference: Autoimmune Dis. 2010; 2010: 249842. Published online 2011 February 24. doi: 10.4061/2010/249842. PMCID: PMC3065662. May Diet and Dietary Supplements Improve the Wellness of Multiple Sclerosis Patients? A Molecular Approach. Paolo Riccio,Rocco Rossano, and Grazia Maria Liuzzi. Dipartimento di Biologia D.B.A.F., Università degli Studi della Basilicata, 85100 Potenza, Italy. Istituto Nazionale di Biostrutture e Biosistemi (INBB), 00100 Roma,

Italy. Dipartimento di Biochimica e Biologia Molecolare "Ernesto Quagliariello", 70126, Bari, Italy.

Estriol

Matrix metalloproteinases (MMPs) play a crucial role in migration of inflammatory cells into the central nervous system (CNS). Levels of MMP-9 are elevated in multiple sclerosis (MS) and predict the occurrence of new active lesions on magnetic resonance imaging (MRI). This translational study aims to determine whether in vivo treatment with the pregnancy hormone estriol affects MMP-9 levels from immune cells in patients with MS and mice with experimental autoimmune encephalomyelitis (EAE). Peripheral blood mononuclear cells (PBMCs) collected from three female MS patients treated with estriol and splenocytes from EAE mice treated with estriol, estrogen receptor (ER) α ligand, ERβ ligand or vehicle were stimulated ex vivo and analyzed for levels of MMP-9. Markers of CNS infiltration were assessed using MRI in patients and immunohistochemistry in mice. Supernatants from PBMCs obtained during estriol treatment in female MS patients showed significantly decreased MMP-9 compared to pre treatment. Decreases in MMP-9 coincided with a decrease in enhancing lesion volume on MRI. Estriol treatment of mice with EAE reduced MMP-9 in supernatants from autoantigen stimulated splenocytes, coinciding with decreased CNS infiltration by T cells and monocytes. Experiments with selective ER ligands revealed that this effect was mediated via ERα. In conclusion, estriol acting via ERα to reduce MMP-9 from immune cells is one mechanism potentially underlying the estriol-mediated reduction in enhancing lesions in MS and inflammatory lesions in EAE. ***Reference:*** *Lab Invest. Author manuscript; available in PMC 2010 April 1. Published in final edited form as: Lab Invest. 2009 October; 89(10): 1076–1083. Published online 2009 August 10. doi: 10.1038/ labinvest.2009.79. PMCID: PMC2753699. NIHMSID: NIHMS130838. Estrogen treatment decreases matrix metalloproteinase (MMP)-9 in autoimmune demyelinating disease through estrogen receptor alpha (ERα). Stefan M Gold, Manda V Sasidhar, Laurie B Morales, Sienmi Du, Nancy L Sicotte, Seema K. Tiwari-Woodruff, and Rhonda R Voskuhl. Multiple Sclerosis Program, Dept Neurology, David Geffen School of Medicine at UCLA, Los Angeles, CA.*

Testosterone

Background - Multiple sclerosis is a chronic inflammatory disease of the central nervous system with a pronounced neurodegenerative component. It has been suggested that novel treatment options are needed that target both aspects of the disease. Evidence from basic and clinical studies suggests that testosterone has an immunomodulatory as well as a potential neuroprotective effect that could be beneficial in MS. **Methods -** Ten male MS patients were treated with 10 g of gel containing 100 mg of testosterone in a cross-over design (6 month observation period followed by 12 months of treatment). Blood samples were obtained at three-month intervals during the observation and the treatment period. Isolated blood peripheral mononuclear cells (PBMCs) were used to examine lymphocyte subpopulation composition by flow cytometry and ex vivo protein production of cytokines (IL-2, IFNγ, TNFα, IL-17, IL-10, IL-12p40, TGFβ1) and growth factors (brain-derived neurotrophic factor BDNF, platelet-derived growth factor PDGF-BB, nerve growth factor NGF, and ciliary neurotrophic factor CNTF). Delayed type hypersensitivity (DTH) skin recall tests were obtained before and during treatment as an in vivo functional immune measure. **Results -** Testosterone treatment significantly reduced DTH recall responses and induced a shift in peripheral lymphocyte composition by decreasing CD4+ T cell percentage and increasing NK cells. In addition, PBMC production of IL-2 was significantly decreased while TGFβ1 production was increased. Furthermore, PBMCs obtained during the treatment period produced significantly more BDNF and PDGF-BB. **Conclusion -** These results are consistent with an immunomodulatory effect of testosterone treatment in MS. In addition, increased production of BDNF and PDGF-BB suggests a potential neuroprotective effect. *Reference: J Neuroinflammation. 2008; 5: 32. Published online 2008 July 31. doi: 10.1186/1742-2094-5-32. PMCID: PMC2518142. Immune modulation and increased neurotrophic factor production in multiple sclerosis patients treated with testosterone. Stefan M Gold, Sara Chalifoux, Barbara S Giesser, and Rhonda R Voskuhl. Department of Neurology, Neuroscience Research Building, 635 Charles E. Young Drive South, University of California Los Angeles, CA, 90095, USA. Cousins Center, 300 Medical Plaza, University of California Los Angeles, CA, 90095, USA.*

Motoneuron loss is a significant medical problem, capable of causing severe movement disorders or even death. We have previously shown that partial depletion of motoneurons from sexually dimorphic, highly androgen-sensitive spinal motor populations induces dendritic atrophy in remaining motoneurons, and this atrophy is attenuated by treatment with testosterone. To test whether testosterone has similar effects in more typical motoneurons, we examined potential neuroprotective effects in motoneurons innervating muscles of the quadriceps. Motoneurons innervating the vastus medialis muscle were selectively killed by intramuscular injection of cholera toxin-conjugated saporin. Simultaneously, some saporin-injected rats were given implants containing testosterone or left untreated. Four weeks later, motoneurons innervating the ipsilateral vastus lateralis muscle were labeled with cholera toxin-conjugated HRP, and dendritic arbors were reconstructed in 3 dimensions. Compared to intact normal males, partial motoneuron depletion resulted in decreased dendritic length in remaining quadriceps motoneurons, and this atrophy was attenuated by testosterone treatment. To examine the functional consequences of the induced dendritic atrophy, and its attenuation with testosterone treatment, the activation of remaining quadriceps motoneurons was assessed using peripheral nerve recording. Partial motoneuron depletion resulted in decreased amplitudes of motor nerve activity, and these changes were attenuated by treatment with testosterone, providing a functional correlate to the neuroprotective effects of testosterone treatment on quadriceps motoneuron morphology. Together, these findings suggest that testosterone has neuroprotective effects on morphology and function in both highly androgen-sensitive as well as more typical motoneuron populations, further supporting a role for testosterone as a neurotherapeutic agent in the injured nervous system. *Reference: J Comp Neurol. Author manuscript; available in PMC 2010 January 20. Published in final edited form as: J Comp Neurol. 2009 January 20; 512(3): 359–372. doi: 10.1002/cne.21885. NIHMSID: NIHMS72267. Neuroprotective effects of testosterone on the morphology and function of somatic motoneurons following the death of neighboring motoneurons. Christine M. Little, Kellie D. Coons, and Dale R. Sengelaub. Program in Neuroscience and Department of Psychological and Brain Sciences, Indiana University, Bloomington, Indiana 47405.*

Fatty Acids

Essential polyunsaturated fatty acids (PUFAs) are critical nutritional lipids that must be obtained from the diet to sustain homeostasis. Omega-3 and -6 PUFAs are key components of biomembranes and play important roles in cell integrity, development, maintenance, and function. The essential omega-3 fatty acid family member docosahexaenoic acid (DHA) is avidly retained and uniquely concentrated in the nervous system, particularly in photoreceptors and synaptic membranes. DHA plays a key role in vision, neuroprotection, successful aging, memory, and other functions. In addition, DHA displays anti-inflammatory and inflammatory resolving properties in contrast to the proinflammatory actions of several members of the omega-6 PUFAs family. This review discusses DHA signalolipidomics, comprising the cellular/tissue organization of DHA uptake, its distribution among cellular compartments, the organization and function of membrane domains rich in DHA-containing phospholipids, and the cellular and molecular events revealed by the uncovering of signaling pathways regulated by DHA and docosanoids, the DHA-derived bioactive lipids, which include neuroprotectin D1 (NPD1), a novel DHA-derived stereoselective mediator. NPD1 synthesis agonists include neurotrophins and oxidative stress; NPD1 elicits potent anti-inflammatory actions and prohomeostatic bioactivity, is anti-angiogenic, promotes corneal nerve regeneration, and induces cell survival. In the context of DHA signalolipidomics, this review highlights aging and the evolving studies on the significance of DHA in Alzheimer's disease, macular degeneration, Parkinson's disease, and other brain disorders. DHA signalolipidomics in the nervous system offers emerging targets for pharmaceutical intervention and clinical translation. *Reference: Annu Rev Nutr. Author manuscript; available in PMC 2012 July 27. Published in final edited form as: Annu Rev Nutr. 2011 August 21; 31: 321–351. doi: 10.1146/annurev.nutr.012809. 104635. PMCID: PMC3406932. NIHMSID: NIHMS394447. Docosahexaenoic Acid Signalolipidomics in Nutrition: Significance in Aging, Neuroinflammation, Macular Degeneration, Alzheimer's, and Other Neurodegenerative Diseases. Nicolas G. Bazan, Miguel F. Molina, and William C. Gordon. Neuroscience Center of Excellence and Department of Ophthalmology, School of Medicine, Louisiana State University Health Sciences Center, New Orleans, Louisiana 70112.*

In multiple sclerosis (MS), compromised blood-brain barrier (BBB) integrity contributes to inflammatory T cell migration into the central nervous system. Matrix metalloproteinase-9 (MMP-9) is associated with BBB disruption and subsequent T cell migration into the CNS. The aim of this paper was to evaluate the effects of omega-3 fatty acids on MMP-9 levels and T cell migration. Peripheral blood mononuclear cells (PBMC) from healthy controls were pretreated with two types of omega-3 fatty acids, eicosapentaenoic acid (EPA), and docosahexaenoic acid (DHA). Cell supernatants were used to determine MMP-9 protein and activity levels. Jurkat cells were pretreated with EPA and DHA and were added to fibronectin-coated transwells to measure T cell migration. EPA and DHA significantly decreased MMP-9 protein levels, MMP-9 activity, and significantly inhibited human T cell migration. The data suggest that omega-3 fatty acids may benefit patients with multiple sclerosis by modulating immune cell production of MMP-9. *Reference: Autoimmune Dis. 2011; 2011: 134592. Published online 2011 July 20. doi: 10.4061/2011/134592. PMCID: PMC3140187. The Effects of Omega-3 Fatty Acids on Matrix Metalloproteinase-9 Production and Cell Migration in Human Immune Cells: Implications for Multiple Sclerosis. Lynne Shinto, Gail Marracci, Lauren Bumgarner, and Vijayshree Yadav, Department of Neurology, Oregon Health & Science University, 3181 SW Sam Jackson Park Road, CR 120, Portland, OR 97239, USA. Research Division, Department of Veterans Affairs Medical Center, Portland, OR 97239, USA.*

Zinc & Copper

The serum concentrations of zinc and copper were measured in 50 patients with multiple sclerosis. Lower serum zinc levels were found compared to age- and sex-matched controls. In younger patients low serum copper concentrations were noted. Zinc concentrations in CSF were unchanged. The possibility that malabsorption of the metals causes the low serum concentrations is discussed. *Reference: J Neurol Neurosurg Psychiatry. 1982 August; 45(8): 691–698. PMCID: PMC1083158. Zinc and copper in multiple sclerosis. R Palm and G Hallmans.*

Homeostasis of metal ions such as Zn2+ is essential for proper brain function. Moreover, the list of psychiatric and neurodegenerative disorders involving a dysregulation of brain Zn2+-levels is long and steadily growing, including Parkinson's and Alzheimer's disease as well as schizophrenia, attention deficit and hyperactivity disorder, depression, amyotrophic lateral sclerosis, Down's syndrome, multiple sclerosis, Wilson's disease and Pick's disease. Furthermore, alterations in Zn2+-levels are seen in transient forebrain ischemia, seizures, traumatic brain injury and alcoholism. Thus, the possibility of altering Zn2+-levels within the brain is emerging as a new target for the prevention and treatment of psychiatric and neurological diseases. Although the role of Zn2+ in the brain has been extensively studied over the past decades, methods for controlled regulation and manipulation of Zn2+ concentrations within the brain are still in their infancy. Since the use of dietary Zn2+ supplementation and restriction has major limitations, new methods and alternative approaches are currently under investigation, such as the use of intracranial infusion of Zn2+ chelators or nanoparticle technologies to elevate or decrease intracellular Zn2+ levels. Therefore, this review briefly summarizes the role of Zn2+ in psychiatric and neurodegenerative diseases and highlights key findings and impediments of brain Zn2+-level manipulation. Furthermore, some methods and compounds, such as metal ion chelation, redistribution and supplementation that are used to control brain Zn2+-levels in order to treat brain disorders are evaluated. *Reference: Drug Deliv Lett. Author manuscript; available in PMC 2011 November 18. Published in final edited form as: Drug Deliv Lett. 2011 September; 1(1): 13–23. PMCID: PMC3220161. NIHMSID: NIHMS332645. Brain-Delivery of Zinc-Ions as Potential Treatment for Neurological Diseases: Mini Review. Andreas M. Grabrucker, Magali Rowan, and Craig C. Garner. Department of Psychiatry and Behavioral Sciences, Stanford School of Medicine, Stanford University, Stanford, CA, USA.*

Ginkgo Biloba

Multiple sclerosis (MS) is a chronic demyelinating neurological disease afflicting young and middle-aged adults, resulting in problems with coordination, strength, cognition, affect, and sensation. The objective of this study was to determine whether a ginkgo extract (EGb 761) improved functional performance in individuals with MS. This study used a double-blind, placebo-controlled, parallel group design. The end point was change between baseline (ie, preintervention) and follow-up evaluation following a regimen of four tablets per day at 60 mg per tablet for four weeks. The study was conducted in academic and clinical-based settings. 22 individuals with MS were randomly assigned to either the treatment or control condition. Groups did not differ with respect to age, IQ, and education. Half of the subjects received 240 mg per day of ginkgo special extract (EGb 761), and the other half received placebo. The main outcome measures assessed depression (Center for Epidemiologic Studies of Depression Scale [CES-D]), anxiety (State-Trait Anxiety Inventory [STAI]), fatigue (Modified Fatigue Impact Scale [MFIS]); symptom severity (Symptom Inventory [SI]) and functional performance (Functional Assessment of Multiple Sclerosis [FAMS]). The ginkgo group had significantly more individuals showing improvement on four or more measures with improvements associated with significantly larger effect sizes on measures of fatigue, symptom severity, and functionality. The ginkgo group also exhibited less fatigue at follow-up compared with the placebo group. This exploratory pilot study showed that no adverse events or side effects were reported and that ginkgo exerted modest beneficial effects on select functional measures (eg, fatigue) among some individuals with MS. *Reference: The effect of Ginkgo biloba on functional measures in multiple sclerosis: a pilot randomized controlled trial. Explore (NY). 2(1):19-24, 2006. Johnson, S. K., et al. University of North Carolina-Charlotte, Charlotte, NC.*

Ten MS patients were treated for five days with intravenous administration of ginkgolide B (one of the principal active constituents of Ginkgo biloba). Eight patients experienced an improvement in their neurological scores commencing two to six days after the commencement of ginkolide B therapy. For 5 of these patients the improvement was sustained. For 3 of these patients the improvement was transitory. *Reference: Pilot study of ginkgolide B, a PAF-acether specific inhibitor in the treatment of acute multiple sclerosis. Rev Neurol (Paris). 148:299-301, 1992. Brochet, B., et al.*

Ginkgo biloba leaf contains terpenes which are also anti-inflammatories. One such terpene, ginkgolide B, is a potent inhibitor of platelet-activating factor, a well-characterized inflammatory mediator. In this double-blind, placebo-controlled trial, ginkgolide B failed to acutely reduce MS exacerbations. The extremely short period of study - only seven days - limits the meaning of this trial. **Reference:** *Double blind placebo controlled multicentre study of ginkgolide B in treatment of acute exacerbations of multiple sclerosis. J Neurol Neurosur Psychiatr. 58:360-362, 1995. Brochet, B., et al.*

Mineral Transporters
By Hans Nieper, M.D.

Preventive medicine is the most important guideline to follow, requiring less effort and less money for better results in the prevention of illness and the protection of our health. A few of you have already heard of the concepts of active mineral transports in directed therapy. How do mineral transport substances work? They release an ion at a site where we want it to be released. We can write an address on the mineral -- on the potential ion -- and have it go where we want it to go so that it can exercise its function, either by activation of enzymes, by restoring structure or by sealing against potential aggression. It is a very simple, completely harmless, yet vitally active principle. Transportation and absorption of minerals involve complex biochemical systems within all cells in the body. Minerals maintain electrical charges which are vital to body physics. A complete understanding of preventive medicine must incorporate both the chemistry and physics of the human body. Nutrients are only useful when they are readily available at the cellular level. Many nutrients move easily through cell membranes by diffusion. These substances are known to be nonpolar because they lack electrical charges. Positive mineral ions such as calcium, magnesium, and potassium may have more difficulty becoming "bio-available" (available for the body's use) because they have such difficulty passing through cell membranes. For this reason, mineral transporters have been developed to enable a mineral ion to be carried to the cell. First developed was potassium magnesium aspartate in 1957-1958, providing the more active transport of potassium and magnesium into the cell. It became quite successful worldwide as a substance for the protection of myocardial necrosis, enhancement of liver functions and the detoxification of digitalis. It has been established that potassium magnesium aspartate also decreases the death rate from heart attack. Since this was so successful, this concept of active mineral transport was pursued and the mineral which had to be transported was changed as well. The most important transporters we have today are aspartic acid, 2-aminoethylphosphoric acid (2-AEP), the salt of the amino acid arginine and orotic acid. Aspartates are minerals bound to the salt of aspartic acid. This transporter delivers the associated mineral to the inner portion of the cell membrane. Potassium magnesium aspartate activates the formation of energy rich phosphates, especially ATP (adenosine triphosphate), resulting in more energy and more oxygen in the blood. Increasing the formation of ATP is one of the most important factors in overcoming muscular fatigue and the potential risk of muscular necrosis in the myocardium, as well as correcting an overspill of the lactate pool. The ions transported by potassium and magnesium to the inner layer of the outer cell membrane activate the respective enzymes, which then result in the formation of more ATP. 2-AEP is a substance which plays a role as a component in the cell membrane and at the same time has the property to form a complex with minerals. This mineral transporter goes into the outer layer of the outer cell membrane where it releases its associated mineral and is itself metabolized with the structure of the cell membrane. The effect here is an increase of the electrical condenser function of cell membranes to resist toxins and viruses which may otherwise enter the cell and cause cellular degeneration. Calcium 2-AEP is especially effective for repairing cell membrane damage. In Germany, calcium, potassium and magnesium 2-AEP are officially declared as the only active substances for the treatment of multiple sclerosis. The myelin is a multilayer of cell membranes. In the case of multiple sclerosis 2-AEP goes to the myelin, fits as a membrane component in the damaged membrane concurrently releasing the mineral which shields against aggression by antibodies. In a discussion of mineral transporters, it is important as well to stress orotates and arginates. These molecules are mostly taken up by tissue, especially by cartilage tissue, by vessel walls, by the blood brain barrier and by the matrix of the bone. Calcium orotate and calcium arginate perform clinical effects in various diseases connected with decalcification and injury of bones -- osteoporosis, rheumatoid and osteoarthritis -- which can rapidly be improved by means of the application of these active mineral transporters. Another mineral transporter is zinc arginate and aspartate which is officially on the market in Germany and offered as a substance for the improvement in diabetes and of immune defenses. The production of insulin is enhanced by actively transported zinc. Zinc arginate and aspartate activates the thymus gland and the formation to T-informed lymphocytes. Lithium carbonate activates white blood cells, especially those suppressed by chemotherapy. Unfortunately, carbonates are not well absorbed by the body. Use of this form of lithium requires regular blood level checks by a physician to avoid toxic levels. Conversely, while active mineral transporters lithium orotate or lithium arginate also activate white blood cells, at recommended doses of 450 mg. per day blood levels do not need to be checked. The same applies to the use of lithium transporters to treat manic depression. Active mineral transporters are simple to use and harmless. In order for the body to utilize a mineral ion, that mineral must be delivered to the targeted site in the cellular structure. Over 30 years of clinical application all over the world has shown that the aspartates, orotates, arginates, and 2-AEP carriers are active mineral transporters that make minerals readily available to the body. ***Reference:*** *Reprinted with permission from Let's Live magazine. For a subscription to Let's Live, please call (800) 225-6473.*

PARKINSON'S DISEASE

Antioxidants

Mitochondrial dysfunction and oxidative damage are highly involved in the pathogenesis of Parkinson's disease. Some mitochondrial antioxidants / nutrients that can improve mitochondrial function and/or attenuate oxidative damage have been implicated in Parkinson's disease therapy. The present study examined the preventative effects of two mitochondrial antioxidant / nutrients, R-alpha-lipoic acid and acetyl-L-carnitine. We demonstrated that 4-week pretreatment with R-alpha-lipoic acid and/or acetyl-L-carnitine effectively protected SK-N-MC human neuroblastoma cells against rotenone-induced mitochondrial dysfunction, oxidative damage, and accumulation of alpha-synuclein and ubiquitin. Most notably, we found that when combined, R-alpha-lipoic acid and acetyl-L-carnitine worked at 100 to 1000 fold lower concentrations than they did individually. *Reference: Combined R-alpha-lipoic acid and acetyl-L-carnitine exerts efficient preventative effects in a cellular model of Parkinson's disease. J Cell Mol Med. 2008. Zhang H, Jia H, Liu J, Ao N, Yan B, Shen W, Wang X, Li X, Luo C, Liu J. Institute for Nutritional Science, Shanghai Institutes of Biological Sciences, Chinese Academy of Sciences, Shanghai, China.*

Pesticides

Parkinson's disease (PD) has been associated with exposure to a variety of environmental agents, including pesticides, heavy metals, and organic pollutants; and inflammatory processes appear to constitute a common mechanistic link among these insults. Indeed, toxin exposure has been repeatedly demonstrated to induce the release of oxidative and inflammatory factors from immunocompetent microglia, leading to damage and death of midbrain dopamine (DA) neurons. In particular, proinflammatory cytokines such as tumor necrosis factor-α and interferon-γ, which are produced locally within the brain by microglia, have been implicated in the loss of DA neurons in toxin-based models of PD; and mounting evidence suggests a contributory role of the inflammatory enzyme, cyclooxygenase-2. Likewise, immune-activating bacterial and viral agents were reported to have neurodegenerative effects themselves and to augment the deleterious impact of chemical toxins upon DA neurons. The present paper will focus upon the evidence linking microglia and their inflammatory processes to the death of DA neurons following toxin exposure. Particular attention will be devoted to the possibility that environmental toxins can activate microglia, resulting in these cells adopting a "sensitized" state that favors the production of proinflammatory cytokines and damaging oxidative radicals. *Reference: Parkinsons Dis. 2011; 2011: 713517. Published online 2010 December 30. doi: 10.4061/2011/713517. PMCID: PMC3018622. Inflammatory Mechanisms of Neurodegeneration in Toxin-Based Models of Parkinson's Disease. Darcy Litteljohn, Emily Mangano, Melanie Clarke, Jessica Bobyn, Kerry Moloney, and*

Shawn Hayley. Institute of Neuroscience, Carleton University, 1125 Colonel By Drive, Ottawa, ON, Canada K1S 5B6.

Pesticides are widely used in agricultural and other settings, resulting in continued human exposure. Pesticide toxicity has been clearly demonstrated to alter a variety of neurological functions. Particularly, there is strong evidence suggesting that pesticide exposure predisposes to neurodegenerative diseases. Epidemiological data has suggested a relationship between pesticide exposure and brain neurodegeneration. However, an increasing debate has aroused regarding this issue. Paraquat is a highly toxic quaternary nitrogen herbicide which has been largely studied as a model for Parkinson's disease providing valuable insight into the possible mechanisms involved in the toxic effects of pesticides and their role in the progression of neurodegenerative diseases. In this work, we review the molecular mechanisms involved in the neurotoxic actions of pesticides, with a particular emphasis on the mechanisms associated with the induction neuronal cell death by paraquat as a model for Parkinsonian neurodegeneration. *Reference: Chem Biol Interact. Author manuscript; available in PMC 2011 November 5. Published in final edited form as: Chem Biol Interact. 2010 November 5; 188(2): 289–300. Published online 2010 June 11. doi: 10.1016/j.cbi.2010.06.003. PMCID: PMC2942983. NIHMSID: NIHMS213625. Molecular Mechanisms of Pesticide-induced Neurotoxicity: Relevance to Parkinson's Disease. Rodrigo Franco, Sumin Li, Humberto Rodriguez-Rocha, Michaela Burns, and Mihalis I. Panayiotidis. Redox Biology Center and School of Veterinary Medicine and Biomedical Sciences. University of Nebraska-Lincoln. Lincoln, NE 68583. Department of Pathology, Medical School, University of Ioannina, University Campus, Ioannina, 45110 Greece. School of Community Health Sciences, University of Nevada, Reno, NV 89557.*

Nicotine

There exists a remarkable diversity of neurotransmitter compounds in the striatum, a pivotal brain region in the pathology of Parkinson's disease, a movement disorder characterized by rigidity, tremor and bradykinesia. The striatal dopaminergic system, which is particularly vulnerable to neurodegeneration in this disorder, appears to be the major contributor to these motor problems. However, numerous other neurotransmitter systems in the striatum most likely also play a significant role, including the nicotinic cholinergic system. Indeed, there is an extensive anatomical overlap between dopaminergic and cholinergic neurons, and acetylcholine is well known to modulate striatal dopamine release both in vitro and in vivo. Nicotine, a drug that stimulates nicotinic acetylcholine receptors (nAChRs), influences several functions relevant to Parkinson's disease. Extensive studies in parkinsonian animals show that nicotine protects against nigrostriatal damage, findings that may explain the well-established decline in Parkinson's disease incidence with tobacco use. In addition, recent work shows that nicotine reduces L-dopa-induced abnormal involuntary movements, a debilitating complication of L-dopa therapy for Parkinson's disease. These combined observations suggest that nAChR stimulation may represent a useful treatment strategy for Parkinson's disease for neuroprotection and symptomatic treatment. Importantly, only selective nAChR subtypes are present in the striatum including the α4β2*, α6β2* and α7 nAChR populations. Treatment with nAChR ligands directed to these subtypes may thus yield optimal therapeutic benefit for Parkinson's disease, with a minimum of adverse side effects. *Reference: Biochem Pharmacol. 2009 October 1; 78(7): 677. Published online 2009 May 9. doi: 10.1016/j.bcp.2009.05.003. NIHMSID: NIHMS142026. Multiple roles for nicotine in Parkinson's disease. Maryka Quik, Luping Z. Huang, Neeraja Parameswaran, Tanuja Bordia, Carla Campos, and Xiomara A. Perez.*

Parkinson's disease is a debilitating neurodegenerative movement disorder characterized by damage to the nigrostriatal dopaminergic system. Current therapies are symptomatic only and may be accompanied by serious side effects. There is therefore a continual search for novel compounds for the treatment of Parkinson's disease symptoms, as well as to reduce or halt disease progression. Nicotine administration has been reported to improve motor deficits that arise with nigrostriatal damage in parkinsonian animals and in Parkinson's disease. In addition, nicotine protects against nigrostriatal damage in experimental models, findings that have led to the suggestion that the reduced incidence of Parkinson's disease in smokers may be due to the nicotine in tobacco. Altogether, these observations suggest that nicotine treatment may be beneficial in Parkinson's disease. Nicotine interacts with multiple nicotinic receptor (nAChR) subtypes in the peripheral and central nervous system, as well as in skeletal muscle. Work to identify the subtypes affected in Parkinson's disease is therefore critical for the development of targeted therapies. Results show that striatal α6β2-containing nAChRs are particularly susceptible to nigrostriatal damage, with a decline in receptor levels that closely parallels losses in striatal dopamine. In contrast, α4β2-containing nAChRs are decreased to a much smaller extent under the same conditions. These observations suggest that development of nAChR agonists or antagonists targeted to α6β2-containing nAChRs may represent a particularly relevant target for Parkinson's disease therapeutics. *Reference: Biochem Pharmacol. 2007 October 15; 74(8): 1224– 1234. Published online 2007 June 17. doi: 10.1016/j.bcp.2007.06.015. NIHMSID: NIHMS32016. Nicotinic receptors as CNS targets for Parkinson's disease. Maryka Quik, Tanuja Bordia, and Kathryn O'Leary. The Parkinson's Institute, 1170 Morse Ave, Sunnyvale, CA 94089.*

Diet

Motor fluctuations and non-response to carbidopa-levodopa (Sinemet) therapy are major problems in the long-term management of Parkinson's disease. Levodopa manipulation, addition of adjuvants, and drug holidays are often unsuccessful. Others have shown that the clinical state of stabilized Parkinsonians can be reversed with intravenous administration of large neutral amino acids. Reasoning that dietary protein might precipitate motor oscillations and non-response, a low-protein daytime diet

(7 g) was offered to fifteen patients. Eighty-six percent of this sample demonstrated immediate sensitivity to Sinemet. While on a low-protein diet, patients' clinical function was predominantly choreatic. Eight patients required a 10-60 percent reduction in their daily levodopa dose in order to minimize this choreatic tendency. Discontinuation of adjuvants did not compromise motor independence. Conversely, while on a high-protein diet (160 g), patients were predominantly immobile with markedly elevated plasma amino acid and levodopa levels. Consequently, elimination of dietary protein from breakfast and lunch can offer an effective and easily modified method for the amelioration of motor fluctuations and non-response to Sinemet in Parkinson's disease during working hours. **Reference:** *Yale J Biol Med. 1987 Mar-Apr; 60(2): 133–137. PMCID: PMC2590325. Dietary method for reducing fluctuations in Parkinson's disease. J. H. Pincus and K. M. Barry.*

Results of case-control studies and of a prospective investigation in men suggest that consumption of coffee could protect against the risk of Parkinson's disease, but the active constituent is not clear. To address the hypothesis that caffeine is protective against Parkinson's disease, the authors examined the relationship of coffee and caffeine consumption to the risk of this disease among participants in two ongoing cohorts, the Health Professionals' Follow-Up Study (HPFS) and the Nurses' Health Study (NHS). The study population comprised 47,351 men and 88,565 women who were free of Parkinson's disease, stroke, or cancer at baseline. A comprehensive life style and dietary questionnaire was completed by the participants at baseline and updated every two to four years. During the follow-up (10 years in men, 16 years in women), the authors documented a total of 288 incident cases of Parkinson's disease. Among men, after adjustment for age and smoking, the relative risk of Parkinson's disease was 0.42 (95% CI: 0.23-0.78; p for trend < 0.001) for men in the top one-fifth of caffeine intake compared to those in the bottom one-fifth. An inverse association was also observed with consumption of coffee (p for trend = 0.004), caffeine from non-coffee sources (p for trend < 0.001), and tea (p for trend = 0.02) but not decaffeinated coffee. Among women, the relationship between caffeine or coffee intake and risk of Parkinson's disease was U-shaped, with the lowest risk observed at moderate intakes (1-3 cups of coffee/day, or the third quintile of caffeine consumption). These results support a possible protective effect of moderate doses of caffeine on risk of Parkinson's disease. **Reference:** *Prospective study of caffeine consumption and risk of Parkinson's disease in men and women. Ann Neurol. 50(1):56-63, 2001. Ascherio, A., et al. Department of Nutrition, Harvard School of Public Health, Boston, MA, USA.*

Acetyl-L-Carnitine

During the past two decades, many pharmacological strategies have been investigated for the management of painful neuropathies. However, neuropathic pain still remains a clinical challenge. A combination of therapies is often required, but unfortunately in most cases adequate pain relief is not achieved. Recently, attention has been focused on the physiological and pharmacological effects of L-acetylcarnitine in neurological disorders. There are a number of reports indicating that L-acetylcarnitine can be considered as a therapeutic agent in neuropathic disorders including painful peripheral neuropathies. In this review article, we will examine the antinociceptive and the neuroprotective effects of Lacetylcarnitine as tested in clinical studies and in animal models of nerve injury. **CONCLUSION** - Despite the different etiologies leading to neuropathic pain, increased neuronal excitability is thought to be the underlying mechanism of all forms of painful neuropathies. Therefore, the current pharmacotherapy of neuropathic pain generally involves the use of drugs that either reduce neuronal discharge or increase endogenous antinociceptive systems. Sodium-channel blockers, antiepileptic agents, opiods, tricyclic antidepressants, gabapentin etc., have been employed to treat the painful symptoms of different forms of neuropathies. However, although the main goal is to reduce pain and minimize side effects of drugs, the management of neuropathic pain should also be addressed to counteract the pathological changes that occur in many forms of neuropathies. Loss of small sensory fibers, demyelination and changes in nerve conduction velocity are common features in different forms of neuropathies. In this respect, L-acetylcarnitine is a promising compound for the treatment of painful neuropathies for its dual mechanisms, which include a significant analgesic effect after chronic administration and the ability to promote peripheral nerve regeneration and to improve vibration perception. Moreover, the apparent lack of side effects suggests that this drug might be suitable for long term treatment, an important characteristic for a chronic condition such as neuropathic pain. Thus, the data to date suggest that L-acetylcarnitine could be considered for use in neuropathic pain conditions alone or in combination with other treatments. Further large-scale controlled clinical trials are needed to assess the efficacy of L-acetylcarnitine in various neuropathic pain conditions. *Reference: Curr Neuropharmacol. 2006 July; 4(3): 233–237. L-Acetylcarnitine: A Proposed Therapeutic Agent for Painful Peripheral Neuropathies. S Chiechio, A Copani, F Nicoletti, and RW Gereau IV, Washington University Pain Center and Department of Anesthesiology, Washington University School of Medicine, St. Louis, MO, USA. Department of Pharmaceutical Sciences, University of Catania, Catania, Italy. Department of Human Physiology and Pharmacology, University of Rome 'La Sapienza', Faculty of Medicine, Rome, Italy and Istituto Neurologico Mediterraneo, Neuromed Pozzilli (IS), Pozzilli, Italy.*

Acetyl-levo-carnitine (ALC) protects against 1-methyl, 4-phenyl-1,2,3,6-tetrahydropyridine (MPTP)-induced toxicity in the nonhuman primate. ALC pretreated monkeys do not show signs of parkinsonism or electroretinographic changes typical of dopaminergic deficiency when given MPTP. In addition, pilot neurochemical and morphological data confirm a partial protection effect. While MAO-B inhibitors, like L-Deprenyl, are thought to protect dopaminergic neurons from MPTP-induced cell death by preventing the conversion of MPTP to its toxic metabolite MPP+, ALC is not known to have MAO-B affinity. Converging evidence suggests that ALC may affect directly mitochondrial respiration, which is known to be the target of MPP+ and affected in human neurodegenerative diseases, including Parkinson's disease. The results of this study point to new therapeutic avenues for the treatment of these nosologic entities. *Reference: Acetyl-levo-carnitine protects against MPTP-induced parkinsonism in primates. J Neural Transm Park Dis Diment Sect. 3(1):63-72, 1991. Bodis-Wollner, I., et al. Department of Neurology, Mount Sinai School of Medicine, C.U.N.Y., New York.*

The author recommends the use of ALC for Parkinson's disease due to its role as a mitochondrial energy transporter. In an animal study, ALC protected the suprachiasmatic nucleus from MPP+ induced damage. ALC also enhances dopaminergic transmission. *Reference: Parkinson's disease as multifactorial oxidative neurodegeneration: implications for integrative management. Altern Med Rev. 5(6):502-529, 2000. Kidd, P. M., et al.*

Acetyl-L-carnitine (ALCAR) plays an integral role in the transport of long chain fatty acids across the inner mitochondrial membrane for oxidative phosphorylation. In non-human primates, administration of ALCAR was reported to prevent 1-methyl-4-phenyl-1,2,3,6-tetrahydropyridine (MPTP)-induced neurological injury to the substantia nigra. The present study investigates the effects of ALCAR against the toxicity of 1-methyl-4-phenylpyridinium (MPP(+)), the neurotoxic metabolite of MPTP, in murine brain neuroblastoma cells. MPP(+), a potent mitochondrial toxin, induced a dose-dependent reduction in mitochondrial oxygen consumption and cell viability, corresponding to an accelerated rate of cellular glucose utilization. Treatment with ALCAR, but not L-carnitine, prevented MPP(+) toxicity and partially restored intracellular ATP concentrations, but did not reverse the MPP(+)-induced loss of mitochondrial oxygen consumption. These data indicate that protective effects are independent of oxidative phosphorylation. ALCAR had a substantial glucose sparing effect in both controls and MPP(+)-treated groups, demonstrating a potential role in enhancing glucose utilization through glycolysis. Antagonizing the entry of fatty acids into the mitochondria, with either insulin or malonyl CoA, did not interfere with ALCAR protection against MPP(+). On the contrary, insulin potentiated the protective effects of ALCAR. In conclusion, these data indicate that ALCAR protects against MPP(+) toxicity, independent of mitochondrial oxidative capacity or beta-oxidation of fatty acids. In contrast, the protective effects of ALCAR appear to involve potentiation of energy derived from glucose through anaerobic glycolysis. *Reference: Acetyl-L-carnitine cytoprotection against 1-methyl-4-phenylpyridinium toxicity in neuroblastoma cells. Biochem Pharmacol. 66(2):297-306, 2003. Mazzio, E., et al. College of Pharmacy and Pharmaceutical Sciences, Florida A & M University, Tallahassee, FL, USA.*

Two groups of 10 patients with Parkinson's disease received doses of either 1g acetyl-L-carnitine (ALC) per day for seven days or 2g. The effects of this drug on intermittent luminous stimulation and on nocturnal sleep patterns were studied. In both cases with either dose of ALC the effect was an improvement of the H response, sleep stages and spindling activity. *Reference: Clinical pharmacodynamics of acetyl-L-carnitine in patients with Parkinson's disease. Int J Clin Pharmacol Res. 10(1-2):139-143, 1990. Puca, F. M., et al.*

The authors studied the effect of acetyl-L-carnitine (ALCAR) on dopamine release and the effect of long-term acetyl-L-carnitine treatment on age-related changes in striatal dopamine receptors and brain amino acid levels. In striatal tissue that had been incubated with [3H]dopamine, acetyl-L-carnitine increased the release of [3H]dopamine evoked by electrical stimulation. In striatal tissue from aged mice administered acetyl-L-carnitine for 3 months, the release of [3H]dopamine evoked by electrical stimulation was higher than that of its aged control; the release after a second stimulation was similar in the two groups. There was a significant decline in the number of D1 striatal dopamine receptors with age. The Bmax was 51% lower in 1.5-year-old mice than in 4-month-old animals. Administration of acetyl-L-carnitine for 3 months diminished the reduction in the binding of [3H]SCH-23390. [3H]Spiperone binding to D2 receptors was not decreased with age and was not affected by acetyl-L-carnitine treatment. Age-related decreases in levels of several amino acids were observed in several brain regions. Acetyl-L-carnitine lessened the reduction in the level of taurine only in the striatum. The findings confirm the multiple effects of acetyl-L-carnitine in brain, and suggest that its administration can have a positive effect on age-related changes in the dopaminergic system. *Reference: Effect of acetyl-L-carnitine on the dopaminergic system in aging brain. J Neurosci Res. 30(3):555-559, 1991. Sershen, H., et al. Center for Neurochemistry, Nathan S. Kline Institute for Psychiatric Research, Orangeburg, New York 10962.*

The damage to the central nervous system that is observed after administration of either methamphetamine (METH) or 1-methyl-4-phenylpyridinium (MPP(+)), the neurotoxic metabolite of 1-methyl-4-phenyl-1,2,3,6-tetrahydropyridine (MPTP), is known to be linked to dopamine (DA). The underlying neurotoxicity mechanism for both METH and MPP(+) seem to involve free radical formation and impaired mitochondrial function. The MPP(+) is thought to selectively kill nigrostriatal dopaminergic neurons by inhibiting mitochondrial complex I, with cell death being attributed to oxidative stress damage to these vulnerable DA neurons. In the present study, MPP(+) was shown to significantly inhibit the response to MTT by cultured PC12 cells. This inhibitory action of MPP(+) could be partially reversed by the co-incubation of the cells with the acetylated form of carnitine, acetyl-l-carnitine (ALC). Since at least part of the toxic action of MPP(+) is related to mitochondrial inhibition, the partial reversal of the inhibition of MTT response by ALC could involve a partial restoration of mitochondrial function. The role carnitine derivatives, such as ALC, play in attenuating MPP(+) and METH-evoked toxicity is still under investigation to elucidate the contribution of mitochondrial dysfunction in mechanisms of neurotoxicity. *Reference: Role of mitochondrial dysfunction in neurotoxicity of MPP:+: partial protection of PC12 cells by acetyl-l-carnitine. Ann N Y Acad Sci. 1025:267-273, 2004. Virmani, A., et al. Sigma-tau HealthScience S.p.A., Pomezia, Italy.*

Creatine Monohydrate

Substantial evidence indicates bioenergetic dysfunction and mitochondrial impairment contribute either directly and/or indirectly to the pathogenesis of numerous neurodegenerative disorders. Treatment paradigms aimed at ameliorating this cellular energy deficit and/or improving mitochondrial function in these neurodegenerative disorders may prove to be useful as a therapeutic intervention. Creatine is a molecule that is produced both endogenously, and acquired exogenously through diet, and is an extremely important molecule that participates in buffering intracellular energy stores. Once creatine is transported into cells, creatine kinase catalyzes the reversible transphosphorylation of creatine via ATP to enhance the phosphocreatine energy pool. Creatine kinase enzymes are located at strategic intracellular sites to couple areas of high energy expenditure to the efficient regeneration of ATP. Thus, the creatinekinase/phosphocreatine system plays an integral role in energy buffering and overall cellular bioenergetics. Originally, exogenous creatine supplementation was widely used only as an ergogenic aid to increase the phosphocreatine pool within muscle to bolster athletic performance. However, the potential therapeutic value of creatine supplementation has recently been investigated with respect to various neurodegenerative disorders that have been associated with bioenergetic deficits as playing a role in disease etiology and/or progression which include; Alzheimer's, Parkinson's, amyotrophic lateral sclerosis (ALS), and Huntington's disease. This review discusses the contribution of mitochondria and bioenergetics to the progression of these neurodegenerative diseases and investigates the potential neuroprotective value of creatine supplementation in each of these neurological diseases. In summary, current literature suggests that exogenous creatine supplementation is most efficacious as a treatment paradigm in Huntington's and Parkinson's disease but appears to be less effective for ALS and Alzheimer's disease.

Conclusion - Exogenous creatine supplementation appears to primarily exert its beneficial effects by increasing the PCr pool to improve overall cellular bioenergetics. Additionally, some evidence suggests that creatine may also enhance mitochondrial function and reduce the susceptibility to mitochondrially mediated apoptosis. These beneficial effects of creatine supplementation were initially recognized in muscle tissue where they were shown to prolong contractility and enhance overall athletic performance. The convincing functional improvements in muscle tissue led to the hypothesis that creatine may be useful as a therapeutic intervention to target neurological diseases with metabolic/bioenergetic dysfunction as part of their disease etiology. The evidence presented in this review suggests that creatine supplementation improves bioenergetic deficits and may exert neuroprotective effects in Parkinson's and Huntington's disease. However, current evidence suggests that creatine supplementation is not efficacious in the treatment of AD and ALS (refer to Andres et al. 2008 for an additional/alternative review of the neuroprotective effect of creatine). Further clinical studies investigating the role of creatine in Parkinson's and Huntington's disease over the next several years will certainly provide insight and potentially substantiate the neuroprotective role of creatine in these neurological diseases. In addition to the clinical trials of creatine supplementation in Parkinson's and Huntington's disease, more creatine studies utilizing animal and cell culture models of these diseases are warranted to fully understand and appreciate the exact mechanisms by which creatine exerts its neuroprotective effects. Further insight of the molecular details and/or mechanisms of the neuroprotective effects of creatine supplementation in these diseases may potentially offer novel cellular targets and/or processes for future therapeutic interventions. **Reference:** *Neuromolecular Med. 2008; 10(4): 275–290. Published online 2008 November 13. doi: 10.1007/s12017-008-8053-y. PMCID: PMC2886719. NIHMSID: NIHMS196779. Creatine and Its Potential Therapeutic Value for Targeting Cellular Energy Impairment in Neurodegenerative Diseases. Peter J. Adhihetty and M. Flint Bea. Department of Neurology and Neuroscience, Weill Medical College of Cornell University, 525 East 68th Street, New York, NY 10021, USA.*

Progressive destruction of neurons that produce dopamine in the basal ganglia of the brain, particularly the substantia nigra, is a hallmark of Parkinson's disease. The syndrome of the Parkinsonian phenotype is caused by many etiologies, involving multiple contributing mechanisms. Characteristic findings are pathologic inclusions called Lewy bodies, which are protein aggregates inside nerve cells. Environmental insults are linked with the disease, and a number of associated genes have also been identified. Neuroinflammation, microglia activation, oxidative stress, and mitochondrial dysfunction are central processes producing nerve damage. In addition, protein misfolding, driven by accumulation and condensation of α-synuclein, compounded by inadequate elimination of defective protein through the ubiquitin- proteasome system, promote apoptosis. Current pharmacologic therapy is palliative rather than disease- modifying, and typically becomes unsatisfactory over time. Coenzyme Q10 and creatine, two agents involved in energy production, may be disease-modifying, and able to produce sufficient beneficial pathophysiologic changes in preclinical studies to warrant large studies now in progress. Use of long-chain omega-3 fatty acids and vitamin D in PD are also topics of current interest. **Conclusion** - "Mitochondrial therapy", both preventive and immediate, is a relatively new concept, and inroads have been significant, not only in neurologic disease but also in the intensive care unit, and in cardiology, renal, and other medical disciplines. While advances in the clinical management of PD with drugs have improved the quality of life in patients dramatically in terms of symptoms, there are no disease-modifying agents available. Recent work suggests that inflammation, oxidative, and nitrosative stress, accumulation of abnormally folded and/or aggregated proteins, and defects in the ubiquitin-proteasome system are central molecular events in the pathogenesis of familial and sporadic PD. The possible beneficial disease-modifying effects of CoQ10 and creatine are presented in the context of this current molecular model. In view of the rapid and encouraging recent work concerning omega-3 fatty acids and vitamin D, their supportive practical role in targeted pharmaconutritional therapy of PD deserves clinical consideration. *Reference: Clin Pharmacol. 2010; 2: 185–198. Published online 2010 September 17. doi: 10.2147/CPAA.S12082. Mitochondrial therapy for Parkinson's disease: Neuroprotective pharmaconutrition may be disease-modifying. Richard Kones. Cardiometabolic Research Institute, Houston, TX, USA. Correspondence: Richard Kones, MD, Cardiometabolic Research institute, 8181, Fannin St, U314 Houston, TX 77055, USA, Tel +1 713 790 9100, Fax +1 713 790 9292, Email drrkones@comcast.net.*

Persons with Parkinson disease (PD) exhibit decreased muscular fitness including decreased muscle mass, muscle strength, bioenergetic capabilities and increased fatigability. The purpose of this investigation was to evaluate the therapeutic effects of resistance training with and without creatine supplementation in patients with mild to moderate PD. Twenty patients with idiopathic PD were randomized to receive creatine monohydrate supplementation plus resistance training (CRE) or placebo (lactose monohydrate) plus resistance training (PLA), using a double-blind procedure. Creatine and placebo supplementation consisted of 20 grams/day for the first 5 days and 5 grams/day thereafter. Both groups participated in progressive resistance training (24 sessions, 2 times per week, 1 set of 8-12 repetitions, 9 exercises). Participants performed 1-repetition maximum (1-RM) for chest press, leg extension, and biceps curl. Muscular endurance was evaluated for chest press and leg extension as the number of repetitions to failure using 60% of baseline 1-RM. Functional performance was evaluated as the time to perform 3 consecutive chair rises. Statistical analyses (ANOVA) revealed significant Group x Time interactions for chest press strength and biceps curl strength, and post hoc testing revealed that the improvement was significantly greater for CRE. Chair rise performance significantly improved only for CRE (12%, P=.03). Both PLA and CRE significantly improved 1-RM for leg extension (PLA: 16%; CRE: 18%). Muscular endurance improved significantly for both groups. These findings demonstrate that creatine supplementation can enhance the benefits of resistance training in patients with PD. *Reference: Resistance training with creatine monohydrate improves upper-body strength in patients with Parkinson disease: a randomized trial. Neurorehabil Neural Repair. 21(2):107-115, 2007. Hass, C. J., et al. Department of Biobehavioral Sciences, Teachers College, Columbia University, New York, NY, USA.*

Systemic administration of 1-methyl-4-phenyl-1,2,3, 6-tetrahydropyridine (MPTP) produces parkinsonism in experimental animals by a mechanism involving impaired energy production. MPTP is converted by monoamine oxidase B to 1-methyl-4-phenylpyridinium (MPP+), which blocks complex I of the electron transport chain. Oral supplementation with creatine or cyclocreatine, which are substrates for creatine kinase, may increase phosphocreatine (PCr) or cyclophosphocreatine (PCCr) and buffer against ATP depletion and thereby exert neuroprotective effects. Oral supplementation with either creatine or cyclocreatine produced significant protection against MPTP-induced dopamine depletions in mice. Creatine protected against MPTP-induced loss of Nissl and tyrosine hydroxylase immunostained neurons in the substantia nigra. Creatine and cyclocreatine had no effects on the conversion of MPTP to MPP+ in vivo. These results further implicate metabolic dysfunction in MPTP neurotoxicity and suggest a novel therapeutic approach, which may have applicability for Parkinson's disease. **Reference:** *Creatine and cyclocreatine attenuate MPTP neurotoxicity. Exp Neurol. 157(1):142-149, 1999. Matthews, R. T., et al. Neurology Service, Massachusetts General Hospital, Boston, Massachusetts, USA.*

Although this study involved the treatment of neuromuscular disease patients, researchers speculated that creatine monohydrate may also be helpful in treating Alzheimer's disease. This speculation is based on the theory that creatine monohydrate supplementation may provide additional energy to neurons and muscles that are affected by Parkinson's disease. **Reference:** *Creatine monohydrate increases strength in patients with neuromuscular disease. Neurology. 52(4):854-857, 1999. Tarnopolsky, M., et al.*

Creatine and minocycline were prioritized for testing in Phase II clinical trials based on a systematic evaluation of potentially disease modifying compounds for Parkinson disease (PD). The objective was to test whether creatine and minocycline alter the course of early PD relative to a predetermined futility threshold for progression of PD in a randomized, double-blind, Phase II futility clinical trial. Agents that do not perform better than the futility threshold are rejected as futile and are not considered for further study. Participants had a diagnosis of PD within 5 years, but did not require medications for the management of symptoms. The primary outcome was the change in the total Unified Parkinson's Disease Rating Scale (UPDRS) score from baseline to either the time when there was sufficient disability to warrant symptomatic therapy for PD or 12 months, whichever came first. Subjects were randomized 1:1:1 to receive creatine 10 g/day, minocycline 200 mg/day, or matching placebo. The futility threshold was set as a 30% reduction in UPDRS progression based on the placebo/tocopherol arm of the Deprenyl And Tocopherol Antioxidative Therapy Of Parkinsonism (DATATOP) trial. p Values 0.1 indicate futility. 200 subjects were randomized to the three groups. Neither creatine (p = 0.96) nor minocycline (p = 0.66) could be rejected as futile based on the DATATOP futility threshold. The rate of progression for the calibration placebo group fell outside the 95% CI for the DATATOP historical control. In a sensitivity analysis, based on the threshold derived from the calibration placebo group, again neither drug could be rejected as futile. Tolerability was 91% in the creatine group and 77% in the minocycline group. Common adverse events included upper respiratory symptoms (26%), joint pain (19%), and nausea (17%). Both creatine and minocycline should be considered for definitive Phase III trials to determine if they alter the long term progression of Parkinson disease (PD). Additional factors must be weighed before selecting agents for Phase III trials, including safety, tolerability, activity, cost, and availability of these two agents in comparison with other agents currently in development for PD. *Reference: A randomized, double-blind, futility clinical trial of creatine and minocycline in early Parkinson disease. Neurology. 2006. The NINDS NET-PD Investigators.*

Parkinson's disease (PD) is a neurologic disorder characterized by dopaminergic cell death in the substantia nigra. PD pathogenesis involves mitochondrial dysfunction, proteasome impairment, and α-synuclein aggregation, insults that may be especially toxic to oxidatively stressed cells including dopaminergic neurons. The enzyme methionine sulfoxide reductase A (MsrA) plays a critical role in the antioxidant response by repairing methionine-oxidized proteins and by participating in cycles of methionine oxidation and reduction that have the net effect of consuming reactive oxygen species. Here, we show that MsrA suppresses dopaminergic cell death and protein aggregation induced by the complex I inhibitor rotenone or mutant α-synuclein, but not by the proteasome inhibitor MG132. By comparing the effects of MsrA and the small-molecule antioxidants N-acetyl-cysteine and vitamin E, we provide evidence that MsrA protects against PD-related stresses primarily via methionine sulfoxide repair rather than by scavenging reactive oxygen species. We also demonstrate that MsrA efficiently reduces oxidized methionine residues in recombinant α-synuclein. These findings suggest that enhancing MsrA function may be a reasonable therapeutic strategy in PD. *Reference: Methionine sulfoxide reductase A (MsrA). Free Radic Biol Med. Author manuscript; available in PMC 2009 August 1. Published in final edited form as: Free Radic Biol Med. 2008 August 1; 45(3): 242–255. Published online 2008 April 11. doi: 10.1016/j.freeradbiomed.2008.03.022. PMCID: PMC2518045. NIHMSID: NIHMS56598. Methionine sulfoxide reductase A protects dopaminergic cells from Parkinson's disease-related insults. Fang Liu,a Jagadish Hindupur,a Jamie L. Nguyen,a Katie J. Ruf,a Junyi Zhu,a Jeremy L. Schieler, Connie C. Bonham, Karl V. Wood, V. Jo Davisson, and Jean-Christophe Rochet,a Department of Medicinal Chemistry and Molecular Pharmacology, Purdue University, West Lafayette, Indiana, 47907. Department of Biochemistry, Purdue University, West Lafayette, Indiana, 47907. Department of Chemistry, Purdue University, West Lafayette, Indiana, 47907.*

MsrA (methionine sulphoxide reductase A) is an antioxidant repair enzyme that reduces oxidized methionine to methionine. Moreover, the oxidation of methionine residues in proteins is considered to be an important consequence of oxidative damage to cells. To understand mechanisms of human msrA gene expression and regulation, we cloned and characterized the 5' promoter region of the human msrA gene. Using 5'-RACE (rapid amplification of cDNA ends) analysis of purified mRNA from human cells, we located the transcription initiation site 59 nt upstream of the reference MsrA mRNA sequence, GenBank® accession number BC 054033. The 1.3 kb of sequence located upstream of the first exon of msrA gene was placed upstream of the luciferase reporter gene in a pGL3-Basic vector and transfected into different cell lines. Sequentially smaller fragments of the msrA promoter region were generated by PCR, and expression levels were monitored from these constructs within HEK-293 and MCF7 human cell lines. Analysis of deletion constructs revealed differences in promoter activity in these cell lines. In HEK-293 cells, the promoter activity was constant from the minimal promoter region to the longest fragment obtained. On the other hand, in MCF7 cells we detected a down-regulation in the longest fragment. Mutation of a putative negative regulatory region that is located between −209 and −212 bp (the CCAA box) restored promoter activity in MCF7 cells. The location of the msrA promoter will facilitate analysis of the transcriptional regulation of this gene in a variety of pathological contexts. *Reference: Biochem J. 2006 January 1; 393(Pt 1): 321–329. Published online 2005 December 12. Prepublished online 2005 September 14. doi: 10.1042/BJ20050973. PMCID: PMC1383691. Identification and analysis of the promoter region of the human methionine sulphoxide reductase A gene. Antonella De Luca, Paolo Sacchetta, Carmine Di Ilio, and Bartolo Favaloro. Department of Biomedical Sciences, University of Chieti "G. D'Annunzio" School of Medicine, and Center of Excellence on Aging, "G. D'Annunzio" University Foundation, Chieti, Italy.*

Coenzyme Q10 (CoQ10)

Coenzyme Q(10) (CoQ(10)) and creatine are promising agents for neuroprotection in neurodegenerative diseases via their effects on improving mitochondrial function and cellular bioenergetics and their properties as antioxidants. The authors examined whether a combination of CoQ(10) with creatine can exert additive neuroprotective effects in a MPTP mouse model of Parkinson's disease, a 3-NP rat model of Huntington's disease (HD) and the R6/2 transgenic mouse model of HD. The combination of the two agents produced additive neuroprotective effects against dopamine depletion in the striatum and loss of tyrosine hydroxylase neurons in the substantia nigra pars compacta (SNpc) following chronic subcutaneous administration of MPTP. The combination treatment resulted in significant reduction in lipid peroxidation and pathologic alpha-synuclein accumulation in the SNpc neurons of the MPTP-treated mice. The authors also observed additive neuroprotective effects in reducing striatal lesion volumes produced by chronic subcutaneous administration of 3-NP to rats. The combination treatment showed significant effects on blocking 3-NP-induced impairment of glutathione homeostasis and reducing lipid peroxidation and DNA oxidative damage in the striatum. Lastly, the combination of CoQ(10) and creatine produced additive neuroprotective effects on improving motor performance and extending survival in the transgenic R6/2 HD mice. These findings suggest that combination therapy using CoQ(10) and creatine may be useful in the treatment of neurodegenerative diseases such as Parkinson's disease and Huntington's Disease. *Reference: Combination therapy with coenzyme Q10 and creatine produces additive neuroprotective effects in models of Parkinson's and Huntington's diseases. J Neurochem. 109(5):1427-1439, 2009. Yang, L., et al. Department of Neurology and Neuroscience, Weill Medical College of Cornell University, New York-Presbyterian Hospital, New York, New York, USA.*

A definitive neuropathological diagnosis of Parkinson's disease requires loss of dopaminergic neurons in the substantia nigra and related brain stem nuclei, and the presence of Lewy bodies in remaining nerve cells. The contribution of genetic factors to the pathogenesis of Parkinson's disease is increasingly being recognized. A point mutation which is sufficient to cause a rare autosomal dominant form of the disorder has been recently identified in the alpha-synuclein gene on chromosome 4 in the much more common sporadic, or 'idiopathic' form of Parkinson's disease, and a defect of complex I of the mitochondrial respiratory chain was confirmed at the biochemical level. Disease specificity of this defect has been demonstrated for the parkinsonian substantia nigra. These findings and the observation that the neurotoxin 1-methyl-4-phenyl-1,2,3, 6-tetrahydropyridine (MPTP), which causes a Parkinson-like syndrome in humans, acts via inhibition of complex I have triggered research interest in the mitochondrial genetics of Parkinson's disease. Oxidative phosphorylation consists of five protein-lipid enzyme complexes located in the mitochondrial inner membrane that contain flavins (FMN, FAD), quinoid compounds (coenzyme Q10, CoQ10) and transition metal compounds (iron-sulfur clusters, hemes, protein-bound copper). These enzymes are designated complex I (NADH:ubiquinone oxidoreductase, EC 1.6. 5.3), complex II (succinate:ubiquinone oxidoreductase, EC 1.3.5.1), complex III (ubiquinol:ferrocytochrome c oxidoreductase, EC 1.10.2.2), complex IV (ferrocytochrome c:oxygen oxidoreductase or cytochrome c oxidase, EC 1.9.3.1), and complex V (ATP synthase, EC 3.6.1.34). A defect in mitochondrial oxidative phosphorylation, in terms of a reduction in the activity of NADH CoQ reductase (complex I) has been reported in the striatum of patients with Parkinson's disease. The reduction in the activity of complex I is found in the substantia nigra, but not in other areas of the brain, such as globus pallidus or cerebral cortex. Therefore, the specificity of mitochondrial impairment may play a role in the degeneration of nigrostriatal dopaminergic neurons. This view is supported by the fact that MPTP generating 1-methyl-4-phenylpyridine (MPP(+)) destroys dopaminergic neurons in the substantia nigra. Although the serum levels of CoQ10 is normal in patients with Parkinson's disease, CoQ10 is able to attenuate the MPTP-induced loss of striatal dopaminergic neurons. *Reference: Ubiquinone (coenzyme Q10) and mitochondria in oxidative stress of Parkinson's disease. Biol Signals Recept. 10(3-4):224-253, 2001. Ebadi, M., et al.*

There is increasing evidence that impairment of mitochondrial function and oxidative damage are contributing factors to the pathophysiology of Parkinson's disease (PD). Studies have reported decreased levels of the mitochondrial electron transport chain carrier, coenzyme Q (10) (CoQ (10)) in plasma and platelets from PD patients. Although a deficit in peripheral CoQ (10) has been reported no studies have assessed the CoQ (10) status of the PD brain. In this study the authors investigated the CoQ (10) status of the substantia nigra, cerebellum, cortex and striatum brain regions of both PD patients and age-matched controls. The results of this study indicate a significant reduction (p=0.007) in CoQ (10) concentration in the cortex region of the brain. In conclusion, the results of this study indicate evidence of a deficit in brain CoQ (10) status may be involved in the pathophysiology of PD. *Reference: The coenzyme Q10 status of the brain regions of Parkinson's disease patients. Neurosci Lett. 447(1):17-19, 2008. Hargreaves, I. P., et al. Department of Molecular Neuroscience, Institute of Neurology, Queen Square, London, UK.*

Coenzyme Q10 (CoQ10) and creatine are promising agents for neuroprotection in neurodegenerative diseases via their effects on improving mitochondrial function and cellular bioenergetics and their properties as antioxidants. We examined whether a combination of CoQ10 with creatine can exert additive neuroprotective effects in a MPTP mouse model of Parkinson's disease (PD), a 3-NP rat model of Huntington's disease (HD) and the R6/2 transgenic mouse model of HD. The combination of the two agents produced additive neuroprotective effects against dopamine depletion in the striatum and loss of tyrosine hydroxylase neurons in the substantia nigra pars compacta (SNpc) following chronic subcutaneous administration of MPTP. The combination treatment resulted in significant reduction in lipid peroxidation and pathologic α-synuclein accumulation in the SNpc neurons of the MPTP-treated mice. We also observed additive neuroprotective effects in reducing striatal lesion volumes produced by chronic subcutaneous administration of 3-NP to rats. The combination treatment showed significant effects on blocking 3-NP-induced impairment of glutathione homeostasis and reducing lipid peroxidation and DNA oxidative damage in the striatum. Lastly, the combination of CoQ10 and creatine produced additive neuroprotective effects on improving motor performance and extending survival in the transgenic R6/2 HD mice. These findings suggest that combination therapy using CoQ10 and creatine may be useful in the treatment of neurodegenerative diseases such as PD and HD. *Reference: J Neurochem. Author manuscript; available in PMC 2010 June 1. Published in final edited form as: J Neurochem. 2009 June; 109(5): 1427–1439. Published online 2009 March 28. doi: 10.1111/j.1471-4159.2009.06074.x. PMCID: PMC2866530. NIHMSID: NIHMS106242. Combination Therapy with Coenzyme Q10 and Creatine Produces Additive Neuroprotective Effects in Models of Parkinson's and Huntington's Diseases. Lichuan Yang, Noel Y. Calingasan, Elizabeth J. Wille, Kerry Cormier, Karen Smith, Robert J. Ferrante, and M. Flint Beal. Department of Neurology and Neuroscience, Weill Medical College of Cornell University, New York-Presbyterian Hospital, New York, NY 10021. Geriatric Research Education and Clinical Center, Bedford Veterans Administration Medical Center, Bedford, Massachusetts 01730. Departments of Neurology, Pathology, and Psychiatry, Boston University School of Medicine, Boston, Massachusetts 02118. Correspondence to: M. Flint Beal, M.D. Department of Neurology and Neuroscience Weill Medical College of Cornell University New York Presbyterian Hospital 525 East 68th Street, F610 New York, NY 10021 ; Email: fbeal@med.cornell.edu.*

Recent studies have demonstrated reduced activity of complex I of the electron transport chain in brain and platelets from Parkinson's disease patients. Platelet mitochondria from parkinsonian patients were found to have lower levels of coenzyme Q10 than mitochondria from age/sex-matched controls. There was a strong correlation between the levels of coenzyme Q10 and the activities of complexes I and II/III. Oral coenzyme Q10 was found to protect the nigrostriatal dopaminergic system in one-year-old mice treated with MPTP, a toxin injurious to the nigrostriatal dopaminergic system. It was also found that oral coenzyme Q10 was well absorbed in parkinsonian patients and caused a trend toward increased complex I activity. These data suggest that coenzyme Q10 may play a role in cellular dysfunction found in Parkinson's disease and may be a potential protective agent for parkinsonian patients. **Reference:** *A possible role of coenzyme Q10 in the etiology and treatment of Parkinson's disease. Biofactors. 9(2-4):267-272, 1999. Shults, C. W., et al.*

Parkinson disease (PD) is a degenerative neurological disorder for which no treatment has been shown to slow the progression. The objective of this study was to determine whether a range of dosages of coenzyme Q(10) is safe and well tolerated and could slow the functional decline in PD. This was a multicenter, randomized, parallel-group, placebo-controlled, double-blind, dosage-ranging trial involving 80 subjects with early PD who did not require treatment for their disability. The patients were randomly assigned to placebo or coenzyme Q(10) at dosages of 300, 600, or 1200 mg/d. The subjects underwent evaluation with the Unified Parkinson Disease Rating Scale (UPDRS) at the screening, baseline, and 1-, 4-, 8-, 12-, and 16-month visits. They were followed up for 16 months or until disability requiring treatment with levodopa had developed. The primary response variable was the change in the total score on the UPDRS from baseline to the last visit. The adjusted mean total UPDRS changes were +11.99 for the placebo group, +8.81 for the 300-mg/d group, +10.82 for the 600-mg/d group, and +6.69 for the 1200-mg/d group. The P value for the primary analysis, a test for a linear trend between the dosage and the mean change in the total UPDRS score, was.09, which met our prespecified criteria for a positive trend for the trial. A prespecified, secondary analysis was the comparison of each treatment group with the placebo group, and the difference between the 1200-mg/d and placebo groups was significant (P =.04). Coenzyme Q(10) was safe and well tolerated at dosages of up to 1200 mg/d. Less disability developed in subjects assigned to coenzyme Q(10) than in those assigned to placebo, and the benefit was greatest in subjects receiving the highest dosage. Coenzyme Q(10) appears to slow the progressive deterioration of function in PD, but these results need to be confirmed in a larger study. *Reference: Effects of coenzyme Q10 in early Parkinson disease: evidence of slowing of the functional decline. Archives of Neurology. 59(10):1541-15550, 2002. Schults, C. W., et al. Department of Neurosciences, Mail Code 0662, University of California-San Diego, 9500 Gilman Dr, La Jolla, CA, USA.*

Mitochondrial dysfunction has been well established to occur in Parkinson's disease (PD) and appears to play a role in the pathogenesis of the disorder. A key component of the mitochondrial electron transport chain (ETC) is coenzyme Q10, which not only serves as the electron acceptor for complexes I and II of the ETC but is also an antioxidant. In addition to being crucial to the bioenergetics of the cell, mitochondria play a central role in apoptotic cell death through a number of mechanisms, and coenzyme Q10 can affect certain of these processes. Levels of coenzyme Q10 have been reported to be decreased in blood and platelet mitochondria from PD patients. A number of preclinical studies in in vitro and in vivo models of PD have demonstrated that coenzyme Q10 can protect the nigrostriatal dopaminergic system. A phase II trial of coenzyme Q10 in patients with early, untreated PD demonstrated a positive trend for coenzyme Q10 to slow progressive disability that occurs in PD. *Reference: Therapeutic role of coenzyme Q(10) in Parkinson's disease. Pharmacol Ther. 107(1):120-130, 2005. Shults, C. W. Department of Neurosciences, University of California San Diego, La Jolla, CA, USA.* 1-Methyl-4-phenyl-1,2,5,6-tetrahydropyridine (MPTP) produces Parkinsonism in both experimental animals and in man. MPTP is metabolized to 1-methyl-4-phenylpridinium, an inhibitor of mitochondrial complex I. MPTP administration produces ATP depletions in vivo, which may lead to secondary excitotoxicity and free radical generation. If this is the case then agents which improve mitochondrial function or free radical scavengers should attenuate MPTP neurotoxicity. In the present experiments three regimens of MPTP administration produced varying degrees of striatal dopamine depletion. A combination of coenzyme Q10 and nicotinamide protected against both mild and moderate depletion of dopamine. In the MPTP regimen which produced mild dopamine depletion nicotinamide or the free radical spin trap N-tert-butyl-alpha-(2-sulfophenyl)-nitrone were also effective. There was no protection with a MPTP regimen which produced severe dopamine depletion. These results show that agents which improve mitochondrial energy production (coenzyme Q10 and nicotinamide) and free radical scavengers can attenuate mild to moderate MPTP neurotoxicity. *Reference: Coenzyme Q10 and nicotinamide and a free radical spin trap protect against MPTP neurotoxicity. Exp Neurol. 132(2):279-283, 1995. Schulz, J. B.,et al. Neurochemistry Laboratory, Massachusetts Gen. Hospital, Boston, USA.*

Coenzyme Q10 (CoQ10) and creatine are promising agents for neuroprotection in neurodegenerative diseases via their effects on improving mitochondrial function and cellular bioenergetics and their properties as antioxidants. The authors examined whether a combination of CoQ10 with creatine can exert additive neuroprotective effects in a MPTP mouse model of Parkinson's disease, a 3-NP rat model of Huntington's disease (HD) and the R6/2 transgenic mouse model of HD. The combination of the two agents produced additive neuroprotective effects against dopamine depletion in the striatum and loss of tyrosine hydroxylase neurons in the substantia nigra pars compacta (SNpc) following chronic subcutaneous administration of MPTP. The combination treatment resulted in significant reduction in lipid peroxidation and pathologic alpha-synuclein accumulation in the SNpc neurons of the MPTP-treated mice. The authors also observed additive neuroprotective effects in reducing striatal lesion volumes produced by chronic subcutaneous administration of 3-NP to rats. The combination treatment showed significant effects on blocking 3-NP-induced impairment of glutathione homeostasis and reducing lipid peroxidation and DNA oxidative damage in the striatum. Lastly, the combination of CoQ10 and creatine produced additive neuroprotective effects on improving motor performance and extending survival in the transgenic R6/2 HD mice. These findings suggest that combination therapy using CoQ10 and creatine may be useful in the treatment of neurodegenerative diseases such as Parkinson's disease and HD. *Reference: Combination therapy with coenzyme Q10 and creatine produces additive neuroprotective effects in models of Parkinson's and Huntington's diseases. J Neurochem. 109(5):1427-1439, 2009. Yang, L., et al. Department of Neurology and Neuroscience, Weill Medical College of Cornell University, New York-Presbyterian Hospital, New York, New York, USA.*

N-Acetylccysteine (NAC)

Levels of glutathione are lower in the substantia nigra (SN) early in Parkinson's disease (PD) and this may contribute to mitochondrial dysfunction and oxidative stress. Oxidative stress may increase the accumulation of toxic forms of α-synuclein (SNCA). We hypothesized that supplementation with n-acetylcysteine (NAC), a source of cysteine – the limiting amino acid in glutathione synthesis, would protect against α-synuclein toxicity. Transgenic mice overexpressing wild-type human α-synuclein drank water supplemented with NAC or control water supplemented with alanine from ages 6 weeks to 1 year. NAC increased SN levels of glutathione within 5–7 weeks of treatment; however, this increase was not sustained at 1 year. Despite the transient nature of the impact of NAC on brain glutathione, the loss of dopaminergic terminals at 1 year associated with SNCA overexpression was significantly attenuated by NAC supplementation, as measured by immunoreactivity for tyrosine hydroxylase in the striatum ($p = 0.007$; unpaired, two-tailed t-test), with a similar but nonsignificant trend for dopamine transporter (DAT) immunoreactivity. NAC significantly decreased the levels of human SNCA in the brains of PDGFb-SNCA transgenic mice compared to alanine treated transgenics. This was associated with a decrease in nuclear NFκB localization and an increase in cytoplasmic localization of NFκB in the

NAC-treated transgenics. Overall, these results indicate that oral NAC supplementation decreases SNCA levels in brain and partially protects against loss of dopaminergic terminals associated with overexpression of α-synuclein in this model. *Reference: PLoS One. 2010; 5(8): e12333. Published online 2010 August 23. doi: 10.1371/journal.pone.0012333. PMCID: PMC2925900. Oral N-Acetyl-Cysteine Attenuates Loss of Dopaminergic Terminals in α-Synuclein Overexpressing Mice. Joanne Clark, Elizabeth L. Clore, Kangni Zheng, Anthony Adame, Eliezer Masliah, and David K. Simon. Department of Neurology, Beth Israel Deaconess Medical Center, Boston, Massachusetts, United States of America. Harvard Medical School, Boston, Massachusetts, United States of America. Department of Neuroscience, School of Medicine, University of Southern California, San Diego, California, United States of America.*

Oxidative stress plays an important role in neurodegenerative disorders such as Parkinson's Disease and Alzheimer's Disease. Methamphetamine (METH) is an amphetamine analog that causes degeneration of the dopaminergic system in mammals and subsequent oxidative stress. In our present study, we have used immortalized human brain microvascular endothelial (HBMVEC) cells to test whether N-Acetylcysteineamide (NACA), a novel antioxidant, prevents METH-induced oxidative stress in vitro. Our studies showed that NACA protects against METH-induced oxidative stress in HBMVEC cells. NACA significantly protected the integrity of our blood brain barrier (BBB) model, as shown by permeability and trans-endothelial electrical resistance (TEER) studies. NACA also significantly increased the levels of intracellular glutathione (GSH) and glutathione peroxidase (GPx). Malondialdehyde (MDA) levels increased dramatically after METH exposure, but this increase was almost completely prevented when the cells were treated with NACA. Generation of reactive oxygen species (ROS) also increased after METH exposure, but was reduced to control levels with NACA treatment, as measured by dichlorofluorescin (DCF). These results suggest that NACA protects the BBB integrity in vitro, which could prevent oxidative stress-induced damage; therefore, the effectiveness of this antioxidant should be evaluated for the treatment of neurodegenerative diseases in the future. *Reference: Published in final edited form as: Brain Res. 2009 June 12; 1275: 87–95. Published online 2009 April 15. doi: 10.1016/ j.brainres.2009.04.008. PMCID: PMC2702674. NIHMSID: NIHMS110860. N-Acetylcysteine Amide Protects Against Methamphetamine-Induced Oxidative Stress and Neurotoxicity in Immortalized Human Brain Endothelial Cells. Xinsheng Zhang, Atrayee Banerjee, William A. Banks, and Nuran Ercal. Department of Chemistry, Missouri University of Science & Technology, Rolla MO 65409. Departments of Internal Medicine, Geriatric Division and Pharmacological and Physiological Science, Saint Louis University, Saint Louis, MO 63106.*

Based on the finding of decreased mitochondrial complex I activity in the substantia nigra of patients with Parkinson's disease, the authors propose that the consequent reduction of ATP synthesis and increased generation of reactive oxygen species may be a possible cause of nigrostriatal cell death. Since sulfhydryl groups are essential in oxidative phosphorylation, thiolic antioxidants may contribute to the preservation of these proteins against oxidative damage. The authors hypothesize that treatment with a sulfur-containing antioxidant such as N-acetylcysteine may provide a new neuroprotective therapeutic strategy for Parkinson's disease. *Reference: Hypothesis: can N-acetylcysteine be beneficial in Parkinson's disease? Life Sciences. 64(15):1253-1257, 1999. Martinez, M., et al.*

The results of several in vitro studies have shown that cysteine prodrugs, particularly N-acetylcysteine, are effective antioxidants that increase the survival of dopaminergic neurons. N-acetylcysteine can be systemically administered to deliver cysteine to the brain and is of potential use for providing neuroprotection in the treatment of Parkinson's disease. However, it has also been reported that an excess of cysteine may induce neurotoxicity. In the present study, the authors injected adult rats intrastriatally with 2.5 microl of 6-hydroxydopamine (7.5 microg) and N-acetylcysteine (240 mM) or cysteine (240 mM) or intraventricularly with 6-hydroxydopamine (200 microg) and subcutaneously with N-acetylcysteine (10 and 100 mg/kg). They studied the effects of these compounds on both the nigrostriatal dopaminergic terminals and the surrounding striatal tissue. The tissue was stained with fluoro-jade (a marker of neuronal degeneration) and processed by immunohistochemistry to detect tyrosine hydroxylase, neuronal and glial markers, and the stress protein heme-oxygenase-1. After intrastriatal injection, both cysteine and N-acetylcysteine had clear neuroprotective effects on the striatal dopaminergic terminals, but also led to neuronal degeneration (as revealed by fluoro-jade staining) and astroglial and microglial activation, as well as intense induction of heme-oxygenase-1 in astrocytes and microglial cells. Subcutaneous administration of N-acetylcysteine also induced significant reduction of the dopaminergic lesion (about 30% reduction). However, the authors did not observe appreciable N-acetylcysteine-induced fluoro-jade labeling in striatal neurons or any of the above-mentioned changes in striatal glial cells. The results suggest that low doses of cysteine prodrugs may be useful neuroprotectors in the treatment of Parkinson's disease. *Reference: Systemic administration of N-acetylcysteine protects dopaminergic neurons against 6-hydroxydopamine-induced degeneration. J Neurosci Res. 76(4):551-562, 2004. Munoz, A. M., et al.*

Oxidative stress to dopaminergic neurons is believed to be one of the causes of neurodegeneration in Parkinson's disease (PD). It was investigated whether N-acetylcysteine (NAC) and l-2-oxothiazolidine-4-carboxylate (OTC) have a preventive effect in an oxidative stress-induced model of PD. The authors found that NAC and OTC prevent degradation of PARP during auto-oxidized dopamine- or auto-oxidized L-DOPA-induced apoptosis in PC12 cells. In an animal model study, NAC and OTC showed a preventive effect against MPTP-induced loss of tyrosine hydroxylase-positive neurons, and suppressed the nuclear translocation of c-jun N-terminal kinase (JNK), suggesting that NAC and OTC can prevent MPTP-induced apoptosis by suppressing JNK activation. These results suggest that NAC and OTC can be used as potential agents to prevent the progression of PD. **Reference:** *Preventive effect of antioxidants in MPTP-induced mouse model of Parkinson's disease. Neurosci Lett. 363(3):243-246, 2004. Park, S. W., et al. Department of Biochemistry, College of Medicine, Pusan National University, Busan, South Korea.*

Astaxanthin

Astaxanthin (AST) is a powerful antioxidant that occurs naturally in a wide variety of living organisms. We have investigated the role of AST in preventing 1-methyl-4-phenyl-1,2,3,6-tetrahydropyridine (MPTP)-induced apoptosis of the substantia nigra (SN) neurons in the mouse model of Parkinson's disease (PD) and 1-methyl-4-phenylpyridinium (MPP+)-induced cytotoxicity of SH-SY5Y human neuroblastoma cells. In in vitro study, AST inhibits MPP+-induced production of intracellular reactive oxygen species (ROS) and cytotoxicity in SH-SY5Y human neuroblastoma cells. Preincubation of AST (50 µM) significantly attenuates MPP+-induced oxidative damage. Furthermore, AST is able to enhance the expression of Bcl-2 protein but reduce the expression of α-synuclein and Bax, and suppress the cleavage of caspase-3. Our results suggest that the protective effects of AST on MPP+-induced apoptosis may be due to its anti-oxidative properties and anti-apoptotic activity via induction of expression of superoxide dismutase (SOD) and catalase and regulating the expression of Bcl-2 and Bax. Pretreatment with AST (30mg /kg) markedly increases tyrosine hydroxylase (TH)-positive neurons and decreases the argyrophilic neurons compared with the MPTP model group. In summary, AST shows protection from MPP+/MPTP-induced apoptosis in the SH-SY5Y cells and PD model mouse SN neurons, and this effect may be attributable to upregulation of the expression of Bcl-2 protein, downregulation of the expression of Bax and α-synuclein, and inhibition of the activation of caspase-3. These data indicate that AST may provide a valuable therapeutic strategy for the treatment of progressive neurodegenerative disease such as Parkinson's disease. **Reference:** *Food Chem Toxicol. Author manuscript; available in PMC 2012 January 1. Published in final edited form as: Food Chem Toxicol. 2011 January; 49(1): 271–280. Published online 2010 November 5. doi: 10.1016/ j.fct.2010.10.029. PMCID: PMC3010303. NIHMSID: NIHMS254275. Astaxanthin protects against MPTP/MPP+-induced mitochondrial dysfunction and ROS production in vivo and in vitro. Dae-Hee Lee and Yong J. Lee. Department of Surgery, School of Medicine, University of Pittsburgh, Pittsburgh, Pennsylvania 15213. Department of Pharmacology & Chemical Biology, School of Medicine, University of Pittsburgh, Pittsburgh, Pennsylvania 15213. All correspondence should be addressed to Dr. Yong J. Lee, Department of Surgery, University of Pittsburgh, Hillman Cancer Center, 5117 Centre, Ave. Room 1.46C, Pittsburgh, PA 15213, U.S.A., Tel (412) 623-3268, Fax (412) 623-7709, Email: leeyj@upmc.edu.*

Inflammation is a hot topic in medical research, because it plays a key role in inflammatory diseases: rheumatoid arthritis (RA) and other forms of arthritis, diabetes, heart diseases, irritable bowel syndrome, Alzheimer's disease, Parkinson's disease, allergies, asthma, even cancer and many others. Over the past few decades, it was realized that the process of inflammation is virtually the same in different disorders, and a better understanding of inflammation may lead to better treatments for numerous diseases. Inflammation is the activation of the immune system in response to infection, irritation, or injury, with an influx of white blood cells, redness, heat, swelling, pain, and dysfunction of the organs involved. Although the pathophysiological basis of these conditions is not yet fully understood, reactive oxygen species (ROS) have often been implicated in their pathogenesis. In fact, in inflammatory diseases the antioxidant defense system is compromised, as evidenced by increased markers of oxidative stress, and decreased levels of protective antioxidant enzymes in patients with rheumatoid arthritis (RA). An enriched diet containing antioxidants, such as vitamin E, vitamin C, β-carotene and phenolic substances, has been suggested to improve symptoms by reducing disease-related oxidative stress. In this respect, the marine world represents a largely untapped reserve of bioactive ingredients, and considerable potential exists for exploitation of these bioactives as functional food ingredients. Substances such as n-3 oils, carotenoids, vitamins, minerals and peptides provide a myriad of health benefits, including reduction of cardiovascular diseases, anticarcinogenic and anti-inflammatory activities. New marine bioactives are recently gaining attention, since they could be helpful in combating chronic inflammatory degenerative conditions. The aim of this review is to examine the published studies concerning the potential pharmacological properties and application of many marine bioactives against inflammatory diseases. **Reference:** *Mar Drugs. 2012 April; 10(4): 812–833. Published online 2012 April 5. doi: 10.3390/md10040812. PMCID: PMC3366677. Marine Bioactives: Pharmacological Properties and Potential Applications against Inflammatory Diseases. Nicolantonio D'Orazio, Maria Alessandra Gammone, Eugenio Gemello, Massimo De Girolamo, Salvatore Cusenza, and Graziano Riccioni. Human Nutrition, Department of Biomedical Science, via Dei Vestini, University G. D'Annunzio, Chieti, 66013, Italy. Cardiology Unit, San Camillo De Lellis Hospital, Manfredonia, FG, Italy. Author to whom correspondence should be addressed; Email: ndorazio@unich.it .*

Parkinson's disease (PD) is a neurodegenerative disorder characterized by selective loss of dopaminergic neurons in the substantia nigra pars compacta. Although understanding of the pathogenesis of PD remains incomplete, increasing evidence from human and animal studies has suggested that oxidative stress is an important mediator in its pathogenesis. Astaxanthin (Asx), a potent antioxidant, has been thought to provide health benefits by decreasing the risk of oxidative stress-related diseases. This study examined the protective effects of Asx on 6-hydroxydopamine (6-OHDA)-induced apoptosis in the human neuroblastoma cell line SH-SY5Y. Pre-treatment of SH-SY5Y cells with Asx suppressed 6-OHDA-induced apoptosis in a dose-dependent manner. In addition, Asx strikingly inhibited 6-OHDA-induced mitochondrial dysfunctions, including lowered membrane potential and the cleavage of caspase 9, caspase 3, and poly(ADP-ribose) polymerase. In western blot analysis, 6-OHDA activated p38 MAPK, c-jun NH(2)-terminal kinase 1/2, and extracellular signal-regulated kinase 1/2, while Asx blocked the phosphorylation of p38 MAPK but not c-jun NH(2)-terminal kinase 1/2 and extracellular signal-regulated kinase 1/2. Pharmacological approaches showed that the activation of p38 MAPK has a critical role in 6-OHDA-induced mitochondrial dysfunctions and apoptosis. Furthermore, Asx markedly abolished 6-OHDA-induced reactive oxygen species generation, which resulted in the blockade of p38 MAPK activation and apoptosis induced by 6-OHDA treatment. Taken together, the present results indicated that the protective effects of Asx on apoptosis in SH-SY5Y cells may be, at least in part, attributable to the its potent antioxidative ability. *Reference: Protective effects of astaxanthin on 6-hydroxydopamine-induced apoptosis in human neuroblastoma SH-SY5Y cells. Journal of Neurochemistry. 107(6):1730-1740, 2008. Ikeda, Y., et al. Research Team for Molecular Biomarkers, Tokyo Metropolitan Institute of Gerontology, Tokyo, Japan.*

NADH (Nicotinamide Adenine Dinucleotide Hydrogen)

NADH was used in an open label trial as novel medication in 34 patients with Parkinson's disease, using an intravenous administration technique. In all patients a beneficial clinical effect was observed. 21 patients (61.7%) showed a very good (better than 30%) improvement of disability, 13 patients (38.3%) a moderate (up to 30%) improvement. Concomitant with the improvement of the disability the urine level of homovanillic acid (HVA) increased significantly in all patients (in some patients by more than a 100%). The daily "on phases" of the patients could be increased from 2 up to 9 hours in the individual patients by NADH administration. *Reference: The coenzyme nicotinamide adenine dinucleotide (NADH) improves the disability of parkinsonian patients. J Neural Transm Park Dis Dement Sect. 1(4):297-302, 1989. Birkmayer, W., et al.*

NADH was used as medication in 885 parkinsonian patients in an open label trial. Approximately 50% of the patients received NADH by intravenous infusion, the other part orally by capsules (5 mg per day). In approximately 80% of the patients a beneficial clinical effect was observed: 19.3% of the patients showed a very good (30% - 50%) improvement of disability, 58.8% a moderate (10% - 30%) improvement. 21.8% did not respond to NADH. Statistical analysis of the improvement in correlation with the disability prior to treatment, the duration of the disease and the age of the patients revealed the following results: All these 3 parameters have a significant although weak influence on the improvement. The disability before the treatment has a positive regression coefficient. The duration of the disease has a negative regression coefficient and so has the age a negative regression coefficient. In other words younger patients and patients with a shorter duration of disease have a better chance to gain a marked improvement than older patients and patients with longer duration of the disease. The orally applied form of NADH yielded an overall improvement in the disability which was comparable to that of the parenterally applied form. *Reference: Nicotinamide adenine dinucleotide (NADH) - a new therapeutic approach to Parkinson's disease. Comparison of oral and parenteral application. Acta Neurol Scand Suppl. 146:32-35, 1993. Birkmayer, J. G., et al.*

Forty Parkinson's disease patients were treated with 25 mg of NADH IV per day. 20% of these patients were able to discontinue levodopa therapy and use NADH alone. Treatment of Parkinson's disease with L-dopa (LD) in combination with decarboxylase and monoamine oxidase inhibitors is a pure substitutional therapy designed to correct the lack of dopamine in the brain. The dopamine deficit is caused by the diminished tyrosine hydroxylase (TH) in the substantia nigra. However, catecholamines such as dopamine and its precursor LD inhibit TH via a feedback mechanism. This suggests that application of LD to PD patients may further decrease the already reduced TH activity. Therefore, therapeutic strategies other than substitution have to be considered, e.g., stimulation of endogenous dopamine production in the brain. This may be achieved by activating the LD producing enzyme. This enzyme is an iron-containing protein with tetrahydrobiopterin (H4biopterin) as coenzyme. H4biopterin is reduced in the brain of PD patients and has therefore been used in clinical trials, but with only partial success. On the other hand, it has been shown that the special iron compound oxyferriscorbone(R) is able to improve the symptoms of parkinsonian patients suggesting production of endogenous LD in the brain of parkinsonians. The stimulation of LD biosynthesis is reflected by an increase in the urine level of homovanillic acid (HVA). The authors believe that this occurs by TH activation by the iron compound oxyferriscorbone, because there is no other enzyme except TH which catalyzes LD formation, and it also has been shown that this enzyme can be markedly activated in vitro by iron. Our findings have already been confirmed. After long-term iron medication, however, its effectiveness subsides in some patients. The author chose nicotinamidade-nindinucleotide (NADH), which promotes the formation of H4biopterin, the active coenzyme of tyrosine hydroxylase. Diagnosis and disability scores of the parkinsonian patients were established according to the method of Birkmayer and Neumayr.12 Nicotinamideadenine-dinucleotide, reduced form disodium salt (synonyms: beta-NADH, reduced DPN, beta-DPNH), was purchased from Sigma Diagnostics (St. Louis, Missouri). 25 mg of NADH was dissolved in 100 ml of 0.9% sterile sodium chloride, pH 7.4, and infused intravenously in 30 min. NADH solutions were always prepared fresh immediately prior to use. Disability scores were determined before, 1 hr after, and 4 hrs. after the NADH infusion. Forty patients have been treated so far. All of them exhibited a pronounced drop of their disability score. The patients' ages ranged from 48 to 85, duration of the disease ranged from 2 to 20 years. The overall improvement of the disability of all patients was 46.25%. A very good response was exhibited in 65% of the patients: more than 30% improvement of disability, 35% of the patients a moderate benefit of up to 30%. Walking and pushing ability improved considerably as did posture, speech, and mimics. The action of NADH lasted between 1 and 4 days, depending on the severity of the symptoms. Withdrawal of NADH led to a relapse with worsening of disability. Approximately 20% of the patients did well on NADH alone, and LD-therapy could be omitted. In the other patients the LD dosage could be reduced materially. Fifteen patients have been examined with regard to the duration of the daily pattern of phases. The daily "on" phases could be increased by 6 to 10 hr. In a number of patients so examined, the urine level of the dopamine metabolite HVA was markedly increased. Such HVA increase is also observed after treatment with LD. As NADH is not a precursor of LD, it seems most likely that it stimulates endogenous LD biosynthesis. The beneficial clinical effect of NADH on the disability of parkinsonian patients has been demonstrated. A possible mechanism by which this may occur is shown in the simplified pathway of LD biosynthesis. L-Dopa is formed from tyrosine by the enzyme TH. This is an iron-containing enzyme with H4Biopterin as coenzyme. H4Biopterin provides electrons to reduce molecular oxygen and is in turn oxidized to the quinonoid-H2-pterin. The dihydropteridine reductase (DHPR) regenerates H4biopterin. The cofactor of this enzyme is NADH.13 H4Biopterin in brain and in cerebrospinal fluid of PD patients is reduced. This H4biopterin deficiency could be due either to a decreased biosynthesis or to a lack in the biologically active form of H4biopterin. It could well be that H4biopterin is exhausted in parkinsonian patients because of an enormous consumption, perhaps caused by a toxic agent. The idea is derived from the observation that MPTP (1-methyl-4-phenyl-1,2,3,6-tetrahydropyridine), a neurotoxin that can induce parkinsonism in men and animals, inhibits DHPR, the enzyme which regenerates tetrahydrobiopterin, the coenzyme required for endogenous dopamine formation.14 MPTP seems to be a competitive inhibitor of DHPR with respect to NADH. If this is so, NADH should be able to neutralize the toxic effect of MPTP or other free radical-inducing agents. There are two arguments in favor of the hypothesis. First, the clinical effect of NADH closely resembles that of LD, indicating that this coenzyme stimulates the endogenous LD biosynthesis. Second, the improvement in the clinical symptoms parallels an increase in the urine level of HVA, which also has been found with the standard LD therapy. *Reference: The clinical benefit of NADH as stimulator of endogenous l-dopa biosynthesis in Parkinson's disease patients. Advances in Neurology Volume 53: Parkinson's Disease: Anatomy, Pathology, and Therapy, M.B. Streifler, A.D. Korczyn, E. Melamed, and M.B.H. Youdim (editors), Raven Press, New York. 1990. Birkmayer, W., et al.*

Parkinson's disease patients have up to 50% less NADH activity compared with healthy persons of the same age. The underlying mechanism for NADH's effects on Parkinson's disease is as follows: 1) NADH increases tetrahydrobiopterin levels. 2.) Tetrahydrobiopterin is a cofactor for Tyrosine Hydroxylase. 3) Tyrsosine Hydroxylase catalyzes the conversion of tyrosine to L-dopa. 4) L-dopa is the precursor to dopamine. 5) Dopamine is the neurotransmitter depleted during Parkinson's disease. *Reference: Nicotinamide-adenine dinucleotide (NADH) in Parkinson's disease and Alzheimer's disease. International Journal of Pharmaceutical Compounding. 4(4):276-279, 2000. Glasnapp, A., et al.*

Exogenous application of levodopa is conventionally used to equalize the striatal dopamine deficit in idiopathic Parkinson's disease (PD). The stimulation of endogenous biosynthesis of levodopa via activation of tyrosine hydroxylase (TH) has been proposed as new therapeutic concept in PD. This may be achieved by exogenous supply with the reduced coenzyme nicotinamide adenine dinucleotide (NADH). Aim of this open prospective study was to investigate (1) the efficacy of a new developed, parenteral application form of NADH on Parkinsonian symptoms and (2) the influence of bioavailability of levodopa. 15 patients, suffering from idiopathic PD (11 male, 4 female, age: 61.40[mean] +/- 10.27[SD] range: 44-74 years, Hoehn and Yahr stage: 3.03 +/- 0.69, range 2-4) received intravenous infusions of NADH (10 mg a' 30 min) over a period of 7 days in addition to conventional Parkinsonian pharmacotherapy. Parkinsonian symptoms were scored before (day 1) and after NADH treatment (day 8). Levodopa plasma levels were estimated over a period of four hours on the day before and on the first day of NADH application by HPLC. Parkinsonian patients showed a significant response, evaluated by the Unified Parkinson's Disease Rating Scale Version 3.0 ($p = 0.025$; Wilcoxon test). Moreover application of NADH significantly increased bioavailability of plasma levodopa (AUC, $p = 0.035$; Cmax $p = 0.025$). NADH in used galenic form may be a potent stimulator of endogenous levodopa biosynthesis with clinical benefit for Parkinsonian patients. **Reference:** *Parenteral application of NADH in Parkinson's disease: clinical improvement partially due to stimulation of endogenous levodopa biosynthesis. J Neural Transm. 103(10):1187-1193, 1996. Kuhn, W., et al.*

Melatonin

Molecular oxygen is toxic for anaerobic organisms but it is also obvious that oxygen is poisonous to aerobic organisms as well, since oxygen plays an essential role for inducing molecular damage. Molecular oxygen is a triplet radical in its ground-stage (.O-O.) and has two unpaired electrons that can undergoes consecutive reductions of one electron and generates other more reactive forms of oxygen known as free radicals and reactive oxygen species. These reactants (including superoxide radicals, hydroxyl radicals) possess variable degrees of toxicity. Nitric oxide (NO•) contains one unpaired electron and is, therefore, a radical. NO• is generated in biological tissues by specific nitric oxide synthases and acts as an important biological signal. Excessive nitric oxide production, under pathological conditions, leads to detrimental effects of this molecule on tissues, which can be attributed to its diffusion-limited reaction with superoxide to form the powerful and toxic oxidant, peroxynitrite. Reactive oxygen and nitrogen species are molecular "renegades"; these highly unstable products tend to react rapidly with adjacent molecules, donating, abstracting, or even sharing their outer orbital electron(s). This reaction not only changes the target molecule, but often passes the unpaired electron along to the target, generating a second free radical, which can then go on to react with a new target amplifying their effects. This review describes the mechanisms of oxidative damage and its relationship with the most highly studied neurodegenerative diseases and the roles of melatonin as free radical scavenger and neurocytoskeletal protector. *Reference:* Curr Neuropharmacol. 2008 September; 6(3): 203–214. doi: 10.2174/ 157015908785777201. PMCID: PMC2687933. Cellular and Biochemical Actions of Melatonin which Protect Against Free Radicals: Role in Neurodegenerative Disorders. Genaro G Ortiz, Gloria A Benítez-King, Sergio A Rosales-Corral, Fermín P Pacheco-Moisés, and Irma E Velázquez-Brizuela. Laboratorio de Desarrollo-Envejecimiento, Enfermedades Neurodegenerativas, División de Neurociencias, Centro de Investigación Biomédica de Occidente (CIBO), Instituto Mexicano del Seguro Social, IMSS, Sierra Mojada 800 C.P. 44340 Guadalajara, Jalisco, México. Laboratorio de Neurofarmacología, Instituto Nacional de Psiquiatría, SSA. México, D.F. Departamento de Química, Centro Universitario de Ciencias Exactas e Ingenierías (CUCEI), Universidad de Guadalajara, Guadalajara, Jalisco. México. Address correspondence to this author at Laboratorio de Desarrollo-Envejecimiento, Enfermedades Neurodegenerativas, División de Neurociencias, CIBO-IMSS, Sierra Mojada 800 CP 44340. Guadalajara, Jalisco, México; Tel: (0133) 36-17-00-60 ext. 31951; Fax: (0133) 36175099; E-mail: genarogabriel @yahoo.com.

Oxidative stress plays a key role in the pathogenesis of aging and many metabolic diseases; therefore, an effective antioxidant therapy would be of great importance in these circumstances. Nutritional, environmental, and chemical factors can induce the overproduction of the superoxide anion radical in both the cytosol and mitochondria. This is the first and key event that leads to the activation of pathways involved in the development of several metabolic diseases that are related to oxidative stress. As oxidation of essential molecules continues, it turns to nitrooxidative stress because of the involvement of nitric oxide in pathogenic processes. Once peroxynitrite forms, it damages via two distinctive mechanisms. First, it has direct toxic effects leading to lipid peroxidation, protein oxidation, and DNA damage. This mechanism involves the induction of several transcription factors leading to cytokine-induced chronic inflammation. Classic antioxidants, including vitamins A, C, and E, have often failed to exhibit beneficial effects in metabolic diseases and aging. Melatonin is a multifunctional indolamine that counteracts virtually all pathophysiologic steps and displays significant beneficial actions against peroxynitrite-induced cellular toxicity. This protection is related to melatonin's antioxidative and anti-inflammatory properties. Melatonin has the capability of scavenging both oxygen- and nitrogen-based reactants, including those formed from peroxynitrite, and blocking transcriptional factors, which induce proinflammatory cytokines. Accumulating evidence suggests that this nontoxic indolamine may be useful either as a sole treatment or in conjunction with other treatments for inhibiting the biohazardous actions of nitrooxidative stress. *Reference:* Mol Med. 2009 Jan-Feb; 15(1-2): 43–50. Published online 2008 November 4. doi: 10.2119/molmed.2008.00117. PMCID: PMC2582546. Melatonin: An Established Antioxidant Worthy of Use in Clinical Trials. Ahmet Korkmaz, Russel J Reiter, Turgut Topal, Lucien C Manchester, Sukru Oter, and Dun-Xian Tan. Department of Physiology, School of Medicine, Gulhane Military Medical Academy, Ankara, Turkey. Department of Cellular and Structural Biology, The

University of Texas Health Science Center at San Antonio, San Antonio, Texas, United States of America. Address correspondence and reprint requests to Sukru Oter, Gulhane Askeri Tip Akademisi, Fizyoloji Anabilim Dali, 06018 Ankara, Turkey. Phone: +90-312-3043602; GSM: +90-532-6529178; Fax: +90-312-3043616; E-mail: fizyoter@gmail.com ; Email: oters@gata.edu.tr.

Deprenyl (aka Selegiline)

In an open, uncontrolled study the longterm (9 years) effect of treatment with Madopar alone (n = 377) or in combination with l-deprenyl (selegiline, selective monoamine oxidase type B inhibitor) (n = 564) have been compared in Parkinsonian patients. In patients who lost their response to conventional Madopar therapy the addition of l-deprenyl resulted in a significant recouping of levodopa effect. The survival analysis revealed a significant increase of life expectancy in Madopar--l-deprenyl group regardless of the fact whether or not the significant demographic differences between the two groups were taken into account. Although the mechanism underlying this action of l-deprenyl is not known, the results are interpreted as indicating l-deprenyl's ability to prevent or retard the degeneration of striatal dopaminergic neurons. l-Deprenyl is the first anti-Parkinson drug having such a property. This hypothesis is not far fetched since l-deprenyl selectively prevents the degeneration of striatal dopaminergic neurons induced in animals by the illicit drug 1-methyl-4-phenyl-1,2,3,6-tetrahydropyridine (MPTP). Since latter compound is known to cause Parkinsonism in man and primates or Parkinson-like neurochemical and pathological changes in other animals the implications of the present study involving monoamine oxidase activity and l-deprenyl are apparent. **Reference:** *Increased life expectancy resulting from addition of L-deprenyl to madopar treatment in Parkinson's disease: A long-term study. J Neural Transm. 64(2):119-127, 1985. Birkmayer, W., et al.*

The authors have performed a 14-month, prospective, randomized, double-blind, placebo-controlled study to evaluate the effect of deprenyl and levodopa/carbidopa (Sinemet) on the progression of signs and symptoms in patients with mild Parkinson's disease (PD). 101 untreated PD patients were randomly assigned to one of the following four treatment groups: Group I, deprenyl + Sinemet; Group II, placebo-deprenyl + Sinemet; Group III, deprenyl + bromocriptine; and Group IV, placebo-deprenyl + bromocriptine. The final visit was performed at 14 months, i.e., 2 months after withdrawal of deprenyl or its placebo and 7 days after withdrawal of Sinemet or bromocriptine. Deterioration in Unified Parkinson's Disease Rating Score (UPDRS) between untreated baseline and final visits was used as an index of disease progression. Placebo-treated patients deteriorated by 5.8 +/- 1.4 points, while deprenyl-treated patients deteriorated by 0.4 +/- 1.3 points (p < 0.001). This effect was sufficiently powerful that a significant deprenyl effect could be detected in the subgroup of 41 patients randomized to Sinemet (p < 0.01) as well as in the 23 patients who completed a 14-day washout of Sinemet or bromocriptine (p < 0.05). No difference in the extent of deterioration was detected in patients randomized to Sinemet versus bromocriptine. This study demonstrates that deprenyl attenuates deterioration in UPDRS score in patients with early PD. These findings are not readily explained by the drug's symptomatic effects and are consistent with the hypothesis that deprenyl has a neuroprotective effect. **Reference:** *Olanow, C. W., et al. The effect of deprenyl and levodopa on the progression of Parkinson's disease. Annals of Neurology. 38(5):771-777, 1995. Department of Neurology, Mount Sinai Medical Center, New York, NY, USA.*

Monoamine oxidase inhibitors (MAO-I) belong to the earliest drugs tried in Parkinson's disease (PD). They have been used with or without levodopa (L-DOPA). Non-selective MAO-I due to their side-effect/adverse reaction profile, like tranylcypromine have limited use in the treatment of depression in PD, while selective, reversible MAO-A inhibitors are recommended due to their easier clinical handling. For the treatment of akinesia and motor fluctuations selective irreversible MAO-B inhibitors selegiline and rasagiline are recommended. They are safe and well tolerated at the recommended daily doses. Their main differences are related to (1) metabolism, (2) interaction with CYP-enzymes and (3) quantitative properties at the molecular biological/genetic level. Rasagiline is more potent in clinical practise and has a hypothesis driven more favourable side effect/adverse reaction profile due to its metabolism to aminoindan. Both selegiline and rasagiline have a neuroprotective and neurorestaurative potential. A head-to head clinical trial would be of utmost interest from both the clinical outcome and a hypothesis-driven point of view. Selegiline is available as tablet and melting tablet for PD and as transdermal selegiline for depression, while rasagiline is marketed as tablet for PD. In general, the clinical use of MAO-I nowadays is underestimated. There should be more efforts to evaluate their clinical potency as antidepressants and antidementive drugs in addition to the final proof of their disease-modifying potential. In line with this are recent innovative developments of MAO-I plus inhibition of acetylcholine esterase for Alzheimer's disease as well as combined MAO-I and iron chelation for PD. **Reference:** *Exp Neurobiol. 2011 March; 20(1): 1–17. Published online 2011 March 31. doi: 10.5607/en.2011.20.1.1. PMCID: PMC3213739. MAO-inhibitors in Parkinson's Disease. Peter Riederer and Gerd Laux. Clinic and Policlinic for Psychiatry, Psychosomatic and Psychotherapy, University of Wuerzburg, 97080 Wuerzburg, Germany. Academic Hospital of Psychiatry, Psychosomatic Medicine, Psychotherapy and Neurology, Gabersee, 83512 Wasserburg a. Inn, Germany. To whom correspondence should be addressed. TEL: 49-931-201-77200, FAX: 49-931-201-77220, Email: peter.riederer@ mail.uni-wuerzburg.de.*

Antioxidants are free radical scavengers and protect living organisms against oxidative damage to tissues. Experimental evidence implicates oxygen-derived free radicals as important causative agents of aging and the present study was designed to evaluate the age-related effects of deprenyl on the antioxidant defense in the cerebellum of male Wistar rats. Experimental rats of three age groups (6, 12, and 18 months old) were administered with liquid deprenyl (2 mg/kg body weight/day for a period of 15 days i.p) and levels of diagnostic marker enzymes (alanine aminotransferase, aspartate aminotransferase, lactate dehydrogenase and creatine phosphokinase) in plasma, lipid peroxides, reduced glutathione and activities of glutathione-dependent antioxidant enzymes (glutathione peroxidase and glutathione-S-transferase) and antiperoxidative enzymes (catalase and superoxide dismutase) in the cerebellar tissue were determined. Intraperitonial administration of deprenyl (2 mg/kg body weight/day for a period of 15 days) significantly (p < 0.05) attenuated the age-related alterations noted in the levels of diagnostic marker enzymes plasma of experimental animals. Deprenyl also exerted an antioxidant effect against aging process by hindering lipid peroxidation to an extent. Moderate rise in the levels of reduced glutathione and activities of glutathione-dependent antioxidant enzymes and antiperoxidative enzymes was also observed. The results of the present investigation indicated that the protective potential of deprenyl was probably due to the increase of the activity of the free radical scavenging enzymes or to a counteraction of free radicals by its antioxidant nature or to a strengthening of neuronal membrane by its membrane-stabilizing action. Histopathological observations also confirmed the protective effect of deprenyl against the age-related aberrations in rat cerebellum. These data on the effect of deprenyl on parameters of normal aging provides new additional information concerning the anti-aging potential of deprenyl. *Reference:* *Cell Stress Chaperones. 2010 September; 15(5): 743–751. Published online 2010 March 13. doi: 10.1007/s12192-010-0177-y. PMCID: PMC3006612. Age-related protective effect of deprenyl on changes in the levels of diagnostic marker enzymes and antioxidant defense enzymes activities in cerebellar tissue in Wistar rats. Manju V. Subramanian and T. J. James. Division of Neurobiology and Ageing, Department of Zoology, Sacred Heart College, Kochi, 682013 India. Manju V. Subramanian, Email: manjuvs@yahoo.com.*

Chronic treatment with low doses of the selective monoamine oxidase (MAO) type B inhibitors selegiline [(−)-deprenyl] and rasagiline, causes elevation in extracellular level of 3,4-dihydroxyphenylethylamine (dopamine) in the rat striatum in vivo (Lamensdorf et al., 1996). The present study was carried out to determine whether this effect of selegiline could be the result of an inhibition of the high-affinity dopamine neuronal transport process. Changes in activity of the dopamine transporter (DAT) in vivo following selegiline treatment were evaluated indirectly by microdialysis technique in the rat, from the change in striatal dopamine extracellular concentration following systemic amphetamine administration (4 mg kg−1, i.p.). Striatal levels of the DAT molecule were determined by immunoblotting. Uptake of [3H]-dopamine was determined in synaptosomes from selegiline-treated animals. Amphetamine-induced increase in striatal extracellular dopamine level was attenuated by one day and by chronic (21 days) treatment with selegiline (0.25 mg kg−1, s.c.). Striatal levels of DAT were elevated after 1 and 21 days treatment with selegiline, but were not affected by clorgyline, rasagiline, nomifensine or amphetamine. The increase in DAT expression, and attenuation of amphetamine-induced dopamine release, were not accompanied by a change in [3H]-dopamine uptake in synaptosomes of selegiline-treated animals. The results suggest that a reversible inhibition of dopamine uptake occurs following chronic low dose selegiline treatment in vivo which may be mediated by an increase in endogenous MAO-B substrates such as 2-phenylethylamine, rather than by the inhibitor molecule or its metabolites. Increased DAT expression appears to be a special property of the selegiline molecule, since it occurs after one low dose of selegiline, and is not seen with other inhibitors of MAO-A or MAO-B. The new DAT molecules formed following selegiline treatment appear not to be functionally active. In conclusion, we found functional evidence for a reduction in striatal dopamine uptake in vivo by selegiline, together with increased synthesis of dopamine transporter molecules. The increase in expression of transporter molecules may be a property of selegiline separate from its effect on MAO. From the present results we cannot tell whether the increase in the transporter expression is due to increase in transporter synthesis or reduction in its metabolism. *Reference: Br J Pharmacol. 1999 February; 126(4): 997–1002. doi: 10.1038/sj.bjp.0702389. PMCID: PMC1571229. Effect of low-dose treatment with selegiline on dopamine transporter (DAT) expression and amphetamine-induced dopamine release in vivo. Itschak Lamensdorf, Shai Porat, Rabi Simantov, and John P M Finberg. Rappaport Faculty of Medicine, Technion, POB 9649, Haifa, Israel. Department of Molecular Genetics, Weizmann Institute of Science, Israel.*

Vitamin D

Background - A role for vitamin D deficiency in Parkinson disease (PD) has recently been proposed. **Objective** - To compare the prevalence of vitamin D deficiency in a research database cohort of patients with PD with the prevalence in age-matched healthy controls and patients with Alzheimer disease (AD). **Design** - Survey study and blinded comparison of plasma 25-hydroxyvitamin D (25[OH]D) concentrations of stored samples in a clinical research database at Emory University School of Medicine. **Setting** - Referral center (PD and AD patients), primary care clinics, and community setting (controls). **Participants** - Participants were recruited into the study between May 1992 and March 2007. Every fifth consecutively enrolled PD patient was selected from the clinical research database. Unrelated AD (n=97) and control (n=99) participants were randomly selected from the database after matching for age, sex, race, APOE genotype, and geographic location. **Main Outcome Measures** - Prevalence of suboptimal vitamin D and mean 25(OH)D concentrations. **Results** - Significantly more patients with PD (55%) had insufficient vitamin D than did controls (36%) or patients with AD (41%; P=.02, $\chi2$ test). The mean (SD) 25(OH)D concentration in the PD cohort was significantly lower than in the AD and control cohorts (31.9 [13.6] ng/mL vs 34.8 [15.4] ng/mL and 37.0 [14.5] ng/mL, respectively; P=.03). **Conclusions** - This report of 25(OH)D concentrations in a predominantly white PD cohort demonstrates a significantly higher prevalence of hypovitaminosis in PD vs both healthy controls and patients with AD. These data support a possible role of vitamin D insufficiency in PD.

Further studies are needed to determine the factors contributing to these differences and elucidate the potential role of vitamin D in pathogenesis and clinical course of PD. *Reference: Arch Neurol. Author manuscript; available in PMC 2009 September 17. Published in final edited form as: Arch Neurol. 2008 October; 65(10): 1348–1352. doi: 10.1001/archneur.65.10.1348. PMCID: PMC2746037. NIHMSID: NIHMS105653. Prevalence of Vitamin D Insufficiency in Patients With Parkinson Disease and Alzheimer Disease. Marian L. Evatt, MD, MS, Mahlon R. DeLong, MD, Natasha Khazai, MD, Ami Rosen, MS, Shirley Triche, RN, and Vin Tangpricha, MD, PhD. Author Affiliations: Division of Movement Disorders, Department of Neurology (Drs Evatt and DeLong and Mss Rosen and Triche), and Division of Endocrinology, Diabetes, and Lipids, Department of Medicine (Drs Khazai and Tangpricha), Emory University School of Medicine, Atlanta, Georgia.*

Parkinson's disease (PD) is the second most common form of neurodegeneration in the elderly population. Clinically, it is characterized by tremor, rigidity, slowness of movement, and postural imbalance. A significant association between low serum vitamin D and PD has been demonstrated, suggesting that elevated vitamin D levels might provide protection against PD. Genetic studies have helped identify a number of proteins linking vitamin D to PD pathology, including the major histocompatibility complex (MHC) class II, the vitamin D receptor (VDR), cytochrome P450 2D6 (CYP2D6), chromosome 22, the renin-angiotensin system (RAS), heme oxygenase-1 (HO-1), poly(ADP-ribose) polymerase-1 gene (PARP-1), neurotrophic factor (NTF), and Sp1 transcription factor. Vitamin D has also been implicated in PD through its effects on L-type voltage-sensitive calcium channels (L-VSCC), nerve growth factor (NGF), matrix metalloproteinases (MMPs), prostaglandins (PGs) and cyclooxygenase-2 (COX-2), reactive oxygen species (ROS), and nitric oxide synthase (NOS). A growing body of evidence suggests that vitamin D supplementation may be beneficial for PD patients. Among the different forms of vitamin D, calcitriol (1,25-dihydroxyvitamin D3) is best indicated for PD, because it is a highly active vitamin D3 metabolite with an appropriate receptor in the central nervous system (CNS). *Reference: ISRN Neurol. 2012; 2012: 134289. Published online 2012 March 7. doi: 10.5402/2012/134289. PMCID: PMC3349248. Role of Vitamin D in Parkinson's Disease. Khanh Luong and Lan Nguyen. Vietnamese American Medical Research Foundation, Westminster, CA 92683, USA. Khanh Luong: Email: lng2687765@aol.com. Academic Editors: M.-C. Chartier-Harlin, S. Lorenzl, and G. Meco.*

More than two decades of pre-clinical research and two recent clinical trials have shown that progesterone (PROG) and its metabolites exert beneficial effects after traumatic brain injury (TBI) through a number of metabolic and physiological pathways that can reduce damage in many different tissues and organ systems. Emerging data on 1,25-dihydroxyvitamin D3 (VDH), itself a steroid hormone, have begun to provide evidence that, like PROG, it too is neuroprotective, although some of its actions may involve different pathways. Both agents have high safety profiles, act on many different injury and pathological mechanisms, and are clinically relevant, easy to administer, and inexpensive. Furthermore, vitamin D deficiency is prevalent in a large segment of the population, especially the elderly and institutionalized, and can significantly affect recovery after CNS injury. The combination of PROG and VDH in pre-clinical and clinical studies is a novel and compelling approach to TBI treatment. *Reference: Front Neuroendocrinol. Author manuscript; available in PMC 2011 January 24. Published in final edited form as: Front Neuroendocrinol. 2009 July; 30(2): 158–172. Published online 2009 April 24. doi: 10.1016/j.yfrne.2009.04.002. PMCID: PMC3025702. NIHMSID: NIHMS115041. Combination Treatment with Progesterone and Vitamin D Hormone May Be More Effective than Monotherapy for Nervous System Injury and Disease. Milos Cekic, M.A., Iqbal Sayeed, Ph.D., and Donald G. Stein, Ph.D. Department of Emergency Medicine, Emory University School of Medicine, Atlanta, Georgia, USA. Manuscript correspondence: Donald G. Stein, Ph.D., Emergency Medicine Brain Research Laboratory, Suite 5100, 1365B Clifton Road NE, Emory University, Atlanta, GA 30322, (404) 712-2540 (phone), (404) 727-2388 (fax), Email: dstei04@emory.edu.*

Vitamins C and E

High dosages of a combination of alpha-tocopherol and ascorbate (3,200 IU per day of alpha-tocopherol + 3,000 mg per day of vitamin C) were administered to patients with early Parkinson's disease as an open-labeled trial and pilot study to test the endogenous toxic hypothesis of the etiology of Parkinson's disease. Patients receiving concomitant amantadine and anticholinergics were allowed to participate, but those receiving levodopa or dopamine agonists were not. The study was begun prior to the availability of deprenyl. The primary end point of the trial was progression of the disease until patients needed treatment with levodopa or a dopamine agonist. The time when levodopa became necessary in the treated patients was compared to another group of patients followed elsewhere who did not receive antioxidants. The time when levodopa became necessary was extended by 2.5 years in the group receiving alpha-tocopherol and ascorbate. Results of this pilot study suggest that the progression of Parkinson's disease may be slowed by administration of these antioxidants. Controlled clinical trials using double-blind randomization techniques are required to confirm these results. *Reference: Fahn, S. A pilot trial of high-dose alpha-tocopherol and ascorbate in early Parkinson's disease. Annals of Neurology. 32:S128-S132, 1992. Department of Neurology, Columbia University College of Physicians and Surgeons, New York, NY.*

High dosages of a combination of 3,200 IU per day of alpha-tocopherol and 3,000 mg of ascorbate were administered to patients with early Parkinson's disease as an open-labeled trial and pilot study to test the endogenous toxic hypothesis of the etiology of Parkinson's disease. Patients receiving concomitant amantadine and anticholinergics were allowed to participate, but those receiving levodopa or dopamine agonists were not. The study was begun prior to the availability of deprenyl. The primary end point of the trial was progression of the disease until patients needed treatment with levodopa or a dopamine agonist. The time when levodopa became necessary in the treated patients was compared to another group of patients followed elsewhere who did not receive antioxidants. The time when levodopa became necessary was extended by 2.5 years in the group receiving alpha-tocopherol and ascorbate. Results of this pilot study suggest that the progression of Parkinson's disease may be slowed by administration of these antioxidants. Controlled clinical trials using double-blind randomization techniques are required to confirm these results. *Reference: Fahn, S. A pilot trial of high-dose alpha-tocopherol and ascorbate in early Parkinson's disease. Annals of Neurology. 32(Supplement):S128-S132, 1992. Department of Neurology, Columbia Univ. College of Physicians & Surgeons, New York, NY, USA.*

Though the etiology is not well understood, late-onset Parkinson's disease (PD) appears to result from several key factors including exposure to unknown environmental toxicants, toxic endogenous compounds and genetic alterations. A plethora of scientific evidence suggest that these environmental and endogenous factors cause PD by producing mitochondrial (mito) oxidative stress and damage in the substantia nigra, leading to cell death. Thus assuming a critical role for mito oxidative stress in PD, therapies to treat or prevent PD must target these mito and protect them against oxidative damage. The focus of this article is to briefly review the experimental and clinical evidence for the role of environmental toxicants and mito oxidative stress/damage in PD as well as discuss the potential protective role of mito d-alpha-tocopherol (T) enrichment and vitamin E therapy in PD. New experimental data are presented that supports the enrichment of mito with d-alpha-tocopherol as a critical event in cytoprotection against toxic mito-derived oxidative stress. The authors propose that chronic, high dose vitamin E dietary supplementation or parenteral vitamin E administration (e.g. vitamin E succinate) may serve as a successful therapeutic strategy for the prevention or treatment of PD (by enriching substantia nigra mito with protective levels of d-alpha-tocopherol). *Reference: Fariss, M. W., et al. Vitamin E therapy in Parkinson's disease. Toxicology. 189(1-2):129-146, 2003. Departments of Pharmaceutical Sciences and Pharmacotherapy, College of Pharmacy, Washington State University, Pullman, WA, USA.*

Exposure of cerebellar granule cells (CGCs) to 1-methyl-4-phenyl-pyridinium (MPP+) results in apoptotic cell death, which is markedly attenuated by co-treatment of CGCs with the radical scavenger vitamin E. Analysis of free radical production and mitochondrial transmembrane potential (DeltaPsim), using specific fluorescent probes, showed that MPP+ mediates early radical oxygen species (ROS) production without a loss of DeltaPsim. Exposure to MPP+ also produces an early increase in Bad dephosphorylation and translocation of Bax to the mitochondria. These events are accompanied by cytochrome c release from mitochondria to cytosol, which is followed by caspase 3 activation. Exposure of the neurons to vitamin E maintains Bad phosphorylation and attenuates Bax translocation, inhibiting cytochrome c release and caspase activation. MPP+-mediated cytochrome c release is also prevented by allopurinol, suggesting the participation of xanthine oxidase in the process. Free radicals play an active role in the MPP+-induced early events that culminate with cell death. **Reference:** *Gonzalez-Polo, R. A., et al. Vitamin E blocks early events induced by 1-methyl-4-phenylpyridinium (MPP+) in cerebellar granule cells. J Neurochem. 84(2):305-315, 2003.*

There is strong evidence that oxidative stress participates in the etiology of Parkinson's disease (PD). The authors designed this study to investigate the neuroprotective effect of vitamin E in the early model of PD. For this purpose, unilateral intrastriatal 6-hydroxydopamine (12.5 g/5 l) lesioned rats were pretreated intramuscularly with D-alpha-tocopheryl acid succinate (24 I.U./kg, i.m.) 1 hour before and three times per week for 1 month post-surgery. Apomorphine- and amphetamine-induced rotational behavior was measured postlesion fortnightly. A parallel tyrosine hydroxylase immunoreactivity and wheat germ agglutinin-horse radish peroxidase (WGA-HRP) tract-tracing study was performed to evaluate the vitamin E pretreatment efficacy. Tyrosine hydroxylase-immunohistochemical analyses showed a reduction of 18% in ipsilateral substantia nigra pars compacta (SNC) cell number of the vitamin E-pretreated lesioned (L+E) group comparing with contralateral side. The cell number dropped to 53% in the lesioned (L+V) group. In addition, retrograde-labeled neurons in ipsilateral SNC were reduced by up to 30% in the L+E group and 65% in the L+V group. Behavioral tests revealed that there are 74% and 68% reductions in contraversive and ipsiversive rotations in the L+E group, respectively, as compared with the L+V group. Therefore repeated intramuscular administration of vitamin E exerts a rapid protective effect on the nigrostriatal dopaminergic neurons in the early unilateral model of PD. **Reference:** *Roghani, M., et al. Neuroprotective effect of vitamin E on the early model of Parkinson's disease in rat: behavioral and histochemical evidence. Brain Res. 892:211-217, 2001.*

Iron chelation

Iron is an essential element in the metabolism of all cells. Elevated levels of the metal have been found in the brains of patients of numerous neurodegenerative disorders, including Parkinson's disease (PD). The pathogenesis of PD is largely unknown, although it is thought through studies with experimental models that oxidative stress and dysfunction of brain iron homeostasis, usually a tightly regulated process, play significant roles in the death of dopaminergic neurons. Accumulation of iron is present at affected neurons and associated microglia in the substantia nigra of PD patients. This additional free-iron has the capacity to generate reactive oxygen species, promote the aggregation of α-synuclein protein, and exacerbate or even cause neurodegeneration. There are various treatments aimed at reversing this pathologic increase in iron content, comprising both synthetic and natural iron chelators. These include established drugs, which have been used to treat other disorders related to iron accumulation. This paper will discuss how iron dysregulation occurs and the link between increased iron and oxidative stress in PD, including the mechanism by which these processes lead to cell death, before assessing the current pharmacotherapies aimed at restoring normal iron redox and new chelation strategies undergoing research. *Reference: Int J Cell Biol. 2012; 2012: 983245. Published online 2012 June 13. doi: 10.1155/2012/983245. PMCID: PMC3382398. Chelators in the Treatment of Iron Accumulation in Parkinson's Disease. Ross B. Mounsey and Peter Teismann. School of Medical Sciences, College of Life Sciences and Medicine Institute of Medical Sciences, University of Aberdeen, Foresterhill, Aberdeen AB25 2ZD, UK. Peter Teismann: Email: p.teismann@abdn.ac.uk. Academic Editor: Pier Giorgio Mastroberardino.*

In addition to their well-established role in providing the cell with ATP, mitochondria are the source of iron-sulfur clusters (ISCs) and heme – prosthetic groups that are utilized by proteins throughout the cell in various critical processes. The post-transcriptional system that mammalian cells use to regulate intracellular iron homeostasis depends, in part, upon the synthesis of ISCs in mitochondria. Thus, proper mitochondrial function is crucial to cellular iron homeostasis. Many neurodegenerative diseases are marked by mitochondrial impairment, brain iron accumulation, and oxidative stress – pathologies that are inter-related. This review discusses the physiological role that mitochondria play in cellular iron homeostasis and, in so doing, attempts to clarify how mitochondrial dysfunction may initiate and/or contribute to iron dysregulation in the context of neurodegenerative disease. We review what is currently known about the entry of iron into mitochondria, the ways in which iron is utilized therein, and how mitochondria are integrated into the system of iron homeostasis in mammalian cells. Lastly, we turn to recent advances in our understanding of iron dysregulation in two neurodegenerative diseases (Alzheimer's disease and Parkinson's disease), and discuss the use of iron chelation as a potential therapeutic approach to neurodegenerative disease. *Reference: J Alzheimers Dis. Author manuscript; available in PMC 2011 May 2. Published in final edited form as: J Alzheimers Dis. 2010; 20(Suppl 2): S551–S568. doi: 10.3233/JAD-2010-100354. PMCID: PMC3085540. NIHMSID: NIHMS291523. Mitochondrial Iron Metabolism and Its Role in Neurodegeneration. Maxx P. Horowitza, and J. Timothy Greenamyreb, Medical Scientist Training Program, University of Pittsburgh, Pittsburgh, PA, USA. Center for Neuroscience, University of Pittsburgh, Pittsburgh, PA, USA. Department of Neurology, University of Pittsburgh, Pittsburgh, PA, USA. Pittsburgh Institute for Neurodegenerative Diseases, University of Pittsburgh, Pittsburgh, PA, USA. Correspondence to: University of Pittsburgh, 3501 Fifth Avenue, Suite 7039, Pittsburgh, Pennsylvania 15260, USA. Tel.: +1 412 648 9793; Fax: +1 412 648 9766; Email: jgreena@pitt.edu .*

Parkinson's disease (PD) is a neurological disorder characterized by the progressive impairment of motor skills in patients. Growing evidence suggests that abnormal redox-active metal accumulation, caused by dysregulation, plays a central role in the neuropathology of PD. Redox-active metals (e.g. Fe and Cu) catalyze essential reactions for brain function. However, these metals can also participate in the generation of highly toxic free radicals that can cause oxidative damage to cells and ultimately lead to the death of dopamine-containing neurons. The emergence of redox-active metals as key players in the pathogenesis of PD strongly suggests that metal-chelators could be beneficial in the treatment of this condition. This mini-review summarizes major recent developments on natural, synthetic iron chelating compounds and hydrogen peroxide-triggered prochelators as potential candidates for PD treatment. *Reference: Published in final edited form as: Curr Bioact Compd. 2008 October 1; 4(3): 150–158. doi: 10.2174/157340708786305952. PMCID: PMC2756717. NIHMSID: NIHMS92951. Iron Chelators as Potential Therapeutic Agents for Parkinson's Disease. Carlos A. Perez, Yong Tong, and Maolin Guo. Department of Chemistry and Biochemistry, University of Massachusetts, Dartmouth, MA 02747-2300.*

More than 80 years after iron accumulation was initially described in the substantia nigra (SN) of Parkinson's disease (PD) patients, the mechanisms responsible for this phenomenon are still unknown. Similarly, how iron is delivered to its major recipients in the cell – mitochondria and the respiratory complexes – has yet to be elucidated. Here, we report a novel transferrin/transferrin receptor 2 (Tf/TfR2)-mediated iron transport pathway in mitochondria of SN dopamine neurons. We found that TfR2 has a previously uncharacterized mitochondrial targeting sequence that is sufficient to import the protein into these organelles. Importantly, the Tf/TfR2 pathway can deliver Tf bound iron to mitochondria and to the respiratory complex I as well. The pathway is redox-sensitive and oxidation of Tf thiols to disulfides induces release from Tf of highly reactive ferrous iron, which contributes to free radical production. In the rotenone model of PD, Tf accumulates in dopamine neurons, with much of it accumulating in the mitochondria. This is associated with iron deposition in SN, similar to what occurs in PD. In the human SN, TfR2 is also found in mitochondria of dopamine neurons, and in PD there is a dramatic increase of oxidized Tf in SN. Thus, we have discovered a novel mitochondrial iron transport system that goes awry in PD, and which may provide a new target for therapeutic intervention. *Reference: Neurobiol Dis. Author manuscript; available in PMC 2009 November 29. Published in final edited form as: Neurobiol Dis. 2009 June; 34(3): 417–431. Published online 2009 February 26. doi: 10.1016/j.nbd.2009.02.009. PMCID: PMC2784936. NIHMSID: NIHMS122429. A novel transferrin/TfR2-mediated mitochondrial iron transport system is disrupted in Parkinson's disease. Pier Giorgio Mastroberardino, Eric K. Hoffman, Maxx P. Horowitz, Ranjita Betarbet, Georgia Taylor, Dongmei Cheng, Hye Mee Na, Claire-Anne Gutekunst, Marla Gearing, John Q. Trojanowski, Marjorie Anderson, Charleen T. Chu, Junmin Peng, and J. Timothy Greenamyre. Department of Neurology, University of Pittsburgh, 3501 fifth avenue, Pittsburgh, PA 15260, USA. Pittsburgh Institute for Neurodegenerative Diseases, USA. Medical Scientist Training Program and Center for Neuroscience, University of Pittsburgh, USA. Department of Pathology, University of Pittsburgh, Pittsburgh, PA 15213, USA.*

Department of Neurology, Center for Neurodegenerative Disease, Emory University, Atlanta, GA 30322, USA. Department of Human Genetics, Center for Neurodegenerative Disease, Emory University, Atlanta, GA 30322, USA. Department of Pathology, Center for Neurodegenerative Disease, Emory University, Atlanta, GA 30322, USA. Center for Neurodegenerative Disease Research, University of Pennsylvania, Philadelphia, PA 19104, USA. University of Washington, Department of Rehabilitation Medicine, Seattle, WA 98195, USA. Corresponding author. Department of Neurology, University of Pittsburgh, 3501 fifth avenue, Pittsburgh, PA 15260, USA. Fax: +1 412 648 9766. E-mail address:Email: mastroberardinopg@upmc.edu (P.G. Mastroberardino).

PLAGUE

Berberine

Coptis chinensis Franch. is a natural herb widely used in China for prevention and treatment of infectious diseases. Plague is a deadly disease caused by Yersinia pestis. Coptis chinensis Franch. is considered the therapeutic agent of choice against plague rather than conventional antibiotics because of its low cost and low toxicity. Berberine is the major constituent of a Coptis chinensis Franch. extract. In the present study, DNA microarray was used to investigate the transcription of Y. pestis in response to berberine. The minimal inhibition concentration (MIC) of berberine to Y. pestis was determined with the liquid dilution method. The gene expression profile of Y. pestis was performed by exposing Y. pestis to berberine at a concentration of 10 x MIC for 30 min. Total RNA was extracted and purified from Y. pestis, reverse-transcribed to cDNA, and then labeled with Cy-dye probes. The labeled probes were hybridized to the microarray. The results were obtained by a laser scanner and analyzed with SAM software. A total of 360 genes were differentially expressed in response to berberine: 333 genes were upregulated, and 27 were downregulated. The upregulation of genes that encode proteins involved in metabolism was a remarkable change. In addition to a number of genes of unknown encoding or unassigned functions, genes encoding cellular envelope and transport/binding functions represented the majority of the altered genes. A number of genes related to iron uptake were induced. This study revealed global transcriptional changes of Y. pestis in response to berberine, hence providing insights into the mechanisms of Coptis chinensis Franch. against Y. pestis. **Reference:** *Planta Med. 2009 Mar;75(4):396-8. Epub 2008 Dec 3. Microarray expression profiling of Yersinia pestis in response to berberine. Zhang J, Zuo G, Bai Q, Wang Y, Yang R, Qiu J. Department of Health Laboratory Technology, School of Public Health, Chongqing Medical University, Chongqing, PR China.*

Coumarin

Seven different methods for the extraction of coumarin and corresponding glycosides from Melilotus officinalis L. and furanocoumarins (psoralen and angelicin) from Psoralea cinerea Lindl. were compared. In the case of coumarins, extraction with polar solvents (water, ethanol, methanol) was shown to be the most efficient: water extraction gave the highest total coumarin concentration, especially for the major component β-D-glucosyl cis-O-hydroxycinnamic acid. Free coumarin could also be recovered in large quantity when the extraction was performed with water at room temperature instead of at 100°C. Ethyl acetate, diethyl ether and chloroform extracted the free coumarin poorly and the glycosides hardly at all. In the case of furanocoumarins, the best results were obtained with boiling methanol using either Soxhlet extraction or refluxed solvent. Other extraction methods involving water, methanol at room temperature, ethyl

acetate or chloroform gave essentially similar results. Diethyl ether was the least satisfactory in terms of furanocoumarin concentration, whilst water extraction of furanocoumarins is of particular interest because the extracted quantities can be easily correlated with the methanol method.
Reference: *Extraction of coumarins from plant material (Leguminosae). F. Bourgaud, A. Poutaraud, A. Guckert. Volume 5, Issue 3, pages 127–132, May/June 1994, Article first published online: 2 MAR 2007.*

RHEUMATOID ARTHRITIS

Ginger

This study examined the effect of eugenol and ginger oil on severe chronic adjuvant arthritis in rats. Severe arthritis was induced in the right knee and right paw of male Sprague-Dawley rats by injecting 0.05 ml of a fine suspension of dead Mycobacterium tuberculosis bacilli in liquid paraffin (5 mg/ml). Eugenol (33 mg/kg) and ginger oil (33 mg/kg), given orally for 26 days, caused a significant suppression of both paw and joint swelling. These findings suggest that eugenol and ginger oil have potent anti-inflammatory and/or antirheumatic properties. *Reference:* *Gaby, A. R., Alternative treatments for rheumatoid arthritis. Alternative Medicine Review. 4(6):392-402, 1999. · Sharma, J. N., et al. Suppressive effects of eugenol and ginger oil on arthritic rats. Pharmacology. 49(5):314-318, 1994.*

One of the features of inflammation is increased oxygenation of arachidonic acid which is metabolized by two enzymic pathways--the cyclooxygenase (CO) and the 5-lipoxygenase (5-LO) - leading to the production of prostaglandins and leukotrienes respectively. Amongst the CO products, PGE2 and amongst the 5-LO products, LTB4 are considered important mediators of inflammation. More than 200 potential drugs ranging from non-steroidal anti-inflammatory drugs, corticosteroids, gold salts, disease modifying anti-rheumatic drugs, methotrexate, cyclosporine are being tested. None of the drugs has been found safe; all are known to produce from mild to serious side-effects. Ginger is described in Ayurvedic and Tibb systems of medicine to be useful in inflammation and rheumatism. In all 56 patients (28 with rheumatoid arthritis, 18 with osteoarthritis and 10 with muscular discomfort) used powdered ginger against their afflictions. Amongst the arthritis patients more than three-quarters experienced, to varying degrees, relief in pain and swelling. All the patients with muscular discomfort experienced relief in pain. None of the patients reported adverse effects during the period of ginger consumption which ranged from 3 months to 2.5 years. It is suggested that at least one of the mechanisms by which ginger shows its ameliorative effects could be related to inhibition of prostaglandin and leukotriene biosynthesis, i.e. it works as a dual inhibitor of eicosanoid biosynthesis. *Reference:* *Srivastava, K. C., et al. Ginger (Zingiber officinale) in rheumatism and musculoskeletal disorders. Med Hypotheses. 39(4):342-348, 1992.*

Green Tea

Regulation of IL-6 transsignaling by the administration of soluble gp130 (sgp130) receptor to capture the IL-6/soluble IL-6R complex has shown promise for the treatment of rheumatoid arthritis (RA). However, enhancing endogenous sgp130 via alternative splicing of the gp130 gene has not yet been tested. The authors found that epigallocatechin-3-gallate (EGCG), an anti-inflammatory compound found in green tea, inhibits IL-

1beta-induced IL-6 production and transsignaling in RA synovial fibroblasts by inducing alternative splicing of gp130 mRNA, resulting in enhanced sgp130 production. Results from in vivo studies using a rat adjuvant-induced arthritis model showed specific inhibition of IL-6 levels in the serum and joints of EGCG-treated rats by 28% and 40%, respectively, with concomitant amelioration of rat adjuvant-induced arthritis. The authors also observed a marked decrease in membrane-bound gp130 protein expression in the joint homogenates of the EGCG-treated group. In contrast, quantitative RT-PCR showed that the gp130/IL-6Ralpha mRNA ratio increased by approximately 2-fold, suggesting a possible mechanism of sgp130 activation by EGCG. Gelatin zymography results showed EGCG inhibits IL-6/soluble IL-6R-induced matrix metalloproteinase-2 activity in RA synovial fibroblasts and in joint homogenates, possibly via up-regulation of sgp130 synthesis. The results of these studies provide previously undescribed evidence of IL-6 synthesis and transsignaling inhibition by EGCG with a unique mechanism of sgp130 up-regulation, and thus hold promise as a potential therapeutic agent for rheumatoid arthritis. **Reference:** *Ahmed, S., et al. Epigallocatechin-3-gallate inhibits IL-6 synthesis and suppresses transsignaling by enhancing soluble gp130 production. Proc Natl Acad Sci U S A. 2008. Division of Rheumatology, Department of Internal Medicine, University of Michigan Medical School, Ann Arbor, MI.*

Identification of common dietary substances capable of affording protection or modulating the onset and severity of arthritis may have important human health implications. An antioxidant-rich polyphenolic fraction isolated from green tea (green tea polyphenols, GTPs) has been shown to possess anti-inflammatory and anticarcinogenic properties in experimental animals. In this study the authors determined the effect of oral consumption of GTP on collagen-induced arthritis in mice. Collagen-induced arthritis (CIA) in mice is a widely studied animal model of inflammatory polyarthritis with similarities to rheumatoid arthritis (RA). In three independent experiments mice given GTP in water exhibited significantly reduced incidence of arthritis (33% to 50%) as compared with mice not given GTP in water (84% to 100%). The arthritis index also was significantly lower in GTP-fed animals. Western blot analysis showed a marked reduction in the expression of inflammatory mediators such as cyclooxygenase 2, IFN-gamma, and tumor necrosis factor alpha in arthritic joints of GTP-fed mice. Histologic and immunohistochemical analysis of the arthritic joints in GTP-fed mice demonstrated only marginal joint infiltration by IFN-gamma and tumor necrosis factor alpha-producing cells as opposed to massive cellular infiltration and fully developed pannus in arthritic joints of non-GTP-fed mice. The neutral endopeptidase activity was approximately 7-fold higher in arthritic joints of non-GTP-fed mice in comparison to nonarthritic joints of unimmunized mice whereas it was only 2-fold higher in the arthritic joints of GTP-fed mice. Additionally, total IgG and type II collagen-specific IgG levels were lower in serum and arthritic joints of GTP-fed mice. Taken together these studies suggest that a polyphenolic fraction from green tea that is rich in antioxidants may be useful in the prevention of onset and severity of rheumatoid arthritis. *Reference: Haqqi, T. M., et al. Prevention of collagen-induced arthritis in mice by a polyphenolic fraction from green tea. Proceedings of the National Academy of Sciences. 96(8):4524-4529, 1999. Department of Medicine, Division of Rheumatic Diseases, Case Western Reserve University, 10900 Euclid Avenue, Cleveland, OH, USA.*

Green tea, a product of the dried leaves of Camellia sinensis, is the most widely consumed beverage in the world. The polyphenolic compounds from green tea (PGT) possess anti-inflammatory properties. The authors investigated whether PGT can afford protection against autoimmune arthritis and also examined the immunological basis of this effect using the rat adjuvant arthritis (AA) model of human rheumatoid arthritis (RA). AA can be induced in Lewis rats (RT.1(l)) by immunization with heat-killed Mycobacterium tuberculosis H37Ra (Mtb), and arthritic rats raise a T cell response to the mycobacterial heat-shock protein 65 (Bhsp65). Rats consumed green tea (2-12 g/L) in drinking water for 1-3 wk and then were injected with Mtb to induce disease. Thereafter, they were observed regularly and graded for signs of arthritis. Subgroups of these rats were killed at defined time points and their draining lymph node cells were harvested and tested for T cell proliferative and cytokine responses. Furthermore, the sera collected from these rats were tested for anti-Bhsp65 antibodies. Feeding 8 g/L PGT to Lewis rats for 9 d significantly reduced the severity of arthritis compared with the water-fed controls. Interestingly, PGT-fed rats had a lower concentration of the proinflammatory cytokine interleukin (IL)-17 but a greater concentration of the immunoregulatory cytokine IL-10 than controls. PGT feeding also suppressed the anti-Bhsp65 antibody response. Thus, green tea induced changes in arthritis-related immune responses. The authors suggest further systematic exploration of dietary supplementation with PGT as an adjunct nutritional strategy for the management of RA. *Reference: Kim, H. R., et al. Green tea protects rats against autoimmune arthritis by modulating disease-related immune events. Journal of Nutrition. 138(11):2111-2116, 2008.*

Green tea possibly helps to prevent rheumatoid arthritis. *Reference: Yang, C. S., et al. Effects of tea consumption on nutrition and health. Journal of Nutrition. 130:2409-2412, 2000.*

Fish Oil

The present study investigated the efficacy and safety of parenteral omega-3 fatty acids (omega-3 FA) in patients with active rheumatoid arthritis (RA). The authors performed a double-blind, randomized, placebo-controlled study in 23 patients with moderate to severe RA. Patients received either 0.2 g of fish oil emulsion/kg (active) or 0.9% saline (placebo) infusion intravenously for 14 consecutive days, followed by 20 weeks of 0.05 g of fish oil/kg (active) or paraffin wax (placebo) ingested orally as capsules. A decrease in swollen and tender joint counts was the primary efficacy measure. At baseline, both swollen and tender joint counts were not significantly different between patients in the treatment and placebo groups. Twenty patients completed the infusion portion of the study, and 13 completed the oral portion. Swollen joint count was significantly lower in the omega-3 FA group compared with the placebo group after 1 week of infusion (P = .002) as well as after 2 weeks of infusion (P = .046). Tender joint count also tended to be lower in the omega-3 FA group, although this did not reach statistical significance. Both swollen and tender joint counts were significantly lower in the omega-3 FA group compared with the placebo group during and at the end of oral treatment. This pilot study indicates that parenteral omega-3 FAs are well tolerated and improve clinical symptoms of RA. Subsequent oral administration of omega-3 FAs may prolong the beneficial effects of the infusion therapy. These results warrant validation in larger multicenter studies. *Reference: Alexander, J. W. Immunonutrition: the role of omega-3 fatty acids. Nutrition. 14(7-8):627-633, 1998. Bahadori, B., et al. omega-3 fatty acids infusions as adjuvant therapy in rheumatoid arthritis. JPEN J Parenter Enteral Nutr. 34(2):151-155, 2010. Internal Medicine, State Hospital Muerzzuschlag, Muerzzuschlag, Austria.*

This study evaluated whether supplementation with olive oil could improve clinical and laboratory parameters of disease activity in patients who had rheumatoid arthritis and were using fish oil supplements. Forty-three patients (34 female, 9 male; mean age = 49 +/- 19y) were investigated in a parallel randomized design. Patients were assigned to one of three groups. In addition to their usual medication, the first group (G1) received placebo (soy oil), the second group (G2) received fish oil omega-3 fatty acids (3 g/d), and the third group (G3) received fish oil omega-3 fatty acids (3 g/d) and 9.6 mL of olive oil. Disease activity was measured by clinical and laboratory indicators at the beginning of the study and after 12 and 24 wk. Patients' satisfaction in activities of daily living was also measured. There was a statistically significant improvement (P < 0.05) in G2 and G3 in relation to G1 with respect to joint pain intensity, right and left handgrip strength after 12 and 24 wk, duration of morning stiffness, onset of fatigue, Ritchie's articular index for pain joints after 24 wk, ability to bend down to pick up clothing from the floor, and getting in and out of a car after 24 wk. G3, but not G2, in relation to G1 showed additional improvements with respect to duration of morning stiffness after 12 wk, patient global assessment after 12 and 24 wk, ability to turn faucets on and off after 24 wk, and rheumatoid factor after 24 wk. In addition, G3 showed a significant improvement in patient global assessment in relation to G2 after 12 wk. Ingestion of fish oil omega-3 fatty acids relieved several clinical parameters used in the present study. However, patients showed a more precocious and accentuated improvement when fish oil supplements were used in combination with olive oil. *Reference: Berbert, A. A., et al. Supplementation of fish oil and olive oil in patients with rheumatoid arthritis. Nutrition. 21(2):131-136, 2005. Department of Department of Pathology, Londrina State University, Parana, Brazil.*

In a double blind noncrossover study, dietary supplementation with fish oil (18 g/day), was compared with an olive oil supplement over a 12-week period in patients with rheumatoid arthritis receiving established conventional therapies. An improvement in tender joint score and grip strength was seen at 12 weeks in the fish oil treated group but not in the olive oil treated group. The more subjective measures of mean duration of morning stiffness and analogue pain score improved to a similar extent in both groups, although statistical significance was only achieved in paired analyses in the olive oil treated group. Production of leukotriene B4 by isolated neutrophils stimulated in vitro was reduced by 30% in the fish oil treated group and unchanged in the olive oil treated group. *Reference: Cleland, L. G., et al. Clinical and biochemical effects of dietary fish oil supplements in rheumatoid arthritis. Journal of Rheumatology. 15(10):1471-1475, 1988.*

Fish oils are a rich source of omega-3 long chain polyunsaturated fatty acids (n-3 LC PUFA). The specific fatty acids, eicosapentaenoic acid and docosahexaenoic acid, are homologues of the n-6 fatty acid, arachidonic acid (AA). This chemistry provides for antagonism by n-3 LC PUFA of AA metabolism to pro-inflammatory and pro-thrombotic n-6 eicosanoids, as well as production of less active n-3 eicosanoids. In addition, n-3 LC PUFA can suppress production of pro-inflammatory cytokines and cartilage degradative enzymes. In accordance with the biochemical effects, beneficial anti-inflammatory effects of dietary fish oils have been demonstrated in randomized, double-blind, placebo-controlled trials in rheumatoid arthritis (RA). Also, fish oils have protective clinical effects in occlusive cardiovascular disease, for which patients with RA are at increased risk. Implementation of the clinical use of anti-inflammatory fish oil doses has been poor. Since fish oils do not provide industry with the opportunities for substantial profit associated with patented prescription items, they have not received the marketing inputs that underpin the adoption of usual pharmacotherapies. Accordingly, many prescribers remain ignorant of their biochemistry, therapeutic effects, formulations, principles of application and complementary dietary modifications. Evidence is presented that increased uptake of this approach can be achieved using bulk fish oils. This approach has been used with good compliance in RA patients. In addition, an index of n-3 nutrition can be used to provide helpful feedback messages to patients and to monitor the attainment of target levels. Collectively, these issues highlight the challenges in advancing the use of fish oil amid the complexities of modern management of RA, with its emphasis on combination chemotherapy applied early. *Reference: Cleland, L., et al. The role of fish oils in the treatment of rheumatoid arthritis. Drugs. 63(9):845-853, 2003. Rheumatology Unit, Royal Adelaide Hospital, Adelaide, South Australia, Australia.*

There is a general belief among doctors, in part grounded in experience, that patients with arthritis need nonsteroidal anti-inflammatory drugs (NSAIDs). Implicit in this view is that these patients require the symptomatic relief provided by inhibiting synthesis of nociceptive prostaglandin E2, a downstream product of the enzyme cyclo-oxygenase (COX), which is inhibited by NSAIDs. However, the concept of 'safe' NSAIDs has collapsed following a multiplicity of observations establishing increased risk for cardiovascular events associated with NSAID use, especially but not uniquely with the new COX-2-selective NSAIDs. This mandates greater parsimony in the use of these agents. Fish oils contain a natural inhibitor of COX, reduce reliance on NSAIDs, and reduce cardiovascular risk through multiple mechanisms. Fish oil thus warrants consideration as a component of therapy for arthritis, especially rheumatoid arthritis, in which its symptomatic benefits are well established. A major barrier to the therapeutic use of fish oil in inflammatory diseases is ignorance of its mechanism, range of beneficial effects, safety profile, availability of suitable products, effective dose, latency of effects and instructions for administration. This review provides an evidence-based resource for doctors and patients who may choose to prescribe or take fish oil. **Reference:** *Cleland, L. G., et al. Fish oil: what the prescriber needs to know. Arthritis Res Ther. 8(1):202, 2005. Rheumatology Unit, Royal Adelaide Hospital, North Terrace, Adelaide, Australia.*

This study involved the administration of 3,600 mg of fish oils per day to 32 rheumatoid arthritis patients with elevated interleukin 1 levels. The plasma concentration of interleukin 1 beta was significantly reduced after 12 weeks of dietary supplementation with fish oils. **Reference:** *Espersen, G. T., et al. Decreased interleukin-1 beta levels in plasma from rheumatoid arthritis patients after dietary supplementation with n-3 polyunsaturated fatty acids. Clin Rheumatol. 11(3):393-395, 1992.*

51 rheumatoid arthritis patients were given fish oil (containing 3,600 mg of omega-3 fatty acids) for 12 weeks. Small but significant improvements were observed in morning stiffness and joint tenderness. The effect of dietary supplementation with n-3 polyunsaturated fatty acids (n-3 PUFA) on disease variables in patients with active rheumatoid arthritis was evaluated in a multicentre, randomized and double blind study. 51 patients with active rheumatoid arthritis were included from three Danish hospital Departments of Rheumatology. The patients were allocated to 12 weeks of treatment with either six n-3 PUFA capsules (3.6 g) or six capsules with a fat composition averaging the Danish diet. Small but significant improvements in morning stiffness, joint tenderness and C-reactive protein were observed. There were no serious side-effects. Dietary supplementation with n-3 PUFA in patients with active rheumatoid arthritis has a modest effect on three out of eight disease variables, without effect on other traditional parameters for monitoring disease activity. **Reference:** *Faarving, K. L., et al. [Fish oils and rheumatoid arthritis: a randomized and double-blind study.] Ugeskr Laeger. 156(23):3495-3498, 1994.*

Meta- and mega-analysis of randomized controlled trials indicate reduction in tender joint counts and decreased use of non-steroidal anti-inflammatory drugs with fish-oil supplementation in long-standing rheumatoid arthritis (RA). Since NSAIDs confer cardiovascular risk and there is increased cardiovascular mortality in RA, an additional benefit of fish oil in RA may be reduced cardiovascular risk via direct mechanisms and decreased non-steroidal anti-inflammatory drug use. Potential mechanisms for anti-inflammatory effects of fish oil include inhibition of inflammatory mediators (eicosanoids and cytokines), and provision of substrates for synthesis of lipid suppressors of inflammation (resolvins). Future studies need progress in clinical trial design and need to shift from long-standing disease to examination of recent-onset RA. The authors are addressing these issues in a current randomised controlled trial of fish oil in recent-onset RA, where the aim is to intervene before joint damage has occurred. Unlike previous studies, the trial occurs on a background of drug regimens determined by an algorithm that is responsive to disease activity and drug intolerance. This allows drug use to be an outcome measure whereas in previous trial designs, clinical need to alter drug use was a 'problem'. Despite evidence for efficacy and plausible biological mechanisms, the limited clinical use of fish oil indicates there are barriers to its use. These probably include the pharmaceutical dominance of RA therapies and the perception that fish oil has relatively modest effects. However, when collateral benefits of fish oil are included within efficacy, the argument for its adjunctive use in RA is strong. *Reference: Gaby, A. R., Alternative treatments for rheumatoid arthritis. Alternative Medicine Review. 4(6):392-402, 1999. Harrison, R. A. Fish oils are beneficial to patients with established rheumatoid arthritis. J Rheumatol. 28(11):2563-2565, 2001. James, J., et al. Fish oil and rheumatoid arthritis: past, present and future. Proc Nutr Soc. 2010. Rheumatology Unit, Royal Adelaide Hospital, Adelaide, South Australia, Australia.*

The objective of this non-randomized, double-blind, placebo controlled, crossover trial was to determine the efficacy of fish-oil dietary supplements in active rheumatoid arthritis and their effect on neutrophil leukotriene levels. The study involved 40 volunteers with active, definite or classical rheumatoid arthritis. There was a 14 week treatment period and a 4 week washout period. Patients were permitted to contine their use of NSAIDS. Twenty-one patients began with a daily dosage of 2.7 grams of eicosapaentanoic acid and 1.8 grams of docosahexenoic acid given in 15 MAX-EPA capsules and 19 began with identical-appearing placebos. The background diet was unchanged. The following results favored fish oil over placebo after 14 weeks: mean time to onset of fatigue improved by 156 minutes and number of tender joints decreased by 3.5. Other clinical measures favored fish oil as well but did not reach statistical significance. Neutrophil leukotriene B4 production was correlated with the decrease in number of tender joints. There were no statistically significant differences in hemoglobin levels, sedimentation rate, or presence of rheumatoid factor or in patient-reported adverse effects. An effect from the fish oil persisted beyond the 4 week washout period. The authors concluded that fish oil ingestion results in subjective alleviation of active rheumatoid arthritis and reduction in neutrophil leukotriene B4 production. **Reference:** *Kremer, J. M., et al. Fish-oil supplementation on active rheumatoid arthritis: a double-blinded, controlled cross-over study. Annals of Internal Medicine. 106(4):497-506, 1987.*

This study used Pharmacaps ethyl ester product to deliver 27mg/kg to 20 patients or 54mg/kg of EPA /day for 24 weeks to 17 rheumatoid arthritis patients in a prospective double blind randomised trial. 10g of olive oil per day was given to 12 control patients. Major findings were significantly fewer tender and swollen joints and higher grip strength. Pain was reduced, and clinical state improved. There were also biochemical changes in the fish oil treated groups, indicative of less inflammation. **Reference:** *Kremer, J. M. Dietary fish oil and olive oil supplementation in patients with rheumatoid arthritis. Arth Rheum. 33(6):810-820, 1990.*

As rheumatoid arthritis (RA) patients have been shown to have impaired plasma fibrinolysis and fish oil has been suggested to be useful for RA, this study investigated the effects of fish oil on fibrinolytic parameters in patients with RA. Forty-five RA patients were randomised to receive either fish oil (1.7 gm eicosapentaenoic acid and 1.1 gm docosahexaenoic acid/day) or placebo treatment for at least 6 months. Plasma levels of fibrinogen, tissue-plasminogen activator (t-PA) and plasminogen activator inhibitor (PAI) activity were measured at 3-month intervals. In the fish oil treatment group, plasma levels of fibrinogen and t-PA activity were reduced at 6 months when compared with baseline [fibrinogen: 3.2 (2.85 - 3.53) g/l vs 3.89 (3.56 - 4.22) g/l, mean (95% confidence intervals for mean), $p < 0.02$; t-PA activity 1.4 (1.01 - 1.78) units/ml vs 1.94 (1.55 - 2.33) units/ml, $p < 0.01$]. No significant changes in plasma PAI activity were seen during the treatment period in these patients. Placebo treatment did not significantly alter the plasma levels of fibrinogen or t-PA and PAI activity. Fish oil supplementation does not appear to produce an improvement in plasma fibrinolysis. Plasma fibrinogen levels and t-PA activity were reduced. This could be due to an effect of fish oil on acute phase protein production. Alternatively, as t-PA is produced on an "on demand" basis, its reduction may be related to the lowering of fibrinogen levels following fish oil therapy. **Reference:** *Lau, C. S., et al. Effects of fish oil on plasma fibrinolysis in patients with mild rheumatoid arthritis. Clinical and Experimental Rheumatology. 13(1):87-90, 1995.*

B10.RIII and B10.G mice were transferred from a diet of laboratory rodent chow to a standard diet in which all the fat (5% by weight) was supplied as either fish oil (17% eicosapentaenoic acid [EPA], 12% docosahexaenoic acid [DHA], 0% arachidonic acid [AA], and 2% linoleic acid) or corn oil (0% EPA, 0% DHA, 0% AA, and 65% linoleic acid). The fatty acid composition of the macrophage phospholipids from mice on the chow diet was similar to that of mice on a corn oil diet. Mice fed the fish oil diet for only 1 wk showed substantial increases in macrophage phospholipid levels of the omega-3 fatty acids (of total fatty acid 4% was EPA, 10%

docosapentaenoic acid [DPA], and 10% DHA), and decreases in omega-6 fatty acids (12% was AA, 2% docosatetraenoic acid [DTA], and 4% linoleic acid) compared to corn oil-fed mice (0% EPA, 0% DPA, 6% DHA, 20% AA, 9% DTA, and 8% linoleic acid). After 5 wk this difference between the fish oil-fed and corn oil-fed mice was even more pronounced. Further small changes occurred at 5-9 wk. The authors studied the prostaglandin (PG) and thromboxane (TX) profile of macrophages prepared from mice fed the two diets just before being immunized with collagen. Irrespective of diet, macrophages prepared from female mice and incubated for 24 h had significantly more PG and TX in the medium than similarly prepared macrophages from male mice. The increased percentage of EPA and decreased percentage of AA in the phospholipids of the macrophages prepared from the fish oil-fed mice was reflected in a reduction in the amount of PGE2 and PGI2 in the medium relative to identically incubated macrophages prepared from corn oil-fed mice. When this same fish oil diet was fed to B10.RIII mice for 26 d before immunization with type II collagen, the time of onset of arthritis was increased, and the incidence and severity of arthritis was reduced compared to arthritis induced in corn oil-fed mice. The females, especially those on the fish oil diet, tended to have less arthritis than the males. These alterations in the fatty acid pool available for PG and leukotriene synthesis suggest a pivotal role for the macrophage and PG in the immune and/or inflammatory response to type II collagen. *Reference: Leslie, C. A., et al. Dietary fish oil modulates macrophage fatty acids and decreases arthritis susceptibility in mice. J Exp Med. 162(4):1336-1449, 1985.*

The objective of this study was to assess the fatty acid pattern in plasma and synovial fluid (SF) in rheumatoid arthritis (RA) and to determine clinical factors related to possible abnormalities. 39 patients with RA were included. SF samples were obtained from 9 patients. Disease activity was assessed using the Ritchie Articular Index and erythrocyte sedimentation rate. Fatty acids were assayed with gas liquid chromatography. Decreased levels of eicosapentaenoic acid (p < 0.0001) and total n3 polyunsaturated fatty acids (p < 0.05) were observed in plasma and in joint fluid, respectively. An increase of the substrates of delta-5-desaturase (C20:3n6 and C20:2n6) and decrease of their products (C20:4n6 and C22:4n6) was observed in plasma total lipids and phospholipids. The long chain mono-unsaturated fatty acids (C20: 1n9, C22: 1n9, C24: ln9) were increased in the joint fluid and in plasma phospholipids. Patients with active disease showed a mild decrease of several saturated fatty acids, n3, and n6 polyunsaturated fatty acids. Minor abnormalities or no changes in fatty acid profile were found related to use of steroids, nonsteroidal anti-inflammatory drugs, and gold salts, or malnutrition. The fatty acid pattern found in RA (decreased levels of n3 polyunsaturated fatty acids) may explain the beneficial effect of fish oil. Changes in n6 polyunsaturated fatty acids suggest that delta-5 desaturation is decreased and this might facilitate the anti-inflammatory effect of botanical lipids in RA. *Reference: Navarro, E., et al. Abnormal fatty acid pattern in rheumatoid arthritis. A rationale for treatment with marine and botanical lipids. J Rheumatol. 27(2):298-303, 2000.*

In this study, 51 active rheumatoid arthritis patients were randomly assigned to receive, in double-blind fashion, fish oil (providing 3.6 g omega-3 fatty acids per day) or placebo (a mixture of fatty acids comparable to that found in an average diet) for 12 weeks. In the fish oil group there was a significant reduction in the duration of morning stiffness, whereas there was no change in the placebo group. Joint tenderness improved to a similar degree in both groups. Grip strength increased by 24 percent in the fish oil group and decreased by 8 percent in the placebo group, but no statistical comparison was made between the two groups. **Reference:** *Nielsen, G. L., et al. The effects of dietary supplementation with n-3 polyunsaturated fatty acids in patients with rheumatoid arthritis: a randomized, double blind trial. Eur J Clin Invest. 22:687-691, 1992.*

Animal, tissue culture, and human studies have evaluated the effects of fish oil supplementation in patients with rheumatoid arthritis (RA) over the last two decades. These studies have clearly shown potentially beneficial changes in cytokine and eicosanoid metabolism. The overall clinical improvement, however, has been only moderate. European clinical trials have shown significant pain reduction in patients with RA treated with vitamin E. A recent animal study in RA-prone mice evaluated the effects of vitamin E in addition to omega-3 and omega-6 fatty acids on cytokine and eicosanoid production. The authors suggest that vitamin E might have an additional positive effect on autoimmune disease by decreasing proinflammatory cytokines and lipid mediators. **Reference:** *Tidow-Kebritchi, S., et al. Effects of diets containing fish oil and vitamin E on rheumatoid arthritis. Nutr Rev. 59(10):335-338, 2001.*

In this double-blind study, 16 patients with rheumatoid arthritis were randomly assigned to receive omega-3 fatty acids or placebo (corn oil) for 12 weeks. The dose of omega-3 fatty acids was 130 mg/kg body weight/day, in the form of ethyl esters of eicosapentaenoic and docosahexaenoic acids. In the group taking fish oil there were significant decreases from baseline in the mean number of tender joints, duration of morning stiffness, physicians' and patients' assessment of global arthritis activity, and physicians' evaluation of pain. In the placebo group no clinical parameters improved. **Reference:** *van der Temple, H., et al. Effects of fish oil supplementation in rheumatoid arthritis. Annals Rheum Dis. 49:76-80, 1990.*

Omega-3 (omega-3) fatty acid rich-fish oil (FO) and vitamin E (vit-E) may delay the progress of certain autoimmune diseases. The present study examined the mechanism of action of omega-3 and omega-6 lipids and vit-E on the serum cytokines and lipid mediators in autoimmune-prone MRL/lpr mice (a model for rheumatoid arthritis, RA). The lpr (lymphoproliferative) gene is overexpressed in these mice causing extensive lymphoproliferation, lupus-like symptoms and accelerated aging. Weanling female MRL/lpr and congenic control MRL/++ mice were fed 10% corn oil (CO, omega6) or FO-based semipurified diets containing two levels of vitamin E (vit-E-75, I.U. and vit-E-500 I.U./Kg diet) for four months. At the end of the experiment, serum anti-DNA antibodies, cytokines and lipid mediators levels were determined. The appearance of enlarged lymph nodes was delayed in the mice fed FO, and the FO-500 IU vit-E diet offered further protection against enlargement of lymph nodes. The MRL/lpr mice exhibited significantly higher levels of serum anti-dsDNA antibodies. The FO-fed mice had significantly lower serum IL-6, IL-10, IL-12, TNF-alpha, PGE2, TXB2 and LTB4 levels compared with CO-fed mice. In mice fed 500 IU vit-E diets, the serum IL-6, IL-10, IL-12 and TNF-alpha levels were significantly lower and serum IL-1beta was significantly higher compared to 75 IU-vit-E-fed mice in CO/FO or both. The levels of anti-DNA antibodies, IL-4, IL-6, TNF-alpha, IL-10 and IL-12 were higher in the sera of MRL/lpr mice. The FO diet lowered the levels of these cytokines (except IL-4) and lipid mediators. Adding 500 IU of vit-E to the FO diet further lowered the levels of IL-6, IL-10, IL-12, and TNF-alpha. It is clear that the beneficial effects of FO can be enhanced by the addition of 500 IU of vit-E in the diet. The FO diet containing 500 IU of vit-E may specifically modulate the levels of IL-6, IL-10, IL-12 and TNF-alpha and thereby may delay the onset of autoimmunity in the MRL/lpr mouse model. The observations from this study may form a basis for selective nutrition intervention based on specific fatty acids and antioxidants in delaying the progress of RA. **Reference:** *Venkatraman, J. T., et al. Effects of dietary omega-3 and omega-6 lipids and vitamin E on serum cytokines, lipid mediators and anti-DNA antibodies in a mouse model for rheumatoid arthritis. J Am Coll Nutr. 18(6):602-613, 1999.*

This study measured the efficacy of fish oil derived (n-3) fatty acid supplementation (3-6 capsules/day) in subjects with rheumatoid arthritis (RA) whose (n-6) fatty acid intake in the background diet was < 10 g/day, compared to olive/corn oil capsule supplement over a 15 week period. The study was a placebo controlled, double blind, randomized 15 week study to determine the effect of fish oils supplementation or placebo on clinical variables in 50 subjects (average age 57) with RA (average duration 13.5 years) whose background diet was naturally low (less than 10 grams per day) in (n-6) fatty acids. Fish oil containing 60% (n-3) fatty acids was supplemented at a rate of 40 mg/kg body weight. Analysis of nine clinical variables indicated there was a significant difference between control and treatment groups. Five subjects in the treatment group and 3 in the control group met the American College of Rheumatology 20% improvement criteria. There were no differences between the two groups at four and eight weeks. At 15 weeks, the average measures of the fish oils group had decreased for swollen joint count, duration of early-morning stiffness, pain, health assessment and patient and physician assessment of arthritis severity. Dietary supplementation resulted in a significant increase in eicosapentaenoic acid in plasma and monocyte lipids in the supplemented group. Fish oil supplementation that delivers (n-3) fatty acids at a dose of 40 mg/kg body weight/day, with dietary (n-6) fatty acid intake < 10 g/day in the background diet, results in substantial cellular incorporation of (n-3) fatty acids and improvements in clinical status in patients with RA. *Reference: Volker, D., et al. Efficacy of fish oil concentrate in the treatment of rheumatoid arthritis. J Rheumatol. 27(10):2343-2346, 2000.*

Supplementation with omega-3 fatty acids present in fish oils can modulate the expression and activity of degradative and inflammatory factors that cause cartilage destruction during arthritis. Incorporation of omega-3 fatty acids (but not other polyunsaturated or saturated fatty acids) into articular cartilage chondrocyte membranes results in a dose-dependent reduction in: 1) the activity of proteoglycan degrading enzymes, and 2) the expression of inflammation-inducible cytokines (interleukin (IL)-1 alpha, tumor necrosis factor (TNF)-alpha), and cyclooxygenase (COX-2). These findings provide evidence that omega-3 fatty acid supplementation can specifically affect regulatory mechanisms involved in chondrocyte gene transcription and thus shows a beneficial role for dietary fish oil supplementation in alleviating causes of arthritis. *Reference: Journal of Biological Chemistry. 275(2):721-724, 2000.*

Cherries

The objective was to assess the possible antioxidant and anti-inflammatory activity of cyanidin from cherries on adjuvant induced arthritis (AA) in SD rats. Arthritis was induced by the complete Freud's adjuvant in male Sprague Dauley rats and assessed based on paw swelling. Rats were randomly divided into normal group (NM), adjuvant arthritis group (AA) and three cyanidin-treated groups in high dosage (HA), middle dosage (MA), and low dosage (LA). The morphological changes in the hind limbs were conducted under a light microscope. We detected glutathione (GSH) in whole blood and malonaldehyde (MDA), superoxide dismutase (SOD), total antioxidative capacity (T-AOC) activity in serum by special kits to assess the antioxidant effects of cyanidin on AA. Moreover, the prostaglandin E2 (PGE2) levels in paw tissues were determined by radioimmunoassay and TNF-alpha levels in serum were determined using ELISA kits specific for rat. **RESULT**: The cyanidin could protect against the paws swelling in AA rats. From the day 14 after AA induction, the swellings of the cyanidin treated groups at high dosage and low dosage were significantly reduced compared with the model group ($P < 0.05, 0.01$). Histological examination of sections through the hind limbs revealed alleviation of inflammatory reaction in the joint after the treatment. The cyanidin at high and low dosage could increase the GSH, SOD activity and T-AOC levels in whole blood or serums and decrease MDA in AA rats ($P < 0.01$). The cyanidin could decrease the PGE2 levels in paw tissues and the TNF-alpha levels in serum at high and low dosages ($P < 0.01$). **CONCLUSION**: The cyanidin could protect against the paws swelling in AA rats, and alleviate the inflammatory reaction in the joint, and the mechanism might be via the increase activity of GSH, SOD and T-AOC that improve the total antioxidative capacity and scavenge the free radicals, perhaps as a result of that the levels of the PGE2 in paw tissues and TNF-alpha contents in serum were decreased. The results suggest that the cyanidin from cherries could be one of the potential candidates for the alleviation of arthritis. **Reference:** *Zhongguo Zhong Yao Za Zhi. 2005 Oct;30(20):1602-5. Antioxidant and anti-inflammatory effects of cyanidin from cherries on rat adjuvant-induced arthritis. He YH, Xiao C, Wang YS, Zhao LH, Zhao HY, Tong Y, Zhou J, Jia HW, Lu C, Li XM, Lu AP. Institute of Basic Theory, China Academy of Traditional Chinese Medicine, Beijing 100700, China.*

TUBERCULOSIS (TB)

Aloe Secundiflora

The emergence of resistance to antimicrobials by pathogens has reached crisis levels, calling for identification of alternative means to combat diseases. **Objective:** To determine antimicrobial activity of crude methanolic extract of Aloe secundiflora Engl. from Lake Victoria region of Kenya. **Materials and Methods**: Extract was tested against four strains of mycobacteria (Mycobacterium tuberculosis, M. kansasii, M. fortuitum and M. smegmatis), Salmonella typhi, Staphylococcus aureus, Pseudomonas aeruginosa, Escherichia coli, Klebsiella pneumoniae and a fungus Candida albicans. activity of the extract was determined using BACTEC™ MGIT™ 960 system. General antibacterial and antifungal activity was determined using standard procedures: zones of inhibition, Minimum Inhibitory Concentrations (MICs) and Minimum Bactericidal/Fungicidal Concentrations (MBCs/MFCs). **Results**: The extract was potent against M. fortuitum, M. smegmatis and M. kansasii where it completely inhibited growth (Zero growth units (GUs)) in all the extract concentrations used. It gave strong antimycobacterial activity (157 GUs) against M. tuberculosis. It showed strong antimicrobial activity ($P \leq 0.05$), giving inhibition zones ≥ 9.00 mm against most microorganisms, such as P. aeruginosa (MIC 9.375 mg mL-1 and MBC of 18.75 mg mL-1), E. coli (both MIC and MBC of 18.75 mg mL-1), S. aureus and S. typhi (both with MIC and MBC of 37.5 mg mL-1). Preliminary phytochemistry revealed presence of terpenoids, flavonoids and tannins. **Conclusion:** The data suggests that Aloe secundiflora could be a rich source of antimicrobial agents. The result gives scientific backing to its use by the local people of Lake Victoria region of Kenya, in the management of conditions associated with the tested microorganisms. *Reference: Pharmacognosy Res. 2011 Apr-Jun; 3(2): 95–99. doi: 10.4103/0974-8490.81956. Methanolic extracts of Aloe secundiflora Engl. inhibits in vitro growth of tuberculosis and diarrhea-causing bacteria. Richard M. Mariita, John A. Orodho, Paul O. Okemo, Claude Kirimuhuzya, Joseph N. Otieno, and Joseph J. Magadula.*

Beta-Sitosterol

This is a double-blind study of 43 persons positively infected with pulmonary tuberculosis receiving conventional multi-antibiotic treatment to ascertain if the addition of a plant sterol/sterolin mixture could improve the clinical outcome. The study took place over 6 months and the patients were closely monitored with a variety of lab and radiographic tests. The group receiving the sterol/sterolin mixture showed a significant weight gain over the placebo group. As well, the treatment group showed a significant increase in lymphocytes and eosinophils. The increase in lymphocytes is consistent with previous experiments indicating a T-cell proliferative effect with the oral intake of phytosterols. The increase in eosinophils is difficult to explain, since no previous allergic response has been attributable to the ingestion of the phytosterols. Other data indicate there may be a relationship between the rise of CD4 lymphocytes and eosinophils. Plant sterol/sterolins have been demonstrated elsewhere to selectively increase CD4 lymphocyte counts. Other lab parameters remained the same between the two groups including hemoglobin, hematocrit, neutrophil count, serum globulin, creatinine, and urea. This preliminary study indicates that the plant sterols and sterolins may have a positive role to play in the complementary treatment of immune-compromised patients. *Reference: Donald, P. R., et al. A randomized placebo-controlled trial of the efficacy of beta-sitosterol and its glucoside as adjuvants in the treatment of pulmonary tuberculosis. Int J Tuberc Lung Dis. 1(6):518-522, 1997.*

Astragalus

The herb Astragalus membranaceus is used in traditional Chinese medicine to boost immunity. This study investigated the effects of Astragalus polysaccharides (APS) and astragalosides (AS) on the phagocytosis of Mycobacterium tuberculosis by macrophages. Peritoneal macrophages were obtained by peritoneal lavage from mice stimulated by starch gravy culture medium and cultured with M. tuberculosis and varying concentrations of APS and AS. Phagocytotic activity was measured using a real-time polymerase chain reaction assay to detect M. tuberculosis DNA. Levels of interleukin-1beta, interleukin-6 and tumour necrosis factor-a secreted by activated macrophages in the culture supernatant were determined using an enzyme-linked immunosorbent assay. Macrophage phagocytotic activity and secreted cytokine levels were significantly increased after treatment with APS and AS. This study provides evidence that APS and AS have strong promoting effects on the phagocytosis of M. tuberculosis by macrophages and the secretion of interleukin-lbeta, interleukin-6 and tumour necrosis factor-alpha by activated macrophages. *Reference: J Int Med Res. 2007 Jan-Feb;35(1):84-90. Effects of Astragalus polysaccharides and astragalosides on the phagocytosis of Mycobacterium tuberculosis by macrophages. Xu HD, You CG, Zhang RL, Gao P, Wang ZR. School of Life Science, Lanzhou University, Lanzhou, China.*

Green Tea

The role played by free radicals in pathogenesis of pulmonary tuberculosis and treatment mediated toxicity is well established. Hence, the present study was undertaken to assess the effect of crude green tea catechin in reducing the oxidative stress seen in patients of AFB positive pulmonary tuberculosis. A total of 200 newly diagnosed cases of AFB positive pulmonary tuberculosis, who received CAT I regimen were enrolled consecutively from DOTS center. Out of 200 patients, 100 randomly selected patients received catechin (500 microg) with antitubercular treatment (ATT) (cases) and 100 received starch (500 microg) with ATT (control). Oxidative stress level in blood samples of cases and controls as compared at the time of enrollment and after one and four months of treatment. Oxidative stress was measured in terms of free radicals (lipid peroxidation, nitric oxide), enzymatic antioxidant (catalase, superoxide dismutase, glutathione peroxidase) and non enzymatic antioxidant (total thiol, reduced glutathione) levels. The results showed significant difference in all the parameters among cases and controls. A significant decrease (p< or = 0.001) in LPO level was observed in cases as compare to controls during the follow up while the level of NO was significantly increased (p< or =0.001) in cases as compare to controls. Significant decrease (p< or =0.001) in catalase and GPx level was observed in cases as compare to controls while SOD levels significantly rose (p< or =0.001) in cases as compared to controls. Significant decrease (p< or =0.001) in SH level was observed in cases as compared to controls while the level of GSH was significantly increased (p< or =0.001). These findings suggest that crude catechin extract can play a definite role as adjuvant therapy in management of oxidative stress seen in pulmonary tuberculosis patients. More detailed studies are needed to document use of catechin in reducing the frequency and severity of side effects of treatment. *Reference: Agarwal, A., et al. Effect of green tea extract (catechins) in reducing oxidative stress seen in patients of pulmonary tuberculosis on DOTS Cat I regimen. Phytomedicine. 17(1):23-27, 2010. Department of Microbiology, Chhatrapati Shahuji Maharaj Medical University, Lucknow, UP, India.*

Lack of maturation of phagosomes containing pathogenic Mycobacterium tuberculosis within macrophages has been widely recognized as a crucial factor for the persistence of mycobacterial pathogen. Host molecule tryptophan-aspartate containing coat protein (TACO) has been shown to play a crucial role in the arrest of such a maturation process. The present study was addressed to understand whether or not polyphenols derived from green tea could down-regulate TACO gene transcription. And if yes, what impact TACO gene down-regulation has on the uptake/survival of M. tuberculosis within macrophages. The reverse-transcriptase polymerase chain reaction and reporter assay technology, employed in this study, revealed that the major component of green tea polyphenols, epigallocatechin-3-gallate had the inherent capacity to down-regulate TACO gene transcription within human macrophages through its ability to inhibit Sp1 transcription factor. The authors also found out that TACO gene promoter does contain Sp1 binding sequence using bioinformatics tools. The down-regulation of TACO gene expression by epigallocatechin-3-gallate was accompanied by inhibition of mycobacterium survival within macrophages as assessed through flow cytometry and colony counts. Based on these results, the authors propose that epigallocatechin-3-gallate may be of importance in the prevention of tuberculosis infection. *Reference: Anand, P. K., et al. Green tea polyphenol inhibits Mycobacterium tuberculosis survival within human macrophages. Int J Biochem Cell Biol. 2005. Molecular Biology Unit, Department of Experimental Medicine and Biotechnology, Chandigarh, India.*

The present study has been undertaken to monitor the extent of oxidative stress in mice infected with M tuberculosis and the role of crude green tea extract in repairing the oxidative damage. The mice were divided into three groups of 9 each; normal, infected-untreated and infected-treated. The infected group of animals exhibited significant enhancement of erythrocytic catalase and glutathione peroxidase activities along with elevated levels of erythrocytic total thiols and plasma lipid peroxidation as compared to normal animals. The infected group also exhibited significantly decreased activity of superoxide dismutase and levels of glutathione in erythrocytes. Upon oral administration of green tea extract for seven days the oxidative stress parameters were reverted back to near normal levels as evidenced by a fall in catalase, glutathione peroxidase, total thiol and extent of lipid peroxidation with concomitant increase in the levels of SOD and reduced glutathione in infected animals. The findings thus, portray that there is a high oxidative stress during early stages of tuberculosis and antioxidants such as green tea extract, can play a vital role by reducing stress through adjuvant therapy. *Reference:* Guleria, R. S., et al. *Protective effect of green tea extract against the erythrocytic oxidative stress injury during mycobacterium tuberculosis infection in mice. Mol Cell Biochem. 236(1-2):173-181, 2002. Department of Microbiology, K. G's. Medical College, Lucknow, India.*

Vitamin A

The results of cross-sectional studies indicate that micronutrient deficiencies are common in patients with tuberculosis. No published data exist on the effect of vitamin A and zinc supplementation on antituberculosis treatment. The goal of this study was to investigate whether vitamin A and zinc supplementation increases the efficacy of antituberculosis treatment with respect to clinical response and nutritional status. In this double-blind, placebo-controlled trial, patients with newly diagnosed tuberculosis were divided into 2 groups. One group (n = 40) received 1500 retinol equivalents (5000 IU) vitamin A (as retinyl acetate) and 15 mg Zn (as zinc sulfate) daily for 6 months (micronutrient group). The second group (n = 40) received a placebo. Both groups received the same antituberculosis treatment recommended by the World Health Organization. Clinical examinations, assessments of micronutrient status, and anthropometric measurements were carried out before and after 2 and 6 mo of antituberculosis treatment. At baseline, 64% of patients had a body mass index (in kg/m2) < 18.5, 32% had plasma retinol concentrations < 0.70 µmol/L, and 30% had plasma zinc concentrations < 10.7 µmol/L. After antituberculosis treatment, plasma zinc concentrations were not significantly different between groups. Plasma retinol concentrations were significantly higher in the micronutrient group than in the placebo group after 6 mo (P < 0.05). Sputum conversion (P < 0.05) and resolution of X-ray lesion area (P < 0.01) occurred earlier in the micronutrient group. Vitamin A and zinc supplementation improves the effect of tuberculosis medication after 2 months of antituberculosis treatment and results in earlier sputum smear conversion.

Reference: Karyadi, E., et al. A double-blind, placebo-controlled study of vitamin A and zinc supplementation in persons with tuberculosis in Indonesia: effects on clinical response and nutritional status. American Journal of Clinical Nutrition. 75(4):720-727, 2002.

The objective of this study was to estimate serum vitamin A in pulmonary tuberculosis (PTB) patients at the start and end of anti-tuberculosis treatment. Serum vitamin A was estimated in 47 PTB patients (pre and post treatment), 46 healthy household contacts and 30 healthy 'normals'. Mean serum vitamin A in patients at the start of treatment was 21.2 microg/dl, which was significantly lower than in household contacts (42.2 microg/dl) and healthy 'normals' (48.1 microg/dl). The vitamin A levels in patients increased following treatment. The low vitamin A levels observed in patients returned to normal at the end of anti-tuberculosis treatment without vitamin A supplementation. *Reference: Ramachandran, G., et al. Vitamin A levels in sputum-positive pulmonary tuberculosis patients in comparison with household contacts and healthy 'normals'. Int J Tuberc Lung Dis. 8(9):1130-1133, 2004. Tuberculosis Research Centre (ICMR), Chennai, India.*

Vitamin C

The author administered 100 mg of vitamin C intravenously to tuberculosis patients and noted positive responses in temperature, weight, general well-being, appetite and blood tests. *Reference: Albrecht, E. Vitamin C as an adjuvant therapy of lung tuberculosis. Medizinische Klinic. 34:972-973, 1938.*

The author studied 74 tuberculosis patients. Vitamin C-treated (200 mg per day for ten weeks) patients experienced a marked increase in hemoglobin content and red blood cell counts. *Reference: Babbar, I. Observation of ascorbic acid. Part XI. Therapeutic effect of ascorbic acid in tuberculosis. Indian Medical Gazzette. 83:409-410, 1948.*

The authors experienced good results giving tuberculosis patients 150 – 200 mg vitamin C orally for six weeks. For the first four days of treatment, patients also received 500 mg of intramuscular vitamin C. *Reference: Bakhsh, I., et al. Vitamin C in pulmonary tuberculosis. The Indian Medical Gazette. 74:274-277, 1939.*
The author aministered 15,000 mg of vitamin C to six advanced (near death) tuberculosis patients for 200 days. Five patients survived for at least six months and were no longer bedridden. *Reference: Charpy, J. Ascorbic acid in very large doses alone or with vitamin D2 in tuberculosis. Bulletin de l'academie Nationale de Medecine. 132:421-423, 1948.*

Massive doses of vitamin C will cure tuberculosis by removing the polysaccharide coat from the Mycobacterium tuberculosis bacteria that cause tuberculosis. *Reference: Klenner, F. R., et al. Observations on the dose and administration of ascorbic acid when employed beyond the range of a vitamin in human pathology. Journal of Applied Nutrition. 23(3-4):61-88, 1971.*

The author describes one case of tuberculosis treated with vitamin C (1,000 mg intravenously either every day or every second day for three weeks). The treatment resulted in lowered temperature and the patient ceased having the tuberculosis cough. **Reference:** *McCormick, W. Vitamin C prophylaxis and therapy of infectious diseases. Archives of Pediatrics. 68(1):1-9, 1951.*

Mammals lacking the ability to synthesize vitamin C are the same mammals that are most susceptible to tuberculosis infections. **Reference:** *Osborn, T., et al. Possible relation between ability to synthesize vitamin C and reaction to tubercle bacillus. Nature. 145:974, 1940.*

The author treated children and adult tuberculosis patients with oral vitamin C (150 mg per day). This relatively low dose was found to definitely improve the condition of 61% of 49 treated adults and 88% of 24 treated children. **Reference:** *Petter, C. Vitamin C and tuberculosis. Lancet. 57:221-224, 1937.*

The authors studied 111 tuberculosis patients – some treated, some untreated. Treated patients received either orange juice or 250 mg vitamin C. Both the orange juice treated and vitamin C treated patients showed a more favorable clinical response as measured by red blood cell count, hemoglobin level and other blood tests. **Reference:** *Radford, M., et al. Blood changes following continuous daily administration of vitamin C and orange juice to tuberculosis patients. American Review of Tuberculosis. 35:784-793, 1937.*

The authors examined the effects of 250 mg oral vitamin C per day for ten weeks to pulmonary tuberculosis patients. The treatment improved the overall blood picture of the treated patients. **Reference:** *Rudra, M., et al. Haematological study in pulmonary tuberculosis and the effect upon it of large doses of vitamin C. Tubercle. 27:93-94, 1946.*

Vitamin D

In innate immune responses, activation of Toll-like receptors (TLRs) triggers direct antimicrobial activity against intracellular bacteria, which in murine, but not human, monocytes and macrophages is mediated principally by nitric oxide. The authors report here that TLR-activation of human macrophages up-regulated expression of the vitamin D receptor and the vitamin D1-hydroxylase genes, leading to induction of the antimicrobial peptide cathelicidin and killing of intracellular Mycobacterium tuberculosis. The authors also observed that sera from African-American individuals, known to have increased susceptibility to tuberculosis, had low 25-hydroxyvitamin D and were inefficient in supporting cathelicidin messenger RNA induction. These data support a link between TLRs and vitamin D-mediated innate immunity and suggest that differences in ability of human populations to produce vitamin D may contribute to susceptibility to microbial infection. **Reference:** *Liu, P. T., et al. Toll-like receptor triggering a vitamin D mediated human antimicrobial response. Science. 311(5768): 1770-1773,2006.*

Vitamin D was used to treat tuberculosis in the pre-antibiotic era. Prospective studies to evaluate the effect of vitamin D supplementation on antimycobacterial immunity have not previously been performed. The objective of this study were to determine the effect of vitamin D supplementation on antimycobacterial immunity and vitamin D status. A double-blind randomized controlled trial was conducted in 192 healthy adult tuberculosis contacts in London, UK. Participants were randomized to receive a single oral dose of 2.5 mg vitamin D or placebo and followed up at 6 weeks. The primary outcome measure was assessed with a functional whole blood assay (BCG-lux assay) that measures the ability of whole blood to restrict luminescence, and thus growth, of recombinant reporter mycobacteria in vitro; the read-out is expressed as a luminescence ratio (luminescence post-infection/baseline luminescensce). Interferon-gamma responses to the M. tuberculosis antigens early secretory antigenic target-6 and culture filtrate protein 10 were determined with a second whole blood assay. Vitamin D supplementation significantly enhanced the ability of participants' whole blood to restrict BCG-lux luminescence in vitro compared to placebo (mean luminescence ratio at follow-up 0.57 vs. 0.71 respectively, 95% CI for difference 0.01 to 0.25; $P=0.03$) but did not affect antigen-stimulated Interferon-gamma secretion. A single oral dose of 2.5 mg vitamin D significantly enhanced the ability of participants' whole blood to restrict BCG-lux luminescence in vitro without affecting antigen-stimulated Interferon-gamma responses. Clinical trials should be performed to determine whether vitamin D supplementation prevents reactivation of latent tuberculosis infection. **Reference:** *Martineau, A. R., et al. A single dose of vitamin D enhances immunity to Myco-bacteria. Am J Respir Crit Care Med. 2007. Queen Mary's School of Medicine and Dentistry, Barts and The London, Centre for Health Sciences, London, United Kingdom.*

The objective of this study was to explore the association between low serum vitamin D and risk of active tuberculosis in humans. This was a systematic review and meta-analysis that used observational studies published between 1980 and July 2006 (identified through Medline) that examined the association between low serum vitamin D and risk of active tuberculosis. For the review, seven papers were eligible from 151 identified in the search. The pooled effect size in random effects meta-analysis was 0.68 with 95% CI 0.43-0.93. This 'medium to large' effect represents a probability of 70% that a healthy individual would have higher serum vitamin D level than an individual with tuberculosis if both were chosen at random from a population. There was little heterogeneity between the studies. Low serum vitamin D levels are associated with higher risk of active tuberculosis. Although more prospectively designed studies are needed to firmly establish the direction of this association, it is more likely that low body vitamin D levels increase the risk of active tuberculosis. In view of this, the potential role of vitamin D supplementation in people with tuberculosis and hypovitaminosis D-associated conditions like chronic kidney disease should be evaluated. *Reference: Nnoaham, K. E., et al. Low serum vitamin D levels and tuberculosis: a systematic review and meta-analysis. Int J Epidemiol. 37(1):113-119, 2008. Department of Public Health, Oxfordshire Primary Care Trust, Headington, Oxford, UK.*

The aim of this study was to compare the vitamin D group of pulmonary tuberculosis patients with a placebo group in terms of clinical improvement, nutritional status, sputum conversion, and radiological improvement. 67 tuberculosis patients visiting the Pulmonary Clinic, of Cipto Mangunkusumo Hospital, Jakarta, from January 1st to August 31st, 2001 were included in this study. The subjects were randomized to receive vitamin D (0.25 mg/day = 10,000 IU) or placebo in a double blind method, during the 6th initial week of Tb treatment. The rate of sputum conversion, complete blood counts, blood chemistry as well as radiologic examination were evaluated. There were more male patients than females (39:28), 78.7% were in the productive age group, 71.6% had low nutritional status, 62.4% with low education level, and 67.2% with low income. One hundred percent of the vitamin D group and only 76.7% of the placebo group had sputum conversion. This difference is statistically significant (p=0.002). The sputum conversion had no correlation with the hemoglobin level, blood clotting time, calcium level, lymphocyte count, age, sex, and nutritional status. There were more subjects with radiological improvement in the vitamin D group. *Reference: Nursyam, E. W., et al. The effect of vitamin D as supplementary treatment in patients with moderately advanced pulmonary tuberculous lesion. Acta Med Indones. 38(1):3-5, 2006. Departement of Internal Medicine, Faculty of Medicine, University of Indonesia-dr.Cipto Mangunkusumo Hospital.*

The objectives of this studey were to determine the normal level of 25 hydroxyvitamin D in healthy individuals, and to seek evidence of vitamin D deficiency in patients with active tuberculosis. There were 35 cases of pulmonary and extra-pulmonary tuberculosis and 16 controls, whose clinical characteristics, dietary intake of vitamin D and biochemical characteristics including serum vitamin D levels were compared. Exclusion criteria: malabsorption, liver or renal disorders, intake of drugs, which can reduce vitamin D levels, HIV infection, diabetes, immune-suppressive treatment, and severe protein energy malnutrition. There was a statistically significant difference (p < 0.005) in mean vitamin D levels between controls (19.5 ng/ml) and study subjects (10.7 ng/ml). Sixteen patients out of 35 had values well below the lower limit of normal (9 ng/ml). No one in the control group had vitamin D level less than 9 ng/ml. However the mean vitamin D level in the control group was less than the mean value quoted in the literature from the West. Sunlight exposure was adequate in those with deficiency but there was reduced dietary intake of vitamin D. Serum 25 hydroxy vitamin D levels less than 9 ng/ml indicates deficiency. Vitamin D deficiency exists in patients with tuberculosis and it is possibly a cause rather than effect of the disease; deficiency is due to decreased dietary intake. Vitamin D deficiency can occur without any symptoms. If symptoms are present, it indicates severe deficiency. Serum calcium and phosphorus values do not often predict the existence of deficiency. **Reference:** *Sasidharan, P. K., et al. Tuberculosis and vitamin D deficiency. J Assoc Physicians India. 50:554-558, 2002. Department of Medicine, Calicut Medical College, Kerala.*

Susceptibility to disease after infection by Mycobacterium tuberculosis (M. tuberculosis) is influenced by environmental and host genetic factors. Vitamin D metabolism leads to activation of macrophages and restricts the intracellular growth of M tuberculosis. This effect may be influenced by polymorphisms at three sites in the vitamin D receptor (VDR) gene. There is a high prevalence of vitamin D deficiency in Gujarati Asians living in London, a population in whom the incidence of tuberculosis is also high. The lowest serum 25-hydroxycholecalciferol concentrations were found in patients with active disease, and the greatest risk of tuberculosis (nearly ten-fold higher) was associated with an undetectable 25-hydroxycholecalciferol concentration. Analysis of vitamin D concentrations during therapy suggests that tuberculosis itself does not lower 25-hydroxycholecalciferol concentrations. In addition, the association between vitamin D concentrations and active tuberculosis showed dose dependency. Although dietary deficiency contributes to the high proportion of vitamin D deficiency in the population, the analysis of indicates that other factors (probably sunlight exposure) are important. The greatest risk of tuberculosis was associated with an undetectable vitamin D concentration, so even moderate supplementation may be useful. **Reference:** *Wilkinson, R. J., et al. Influence of vitamin D deficiency and vitamin D receptor polymorphisms on tuberculosis among Gujarati Asians in west London: a case-control study. Lancet. 355(9204):618-621, 2000.*

Vitamin D can strengthen the immune system to mount a defense against tuberculosis. Vitamin D enhances macrophage phagocytosis of Mycobacterium tuberculosis. Low serum 25(OH)D levels are associated with increased risk of tuberculosis. **Reference:** *Grant, W. B., et al. Benefits and requirements of vitamin D for optimal health: a review. Alternative Medicine Review. 10(2):94-111, 2005.*

ULCERATIVE COLITIS

Aloe vera

Oxygen/nitrogen reactive species (ROS/RNS) are currently implicated in the pathogenesis of ulcerative colitis, drawing attention on the potential prophylactic and healing properties of antioxidants, scavengers, chelators. The authors evaluated the possible protective/curative effects of a natural antioxidant preparation based on Aloe vera and ubiquinol, against intestinal inflammation, lesions, and pathological alterations of the intestinal electrophysiological activity and motility, in a rat model of DSS-induced colitis. 5% dextrane sulfate (DDS) (3 days), followed by 1% DSS (4 days) was administered in drinking water. The antioxidant formulation (25 mg/kg) was delivered with a pre-treatment protocol, or simultaneously or post-colitis induction. Spontaneous and acetylcholine-stimulated electrical activity were impaired in the small intestine and in distal colon, upon exposure to DSS only. Severe inflammation occurred, with increased myeloperoxidase activity, and significant alterations of the oxidant/antioxidant status in colonic tissue and peritoneal cells. Lipoperoxidation, superoxide production, glutathione peroxidase and glutathione-S-transferase activities, and reduced glutathione content increased, whilst superoxide dismutase and catalase activities were sharply suppressed in colon tissue. ROS/RNS formation in peritoneal cells was strongly inhibited. Inflammation, electrical/mechanical impairment in the gut, and a great majority of oxidative stress parameters were improved substantially by pre-treatment with the antioxidant preparation, but not by simultaneous administration or post-treatment.

Reference: Korkina, L., et al. The protective and healing effects of a natural antioxidant formulation based on ubiquinol and Aloe vera against dextran sulfate-induced ulcerative colitis in rats. Biofactors. 18(1-4):255-264, 2003. Department of Molecular Biology, Russian State Medical University, Moscow, Russia.

Oral aloe vera gel is widely used by patients with inflammatory bowel disease and is under therapeutic evaluation for this condition. The aim of this study was to assess the effects of aloe vera in vitro on the production of reactive oxygen metabolites, eicosanoids and interleukin-8, all of which may be pathogenic in inflammatory bowel disease. The anti-oxidant activity of aloe vera was assessed in two cell-free, radical-generating systems and by the chemiluminescence of incubated colorectal mucosal biopsies. Eicosanoid production by biopsies and interleukin-8 release by CaCo2 epithelial cells in the presence of aloe vera were measured by enzyme-linked immunosorbent assay. Aloe vera gel had a dose-dependent inhibitory effect on reactive oxygen metabolite production; 50% inhibition occurred at 1 in 1000 dilution in the phycoerythrin assay and at 1 in 10-50 dilution with biopsies. Aloe vera inhibited the production of prostaglandin E2 by 30% at 1 in 50 dilution (P = 0.03), but had no effect on thromboxane B2 production. The release of interleukin-8 by CaCo2 cells fell by 20% (P < 0.05) with aloe vera diluted at 1 in 100, but not at 1 in 10 or 1 in 1000 dilutions. The anti-inflammatory actions of aloe vera gel in vitro provide support for the proposal that it may have a therapeutic effect in inflammatory bowel disease. *Reference: Langmead, L., et al. Anti-inflammatory effects of aloe vera gel in human colorectal mucosa in vitro. Aliment Pharmacol Ther. 19(5):521-527, 2004. Centre for Adult and Paediatric Gastroenterology, Institute of Cellular and Molecular Science, Barts & the London, Queen Mary School of Med & Dentistry, London, UK.*

The herbal preparation, aloe vera, has been claimed to have anti-inflammatory effects and, despite a lack of evidence of its therapeutic efficacy, is widely used by patients with inflammatory bowel disease. The aim of this study was to perform a double-blind, randomized, placebo-controlled trial of the efficacy and safety of aloe vera gel for the treatment of mildly to moderately active ulcerative colitis. Forty-four evaluable hospital out-patients were randomly given oral aloe vera gel or placebo, 100 mL twice daily for 4 weeks, in a 2:1 ratio. The primary outcome measures were clinical remission (Simple Clinical Colitis Activity Index </= 2), sigmoidoscopic remission (Baron score </= 1) and histological remission (Saverymuttu score </= 1). Secondary outcome measures included changes in the Simple Clinical Colitis Activity Index (improvement was defined as a decrease of >/= 3 points; response was defined as remission or improvement), Baron score, histology score, haemoglobin, platelet count, erythrocyte sedimentation rate, C-reactive protein and albumin. Clinical remission, improvement and response occurred in nine (30%), 11 (37%) and 14 (47%), respectively, of 30 patients given aloe vera, compared with one (7%) [P = 0.09; odds ratio, 5.6 (0.6-49)], one (7%) [P = 0.06; odds ratio, 7.5 (0.9-66)] and two (14%) [P < 0.05; odds ratio, 5.3 (1.0-27)], respectively, of 14 patients taking placebo. The Simple Clinical Colitis Activity Index and histological scores decreased significantly during treatment with aloe vera (P = 0.01 and P = 0.03, respectively), but not with placebo. Sigmoidoscopic scores and laboratory variables showed no significant differences between aloe vera and placebo. Adverse events were minor and similar in both groups of patients. Oral aloe vera taken for 4 weeks produced a clinical response more often than placebo; it also reduced the histological disease activity and appeared to be safe. Further evaluation of the therapeutic potential of aloe vera gel in inflammatory bowel disease is needed. *Reference: Langmead, L., et al. Randomized, double-blind, placebo-controlled trial of oral aloe vera gel for active ulcerative colitis. Aliment Pharmacol Ther. 19(7):739-747, 2004. Centre for Gastroenterology, Institute of Cellular and Molecular Science, Barts and The London, Queen Mary School of Medicine and Dentistry, London, UK.*

American Ginseng

Ulcerative colitis (UC) is a dynamic, idiopathic, chronic inflammatory condition associated with a high colon cancer risk. American ginseng has anti-oxidant properties, and targets many of the players in inflammation. The aim of this study was to test whether American ginseng extract prevents and treats colitis. Colitis in mice was induced by the presence of 1% dextran sulfate sodium (DSS) in the drinking water, or by 1% oxazolone rectally. American ginseng extract was mixed in the chow at levels consistent with that currently consumed by humans as a supplement (75 ppm, equivalent to 58 mg daily). To test prevention of colitis, American ginseng extract was given prior to colitis induction. To test treatment of colitis, American ginseng extract was given after the onset of colitis. In vitro studies were performed to examine mechanisms. Results indicate that American ginseng extract not only prevents, but it treats colitis. iNOS and Cox-2 (markers of inflammation) and p53 (induced by inflammatory stress) are also down-regulated by American ginseng. Mucosal and DNA damage associated with colitis is at least in part a result of an oxidative burst from overactive leukocytes. The authors therefore tested the hypothesis that American ginseng extract can inhibit leukocyte activation, and subsequent epithelial cell DNA damage in vitro and in vivo. Results are consistent with this hypothesis. The use of American ginseng extract represents a novel therapeutic approach for the prevention and treatment of ulcerative colitis. **Reference:** *Jin, Y., et al. American ginseng suppresses inflammation and DNA damage associated with mouse colitis. Carcinogenesis. 2008. Department of Pharmaceutical and Biomedical Sciences, South Carolina College of Pharmacy, University of South Carolina, SC USA.*

Ulcerative colitis is a dynamic, chronic inflammatory condition associated with an increased colon cancer risk. Inflammatory cell apoptosis is a key mechanism regulating ulcerative colitis. American ginseng (AG) is a putative antioxidant that can suppress hyperactive immune cells. The authors have recently shown that AG can prevent and treat mouse colitis. Because p53 levels are elevated in inflammatory cells in both mouse and human colitis, the authors tested the hypothesis that AG protects from colitis by driving inflammatory cell apoptosis through a p53 mechanism. They used isogenic p53(+/+) and p53(-/-) inflammatory cell lines as well as primary CD4(+)/CD25(-) effector T cells from p53(+/+) and p53(-/-) mice to show that AG drives apoptosis in a p53-dependent manner. The authors used a dextran sulfate sodium (DSS) model of colitis in C57BL/6 p53(+/+) and p53(-/-) mice to test whether the protective effect of AG against colitis is p53 dependent. Data indicate that AG induces apoptosis in p53(+/+) but not in isogenic p53(-/-) cells in vitro. In vivo, C57BL/6 p53(+/+) mice are responsive to the protective effects of AG against DSS-induced colitis, whereas AG fails to protect from colitis in p53(-/-) mice. Furthermore, terminal deoxynucleotidyl transferase-mediated dUTP nick end labeling of inflammatory cells within the colonic mesenteric lymph nodes is elevated in p53(+/+) mice consuming DSS + AG but not in p53(-/-) mice consuming DSS + AG. Results are consistent with in vitro data and with the hypothesis that AG drives inflammatory cell apoptosis in vivo, providing a mechanism by which AG protects from colitis in this DSS mouse model. **Reference:** *Jin, Y., et al. American Ginseng suppresses colitis through p53-mediated apoptosis of inflammatory cells. Cancer Prev Res. 2010.*

Ginkgo Biloba

It has been hypothesized that the mechanism responsible for Ginkgo biloba's effect in ulcerative colitis patients who improved or attained remission was due to Ginkgo biloba extract's inhibition of platelet-activating factor (PAF), which mediates mucosal inflammation. *Reference: Head, K. A., et al. Inflammatory bowel disease part I: ulcerative colitis – pathophysiology and conventional and alternative treatment. Alternative Medicine Review. 8(3):247-283, 2003.*

Intestinal inflammatory states, regardless of specific initiating events, share common immunologically mediated pathways of tissue injury and repair. The efficacy of various drugs used to treat ulcerative colitis (UC) was investigated. The aim of the present study is to evaluate the effects of ginkgo biloba extract on the extent and severity of UC caused by intracolonic administration of acetic acid in rats. The inflammatory response was assessed by histology and measurement of myeloperoxidase activity (MPO), reduced glutathione (GSH), tumor necrosis factor (TNF-alpha) and interleukin-1beta (IL-1beta) levels in colon mucosa. Oral pretreatment with Ginkgo biloba in doses of (30, 60, 120mgkg(-1) body weight) and sulfasalazine in a dose of (500mgkg(-1) body weight used as reference) for 2 days before induction of colitis and continued for 5 consecutive days, significantly decreased colonic MPO activity, TNF-alpha, and IL-1beta levels and increased GSH concentration. Moreover, Ginkgo biloba attenuated the macroscopic colonic damage and the histopathological changes-induced by acetic acid. These results suggest that Ginkgo biloba may be effective in the treatment of UC through its scavenging effect on oxygen-derived free radicals. *Reference: Mustafa, A., et al. Ginkgo biloba attenuates mucosal damage in a rat model of ulcerative colitis. Pharmacol Res. 2006. Department of Pharmacology, College of Medicine & KKUH, King Saud University, Riyadh, Saudi Arabia.*

URINARY TRACT INFECTION (UTI)

Nasturtium & Horseradish

PATIENTS AND METHODS: In a prospective cohort study from 251 centers in Germany patients with age of 4 years or above who were treated due to acute sinusitis, bronchitis or urinary tract infections (UTI) in the period from 1st March 2004 - 30th July 2005, were elected. They were included in the study analysis, if they had no exclusion criteria (severe diseases, need for antibiotic therapy, participation in another trial) and came to the final investigation. The patients were treated either with the nasturtium herb and horseradish root containing herbal drug Angocin Anti-Infekt N (test group, n = 1223) or with standard antibiotic therapy (control group, n = 426). Treatment, dosage and treatment duration were determined by the physician in accordance with the patient. 536 subjects (408 test, 128 control patients) suffered from acute sinusitis, 634 subjects (469 test, 165 control patients) from acute bronchitis and 479 subjects (346 test, 133 control patients) from UTI. At study start and end the severity of the symptoms were judged by the investigator and quantified with 4 scores (0 = no symptom, 3 severe symptom). During the treatment information on use of medication, concomitant procedures and adverse events (AEs) in a patient diary. At the end of the study (disease free or after 7-14 days) the patient returned to the investigator, who recorded the vital parameters, finally judged the treatment efficacy and potential persisting symptoms on the basis of score values. Primary efficacy criterion was the change of the complaints quantified by the change of the relative symptom score averaged over all symptoms and related to the baseline value. **RESULTS:** In patients with acute sinusitis the mean relative reduction of the averaged symptom score was 81.3% for the test group and 84.6% for the control group, in patients with acute bronchitis the mean reduction was 78.3% for the test group and 80.3% for the control group, in patients with UTI 81.2% for the test group and 87.9% for the control group. The 95% confidence interval for the difference of the expected reductions between test and control group was -8.5% to 1.8% for acute sinusitis, 7.6% to 3.6% for acute bronchitis and -13.1% to -0.1% for UTI. Non-inferiority of the test treatment, i.e. if the lower limit of the 95% confidence interval is greater than 10%, could be stated for acute sinusitis and bronchitis. In UTI the non-inferiority level was exceeded only by 3%. Complementary procedures were less in the test group than in the control group. For 1.5 % of test patients and 6.8% of control patients AEs were observed. **CONCLUSION:** Therapy with the herbal drug in the indications acute sinusitis, acute bronchitis und acute urinary tract infection is - with regard to its efficacy comparable to the treatment with standard antibiotics. The application of supportive procedures and the administration of concurrent medication were less expressed in the group treated with the herbal drug. In the above mentioned indications the group treated with the herbal drug displayed a clear advantageous safety profile compared to the group treated with standard antibiotics. **Reference:** *Arzneimittelforschung. 2006;56(3):249-57. [Efficacy and safety profile of a herbal drug containing nasturtium herb and horseradish root in acute sinusitis, acute bronchitis and acute urinary tract infection in comparison with other treatments in the daily practice/results of a prospective cohort study]. Goos KH, Albrecht U, Schneider B. Repha GmbH, Biologische Arzneimittel, Langenhagen.*

OBJECTIVE: To evaluate the in-vitro antimicrobial properties of a commercialized preparation (Angocin Anti-Infekt N) containing a combination of the haulm of nasturtium (Tropaeoli majoris herba; N) and of the roots of horseradish (Armoraciae rusticanae radix; H). This preparation can be used to treat upper respiratory tract (URTI) and urinary tract infections (UTI). The active ingredients are volatile mustard oils, which are activated in the gastrointestinal tract after oral intake. Previous research has shown mustard oils derived from either N or H to possess antibacterial activity. **METHODS:** In order to assess the antimicrobial capacity of phytotherapeutic compounds containing volatile mustard oils, a modified gas-test was used. Native preparations of N and H were applied to the lids of Columbia agar plates (ratio N:H = 2.5:1) and mixed with sterile H20. Thirteen different bacterial species including Haemophilus influenzae, Moraxella catarrhalis, Escherichia coli, Pseudomonas aeruginosa, Streptococcus pyogenes, methicillin-susceptible and resistant Staphylococcus aureus (MSSA, MRSA) were tested (20 isolates each). The test organisms were plated onto the blood agar plates and placed above the native preparations. The plates were sealed with adhesive tape and incubated at 37 degrees C. Following incubation of 24 h and 92 h, colony forming units (CFU) were counted and the minimal inhibitory concentrationg (MIC90) was determined for each bacterial species. **RESULTS:** Relevant antimicrobial activities of the combined native preparations were found against H. influenzae (MIC90 50 mg N / 20 mg H), M. catarrhalis (100 mg N / 40 mg H), E. coli (400 mg N / 160 mg H), P aeruginosa (400 mg N / 160 mg H), MSSA (400 mg N 1 160 mg H), MRSA (400 mg N / 160 mg H), and S. pyogenes (400 mg N / 160 mg H). **CONCLUSION**: Antimicrobial testing of a combination of N and H revealed broad antibacterial activities against clinically relevant pathogens covering both gram-positive and gram-negative organisms, thus confirming previous reports of the antibacterial properties of mustard oils. Additionally, this study demonstrated that the combination of N and H leads to synergistic activity in terms of improved Pseudomonas-susceptibility compared to the previous reported activities of the single compounds. Thus, these results prove that there is a rational basis for treatment of URTI and UTI with a combination of N and H. **Reference:** *Arzneimittelforschung. 2006;56(12):842-9. [In vitro study to evaluate the antibacterial activity of a combination of the haulm of nasturtium (Tropaeoli majoris herba) and of the roots of horseradish (Armoraciae rusticanae* *radix)]. Conrad A, Kolberg T, Engels I, Frank U. Institut für Umweltmedizin und Krankenhaushygiene, Universitäitsklinikum Freiburg, Breisacher Strasse 115B, 79106 Freiburg/Brsg., Germany. andreas.conrad@uniklinik-freiburg.de*

Cranberry

Urinary tract infection (UTI) refers to the presence of clinical signs and symptoms arising from the genitourinary tract plus the presence of one or more micro-organisms in the urine exceeding a threshold value for significance (ranges from 102 to 103 colony-forming units/mL). Infections are localized to the bladder (cystitis), renal parenchyma (pyelonephritis) or prostate (acute or chronic bacterial prostatitis). Single UTI episodes are very common, especially in adult women where there is a 50-fold predominance compared with adult men. In addition, recurrent UTIs are also common, occurring in up to one-third of women after first-episode UTIs. Recurrences requiring intervention are usually defined as two or more episodes over 6 months or three or more episodes over 1 year (this definition applies only to young women with acute uncomplicated UTIs). A cornerstone of prevention of UTI recurrence has been the use of low-dose once-daily or post-coital antimicrobials; however, much interest has surrounded non-antimicrobial-based approaches undergoing investigation such as use of probiotics, vaccines, oligosaccharide inhibitors of bacterial adherence and colonization, and bacterial interference with immunoreactive extracts of Escherichia coli. Local (intravaginal) estrogen therapy has had mixed results to date. Cranberry products in a variety of formulations have also undergone extensive evaluation over several decades in the management of UTIs. At present, there is no evidence that cranberry can be used to treat UTIs. Hence, the focus has been on its use as a preventative strategy. Cranberry has been effective in vitro and in vivo in animals for the prevention of UTI. Cranberry appears to work by inhibiting the adhesion of type I and P-fimbriated uropathogens (e.g. uropathogenic E. coli) to the uroepithelium, thus impairing colonization and subsequent infection. The isolation of the component(s) of cranberry with this activity has been a daunting task, considering the hundreds of compounds found in the fruit and its juice derivatives. Reasonable evidence suggests that the anthocyanidin/proanthocyanidin moieties are potent antiadhesion compounds. However, problems still exist with standardization of cranberry products, which makes it extremely difficult to compare products or extrapolate results. Unfortunately, most clinical trials have had design deficiencies and none have evaluated specific key cranberry-derived compounds considered likely to be active moieties (e.g. proanthocyanidins). In general, the preventive efficacy of cranberry has been variable and modest at best. Meta-analyses have established that recurrence rates over 1 year are reduced approximately 35% in young to middle-aged women. The efficacy of cranberry in other groups (i.e. elderly, paediatric patients, those with neurogenic bladder, those with chronic indwelling urinary catheters) is questionable. Withdrawal rates have been quite high (up to 55%), suggesting that these products may not be acceptable over long periods. Adverse events include gastrointestinal intolerance, weight gain (due to the excessive calorie load) and drug-cranberry interactions (due to the inhibitory effect of flavonoids on cytochrome P450-mediated drug metabolism). The findings of the Cochrane Collaboration support the potential use of cranberry products in the prophylaxis of recurrent UTIs in young and middle-aged women. However, in light of the heterogeneity of clinical study designs and the lack of consensus regarding the dosage regimen and formulation to use, cranberry products cannot be recommended for the prophylaxis of recurrent UTIs at this time. **Reference:** *Drugs. 2009;69(7):775-807. doi: 10.2165/00003495-200969070-00002. Cranberry and urinary tract infections. Guay DR. Department of Experimental and Clinical Pharmacology, College of Pharmacy, University of Minnesota, Minneapolis, Minnesota 55455, USA. guayx001@umn.edu.*

WHOOPING COUGH
(AKA PERTUSSIS)

Antibiotics

BACKGROUND: Whooping cough is a highly contagious disease. Infants are the population at highest risk of severe disease and death. Erythromycin for 14 days is recommended for treatment and contact prophylaxis but this regime is considered inconvenient and prolonged. The value of contact prophylaxis is uncertain. **OBJECTIVES:** To study the benefits and risks of antibiotic treatment of and contact prophylaxis against whooping cough. **SEARCH STRATEGY:** The Cochrane Central Register of Controlled Trials (CENTRAL) (The Cochrane Library Issue 1, 2004); MEDLINE (January 1966 to February 2004); EMBASE (January 1974 to August 2003); conference abstracts and reference lists of articles were searched. Study investigators and pharmaceutical companies were approached for additional information (published or unpublished studies). There were no constraints based on language or publication status. **SELECTION CRITERIA:** All randomised and quasi-randomised controlled trials of antibiotics for treatment of and contact prophylaxis against whooping cough were included in the systematic review. **DATA COLLECTION AND ANALYSIS:** At least three reviewers independently extracted data and assessed the quality of each trial. **MAIN RESULTS:** Twelve trials with 1,720 participants met the inclusion criteria. Ten trials investigated treatment regimens and two investigated prophylaxis regimens. The quality of the trials was variable. Results showed that short-term antibiotics (azithromycin for three days, clarithromycin for seven days, or erythromycin estolate for seven days) were equally effective with long-term antibiotic treatment (erythromycin estolate or erythromycin for 14 days) in the microbiological eradication of Bordetella pertussis (B. pertussis) from the nasopharynx. The relative risk (RR) was 1.02 (95% confidence interval (CI) 0.98 to 1.05). Side effects were fewer with short-term treatment (RR 0.66; 95% CI 0.52 to 0.83). There were no differences in clinical improvement or microbiological relapse between short and long-term treatment regimens. Contact prophylaxis (of contacts older than six months of age) with antibiotics did not significantly improve clinical symptoms or the number of cases that developed culture positive B. pertussis. **AUTHORS' CONCLUSIONS:** Antibiotics are effective in eliminating B. pertussis from patients with the disease, rendering them non-infectious, but do not alter the subsequent clinical course of the illness. Effective regimens include: three days of azithromycin, seven days of clarithromycin, seven or 14 days of erythromycin estolate, and 14 days of erythromycin ethylsuccinate. Considering microbiological clearance and side effects, three days of azithromycin or seven days of clarithromycin are the best regimens. Seven days of trimethoprim/sulfamethoxazole also appeared to be effective for the eradication of B. pertussis from the nasopharynx and may serve as an alternative antibiotic treatment for patients who cannot tolerate a macrolide. There is insufficient evidence to determine the benefit of prophylactic treatment of pertussis contacts. *Reference: Cochrane Database Syst Rev. 2005 Jan 25;(1):CD004404. Antibiotics for whooping cough (pertussis). Altunaiji S, Kukuruzovic R, Curtis N, Massie J. Source. Zayed Military Hospital, Zayed Street, PO Box 3740, Abu Dhabi, United Arab Emirates. saltunaiji@hotmail.com. Update in Cochrane Database Syst Rev. 2007;(3):CD004404.*

Vitamin C

The treatment of pertussis in the last 30 years has not shown noticeable progress, and it is worthwhile to regard treatment and prophylaxis from a new viewpoint. I found that specific relationships exist between vitamin C and bacillus pertussis. A part of these investigations has already been published in Japanese. The essentials are reported here: *I. Influence of vitamin C on bacillus pertussis*. **1st.** Bacteria growth: Vitamin C (Redoxon, L-ascorbic acid sodium (PH 6,4 to 6,6]) was added to solid culture medium (PH 7,0) with different pathogenic bacteria like Pneumococcus, influenza bacilli, coliform bacilli, dysentery bacilli, typhus bacilli, diphtheria bacilli, staphylococcus, streptococcus, meningococcus, B. pyocyaneus, B. subtilis, B. prodigiosus, and bacillus pertussis. It was stated that the growth of only the whooping cough bacillus was specifically retarded by vitamin C, while all other bacteria remained almost uninfluenced. The larger the amount of vitamin C, the clearer the disturbance of the growth of the pertussis bacillus; from a gradual alteration of the bacillus body, to the appearance of regressive metamorphosis, and finally to killing. Vitamin C has therefore a bactericidal effect on the pertussis bacillus. The influenza bacilli, which are difficult to differentiate bacteriologically, were compared in detail to the pertussis bacillus. No development disturbances by vitamin C of the bacillus could be observed, also no regressive modifications or other influences. The fact that the two types of bacteria indicate a clear difference in the influence of vitamin C, can be regarded as method for distinction. **2nd.** Virulence: It could be proven by bioassay [animal studies] that pertussis bacillus modified in culture to which vitamin C had been added (1,2—1,8 mg Redoxon per 1 ccm), possessed a strongly reduced virulence compared to pertussis bacillus serving as a control. **3rd.** blood picture: The investigation of the blood picture of rabbits injected intravenously with pertussis bacillus showed strong leukocytosis 3 days after the injection, with relative lymphocytosis (60—80%), returning to normal after a week. On the other hand the blood picture showed probable leukocytosis after treatment with modified pertussis bacillus, but no lymphocytosis. The lymphocytes amounted to only 35—50% and only moderate neutropolynuclear leukocytosis appeared. *II. Influence of vitamin C on the pertussis toxin*. The toxin received from my pertussis bacteria culture possesses sufficient toxicity that after intracutaneous injection trials with rabbits and guinea pigs causes clear development of inflammation. This reaction can clearly be suppressed, however, by prior addition of vitamin C to a certain quantity of toxin. The larger the quantity of vitamin C, the larger the detoxification effect. Furthermore, this intracutaneous reaction to the pertussis toxin is clearly reduced in animals pre-treated with vitamin C injections in comparison to controls. Based on these test results, I used vitamin C in the treatment of children sick with pertussis, and to be sure with very good success. It concerns 81 children. **Investigation method.** Patients diagnosed with pertussis at the health center and pediatric clinic of the Kyoto Imperial University were examined. Among them were simple cases of pertussis, cases of pertussis with bronchitis and pertussis with pneumonia, and more such accompanied by assorted other complications The observation of the children was carried out in different stages. For the treatment of pertussis I used vitamin C Redoxon "Roche" (L-ascorbic acid sodium) in injectable solution, 0.1 g per Ampoule. Those sick only with pertussis were treated exclusively with the vitamin C preparation. Also with patients with pertussis complicated by bronchitis or pneumonia, every other specific handling of the pertussis was discontinued and only the generally symptomatic treatment was performed. Accounting for the degree of illness and the age of the children, intravenous or intramuscular injections [were given as follows:] in light cases 50—100 mg; in moderately severe 100—150 mg; and in severe over 200 mg once daily (sometimes twice). Injections started at first daily; after improvement of the symptoms, each 2nd day; in all 5—6—12 injections. After progress of about 1—3 weeks the symptoms picture was determined and the blood picture was examined. Attention was particularly paid to: strength of the convulsive cough, lip cyanosis during coughing, attacks with breathing difficulty, occurrence of vomiting, as well as degree of the recurrence and number of the cough attacks; furthermore on general symptoms: liveliness, appetite, sleep and disposition. The blood picture was examined at least 3 times. **Results -** The observation of 81 children yields that in 66 cases, at the earliest 4—5 and at the latest after 6—8 injections, i.e. 1—2 weeks after start of the treatment: reduction of lip cyanosis in coughing attacks; attacks with breathing difficulty, vomiting and recurrence disappeared; also the number of cough attacks diminished. Patients became lively, had good appetite and the convalescence progressed very satisfactorily. The best therapeutic successes concerned complication-free cases; above all the therapy was successful with relatively promptly handled patients, i.e. about 1 week after transition to the convulsive stage. Also in patients taken later in treatment, a good result was observed. With the children treated in the early catarrhal stage, the convulsion stage usually still developed, but was shortened compared to the normal progression. Of special mention were 3 serious cases of pertussis pneumonia in artificially nourished babies, for which previous treatment methods, vaccine treatments etc., are rarely successful, and which were deemed as having lethal outcome. Through our therapy, the children were clearly improved after 2—3 weeks and finally healed. The blood picture of patients with pertussis (or pertussis and bronchitis), that showed before treatment a 60 to 90 percent lymphocytosis, displayed 1 week to 10 days after start of the vitamin C injections a reduction of the lymphocytes of 40—60% and a percent increase of the neutronuclear leukocytes and low-grade neutrophily. The leukocyte count showed slight increase in cases of the early convulsion stage after this treatment, but in the majority of the cases in the 2nd week of the convulsion stage, a reduction was found. The blood picture of the pertussis patients with pneumonia was somewhat different, namely that the treatment gradually lowered the leukocyte count and the percentage of the polynuclear leukocytes. The transition to lymphocytosis was approached; in other words, one found an approximately normal blood picture. The few cases in which no therapeutic success was observed were usually concerning those with other complications. Either it emerged from the children's family history that cases with asthma, tuberculosis etc. were present, or even that the children had allergic illnesses, an asthmatic, exudative and scrofulous constitution, tuberculosis, measles, influenza, severe tonsillitis, or it concerned children with innate nervousness.

Summary - Among 81 cases with which vitamin C therapy was tried, in 34 cases a clear improvement of the symptoms or perfect healing was obtained, in 32 cases improvement of the symptoms, while in 15 cases effects were indeterminate. Accordingly the vitamin C therapy can be viewed as an effective specific therapy. This therapy, which even with the use of excess vitamin C doses exhibits no side effects compared to other treatments has the advantage that it can be applied to pertussis in infancy, where so far success with specific vaccine injections is achieved with difficulty because of insufficient production of immune bodies. The explanation of the clinical success of the vitamins C therapy lies in the fact that among the different pathogenic bacteria the growth of B. pertussis is suppressed specifically by vitamin C and is finally killed; also that vitamin C will detoxify the pertussis bacterial toxin. Whether secondary modifications in the organism resulting from vitamin C injections additionally promote healing, is yet to be examined. In summary I would like to report on investigations of the prophylaxis of pertussis. Although the toxicity of pertussis bacillus grown on media with added vitamin C is clearly reduced compared to the original bacterial culture, and in animal trials and in blood picture variations appear as described in the treatment of pertussis, yet sufficient immunity could be obtained thereby. The serological investigation of the rabbit immune serum of the weakened bacteria showed that the agglutination- and complement linkage reactions were the same as the original bacteria. Animals which were injected several times with the weakened pertussis bacteria, could be received alive. Even our injection of the animals with weakened bacilli in multiples of the minimal lethal dose of original bacilli did not lead to the death of the animals, which speaks clearly for the antitoxin action of the weakened pertussis bacteria and which can be regarded as a pilot test of the prophylaxis of the animal infection. Investigations of immunity through these altered pertussis bacteria after incorporation of living bacilli are under way. *Reference: CONCERNING THE VITAMIN C THERAPY OF WHOOPING-COUGH. By Dr. TOSHIO OTANI. From the children's clinic of the Imperial University of Kyoto. (Presented: Prof. S. HATTORI).*

The treatment of whooping cough has been a major problem particularly to those interested in the illnesses of children and to the general practitioner for at least the past four centuries. The disease is at times difficult to diagnose and usually difficult to treat. Many of the recommended procedures seem to be effective in a few cases, but few if any give constant results in all cases. One who has tried the various forms of treatment recommended is still searching for an effective agent. Otani 1 in 1936 treated eighty-one cases of whooping cough with large amounts of vitamin C intravenously and found that thirty-four were greatly benefited, thirty-two moderately benefited, and fifteen unaffected. Ormerod and Unkauf 2 of Winnipeg, working without knowledge of Otani's findings reported ten cases treated with ascorbic acid given orally; confirming the work of Otani and concluding that ascorbic acid definitely shortened the paroxysmal stage of the disease if large amounts were used early in the course of the disease. In a later report by Ormerod, Unkauf and White 3 nineteen additional cases were reported with similar findings. These papers stimulated us to use cevitamic acid in our own cases. We are reporting the following twenty-six cases, all of which had a definite clinical picture confirmed in most cases by a high leucocytosis and lymphocytosis. The first sixteen cases were given fifteen mg. tablets of cevitamic acid, ten tablets daily the first three days, eight tablets daily the next three days, and six daily until symptoms entirely subsided. This medication is palatable, dissolves readily, can be given in food or drinks, is non toxic and has no objectionable features. **Case No. 1.** Baby B. Age four months, coughing ten days. Definite exposure. Symptoms free after ten days of treatment. **Case No. 2.** Baby F. Age six weeks. W B C 22,500. Lymphocytes fifty-two per cent. Coughing two weeks, whooping and vomiting. Symptoms subsided rapidly, disappearing in ten days. **Case No. 3.** M. I. Age three years. Coughing three weeks. W B C 10,950. Lymphocytes fifty-six per cent. Whooping and vomiting disappeared within seven days. **Case No. 4.** M. 11. Age five years. Coughing two weeks. W B C 16,000. Lymphocytes fifty-two per cent. Whooping and vomiting subsided gradually disappearing in two weeks. A Preliminary Report on the Use of Cevitamic Acid in the Treatment of Whooping Cough. **Case No. 5.** D. K. Age four years. Coughing, whooping and vomiting for four weeks. W B C 12,000. Lymphocytes thirty-eight per cent. Symptoms subsided gradually for three weeks. The cevitamic acid not being considered very effective in this case. **Case No. 6**. J. E. Age six years. Coughing for two weeks. Occasional whooping and vomiting. W B C 14,650. Lymphocytes sixty-six per cent. Complete disappearance of symptoms in seven days. **Case No. 7.** F. E. Age four years. Coughing, whooping and vomiting for fourteen days. W B C 21,300. Lymphocytes forty-five per cent. Symptoms disappeared in ten days. **Case No. 8.** J. E. Age two years. Coughing, vomiting and whooping for ten days. W B C 28,3302. Lymphocytes sixty-two per cent. Symptoms subsided gradually during fourteen days. **Case No. 9.** E. J. Age six years. Cough, no whooping or vomiting but with definite exposure. W B C 9,600. Lymphocytes sixty-two per cent. Cough disappeared in six days. **Cases No. 10**. B. O. Age eight years. Coughing and vomiting eight days. W B C

17,200. Lymphocytes sixty percent. Cough subsided in two weeks.* **Case No. 11**. M. W. Age two years. Coughing, whooping and vomiting ten days. W B C 7,700. Lymphocytes sixty per cent. Symptoms subsided abruptly on the fourth day. **Case No. 12.** Baby S. Age two and one-half years. Coughing ten days. Definite exposure. W B C 9,500. Lymphocytes forty-three per cent. Cough subsided abruptly on the sixth day.* **Case No. 13**. H. H. Age two years. WBC 24,000. Lymphocytes forty-eight per cent. Severe whooping cough for seven weeks. Symptoms disappeared completely on the fifth day. **Case No. 14**. J. C. Age seven years. Coughing, whooping and vomiting for two weeks. W B C 19,950. Lymphocytes forty-four per cent. Symptoms subsided gradually for ten days. **Case No. 15.** Baby S. Age ten months. Coughing, whooping and vomiting for two weeks. Definite exposure. Symptom-free at the end of four days. **Case No. 16.** W. O. Age seven years. Night cough for two weeks. Occasional vomiting. W B C 6,600. Lymphocytes sixty-two per cent. Symptom-free in six days. *These cases had previously had Sauer's whooping cough vaccine. The succeeding ten cases were treated with different individual dosage using twenty-five mg. tablets. ***(Cevitamic acid used in the last ten cases was Parke, Davis & Company brand, twentyfive mg. tablet.) **Case No. 17.** Baby P. Male, age two and one-half years. Ten days cough. W B C 26,400. Lymphocytes seventy-three per cent. Given one tablet t. i. d. Symptoms fifty per cent ameliorated in four days. Then developed an acute bronchitis with high fever. Subsequent recovery slow but no spasmodic coughing. **Case No. 18**. Baby Z. Female, age two and one-half years. fourteen days cough and whooping three or four times a night waking for one hour each time. W B C 13,400. Lymphocytes sixty-six per cent. Given one tablet t. i. d. On third night of treatment cough not severe enough to awaken the patient. Free from cough in two weeks. A Preliminary Report on the Use of Cevitamic Acid in the Treatment of Whooping Cough. **Case No. 19.** Baby F. Age nine months. Cough two weeks, whooping. No blood count. Three tablets daily and completely symptom free by the fourth day. **Case No. 20**. D. J. L. Female, age six and one-half years. Coughing and vomiting for three weeks. One tablet t. i. d. Vomiting for two weeks but not so often. Then symptoms rapidly cleared. **Case No. 21**. B. W. Female, age four years. Coughing six days. W B C 13,200. Lymphocytes fiftyone per cent. One tablet t. i. d. Symptoms improved by third day, almost gone on the eighth day, completely gone few days later. Never whooped or vomited. **Case No. 22.** D. J. L. Female. Age five years. Coughing four weeks, last two weeks of which she showed improvement on large amounts of orange juice. W B C 10,800. Lymphocytes fifty-one per cent. One tablet t. i. d. Gave almost immediate complete relief. **Case No. 23.** M.. B. Male. Age twelve years. Two weeks coughing. W B C 13,400. Lymphocytes fifty two per cent. Given three to nine tablets daily. After three days of treatment cough almost completely checked having nine paroxysms in the next ten days where previous to treatment had had nine to twelve paroxysms daily. **Case No. 24**. B. L. Female. Age eleven years. Coughing two weeks. Eight to ten paroxysms daily. W B C 12,000. Lymphocytes sixty per cent. Three to nine tablets daily, after three days one paroxysm at night and one daily. Continued an occasional cough for three weeks. **Case No. 25.** C. D. Female. Age nine years. Sister to above two cases. Had similar symptoms. No blood count taken. Given three to nine tablets daily. Showed little improvement, running usual course of six to seven weeks. **Case No. 26.** D. C. Male. Age three years. Whooping and coughing for five weeks. Had had x-ray treatments with little success. Given one tablet four times a day. Showed immediate remarkable relief. No cough at the end of one week. **CONCLUSIONS** - In this small series of twenty-six cases of whooping cough, cevitamic acid seemed to be strikingly effective in relieving and checking the symptoms in all but two of the cases which apparently received little if any relief. It is our opinion that it should be given further trial in all cases of whooping cough regardless of the age of the patient, or the length of time already elapsed since the original symptoms. *References: 1. Otani, T.: Vitamin C Therapy of Whooping Cough. Klin. Wochnschr. 1936, 15: 1884 (Quoted by Ormerod & Unkauf.) 2. Ormerod, K. J. and Unkauf, B. K: Ascorbic Acid (Vit. C) Treatment of Whooping Cough. Canadian Medical Association Journal 1937, Page 134. 3. Ormerod, K. J., Unkauf, B. M. and White. F. D.: A Further Report on the Ascorbic Acid Treatment of Whooping Cough. Canadian Medical Association Journal September 1937, 268. From The Journal of The Kansas Medical Society , Volume XXXIX, November 1938, Number 11, pp. A Preliminary Report on the Use of Cevitamic Acid in the Treatment of Whooping Cough. **Primary Reference:** A Preliminary Report on the Use of Cevitamic Acid in the Treatment of Whooping Cough. E. L Vermillion, M.D., and George E. Stafford, M.D. Salina, Kansas.* www.seanet.com/~alexs/ascorbate/193x/vermillion-el-etal-kansas_city_med_j-1938-v39-n11-p469.htm

In 2000 the RDA was published for the first time, with 2000 mg as the recommended upper level of supplementation for vitamin C. This level was established in order to prevent most adults from experiencing gastrointestinal problems or diarrhea. This is definitely not a true upper limit due to the fact that many people are taking well in excess of 2000 mg/day without any problems at all. It must also be remembered that reducing the intake of any level that is causing a problem will disappear when the dosage is decreased or stopped. Vitamin C is actually extremely safe. Vitamin C is water soluble, so that excess with dietary excesses not absorbed, and excesses in the blood rapidly excreted in the urine. It exhibits remarkably low toxicity. The LD50 (the dose that will kill 50% of a population) in rats is generally accepted to be 11.9 grams per kilogram of body weight when given by forced gavage (orally). The mechanism of death from such doses (1.2% of body weight, or 0.84 kg for a 70 kg human) is unknown, but may be more mechanical than chemical.[122] The LD50 in humans remains unknown, given lack of any accidental or intentional poisoning death data. However, as with all substances tested in this way, the rat LD50 is taken as a guide to its toxicity in humans. *Reference: Javert CT, Stander HJ (1943). "Plasma Vitamin C and Prothrombin Concentration in Pregnancy and in Threatened, Spontaneous, and Habitual Abortion". Surgery, Gynecology, and Obstetrics 76: 115–122.*

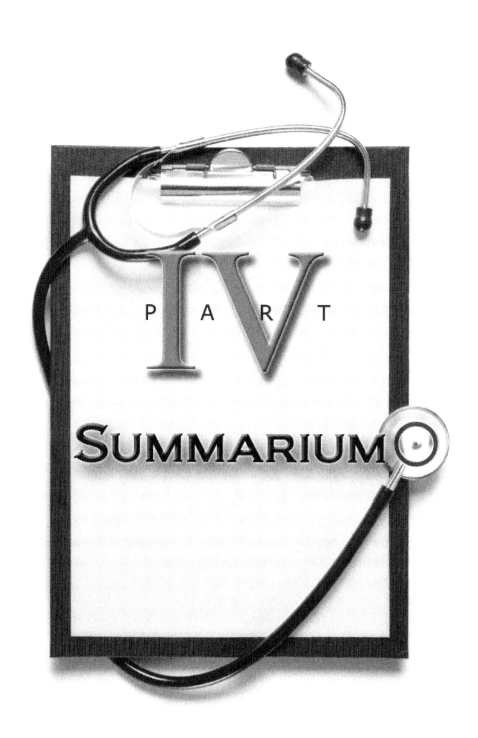

PART

IV

SUMMARIUM

CONCLUSION

During the course of writing this book, the state of medical care has become more and more challenging for the physician that wishes to provide comprehensive medicine versus symptomatic, pharmaceutical based medicine. Physicians that are motivated to continue to evolve and learn are being shackled by both state and federal government regulations that are limiting their choices in care options. Many of the best caregivers are moving to states that offer them the most medical freedom to provide the care they aspire to give their patients. In many cases, their patients actually follow them or travel to them to get the care they need and to which they have grown accustomed.

It is our fear that time is growing short for those of you that wish to establish a working relationship with your primary caregiver. With the rapidly changing country we live in, we believe it would be wise and time well spent to endeavor to find a healthcare provider that is willing and able to work with you and be open to a more comprehensive approach. For those that are able, it is also time to begin to stand together to preserve the freedom to choose for both your caregiver and yourself. If you do not stand as a majority to defend the right to decide your healthcare for yourself, you will certainly lose that right to an ever growing and dictating government that is largely controlled by the pharmaceutical companies' continuing campaign contributions and its influence on the FDA.

Always remember this single truth: **there is far more profit to be made by treating a disease than by curing it.** Pharmaceutical companies have been working by this model for many decades now. They have become so entwined with the medical schools through the reliance developed with their research grants that little unbiased truth remains. That is why the drug companies acquire such wealth. They work diligently to keep developing more and more drugs to treat symptoms, including longer acting and much more addictive pain drugs as well as their extremely long lasting corticosteroids that make you feel better while your disease progresses more rapidly.

As a relatively current example, recent research was released with the headline "*organic foods are no more nutritious than non-organic.*" Why would the news report be so slanted and inaccurate? It is because the networks and newspapers receive tens of millions of dollars in advertising from pharmaceutical companies and companies such as Monsanto. The media is **owned** by "big pharma" interests and Monsanto, thus honest reporting takes a back seat to facts. And without knowing the whole story, the public is now left to make serious decisions without the truth and without being accurately informed. Advertising money has replaced honesty in the press as well as investigative reporting. The whole truth is quite different than the nightly news report, which is nothing more than regurgitation of propaganda spewed by an attractive bobble head.

More accurate reporting would have told the whole story. The organic vs. non-organic story on the news did **not** go into the details or their ramifications. For example, it did not state that the organic food contained slightly more phosphorous than the non-organic products. Or that the organic milk contained more omega-3 fatty acids in the studies that looked at them. Or that more than 33% of conventional produce had detectable pesticide residues, compared with only 7% of organic produce samples. We all know that these residues cause illness. The study also found that organic pork and chicken were 33% less likely to carry bacteria resistant to 3 or more antibiotics than conventionally produced meat. That is a substantial difference and may actually cost you your life if antibiotics do not work on a serious infection and you do not have access to (or knowledge of) alternatives.

Physicians going through this system quickly learn that **memorization**, **subservience** to the authority of their senior professors, and unquestioned **obedience** is the easiest way (and virtually the only way) they can complete medical school in today's system. They are also constantly brainwashed into believing this is the best medicine in the world. Have pity for those that are unable to break from this powerful system, but do **not** settle for them as your trusted partner in medical care. Seek the wisest and strongest that have survived the system and continued to learn a more comprehensive and better way to practice. The good news is that they do still exist.

Our sincere advice for both patients and caregivers alike is to learn the art of reading medical studies. The conclusions that are drawn from the information they collect is very often errant and even ridiculous at times. As an example, a prestigious medical school ran a test to see if testosterone supplementation increased libido in men. They, of course, found that it did. Their conclusion for this portion of the test was fine, but they should have stopped there. They then decided to see if the "female" sex hormone, estradiol, increased libido in women. Already I am sure you are seeing their error. Their final conclusion was that male sex hormones increase male sex drive, but that female sex hormones do not increase the sex drive in women. This shows a completely ignorant finding and conclusion. Estradiol is more dominant than testosterone in females, and estradiol is not just a **female** hormone, it is a human hormone that is higher in women than in men, just as testosterone is higher in men, but both hormones are part of both sexes and is required by both. If they had simply used the same hormone for both tests they would have found that testosterone increases libido in both men **and** women.

Why didn't they do the obvious and test with the same hormone to get its response for both males and females? To put it simply, they had not learned to do an honest study that would actually have meaning. This type of ignorance has led to our current state of inferior medicine. Studies that conclude a drug shrinks a malignant tumor have absolutely nothing to do with improvement of the cancer and most often are detrimental to the patient. But the patient is told that studies have shown the drug to be "effective" against cancer, when in actuality all they are doing is reducing the size or swelling of the tumor. This is often through the destruction of the good cells (such as natural killer cells) that are within the tumor and actively killing the cancer cells.

What is the point we are trying to make? **Learn to read the studies with a jaded eye and look for who is sponsoring the studies, who is getting paid for doing them, and most of all, learn to see through the "smoke and mirrors" to get at the grains of truth.** After all, if you do not take the time to investigate your health issues, who do you expect to do it for you? The medical doctor who is seeing 60 patients a day is not going to be searching for more than his pharmaceutical representative. The medical doctors and naturopaths and homeopaths will expect you to be a participant in your health care, and in order to participate, you must know the rules of the game. Take the time to read actual studies. If you don't understand all of the words, don't be discouraged. Many physicians do not understand all of the words either. In many cases, they are intentionally confusing and difficult to read in order to disguise or obfuscate the true findings. If so, realize there is a reason, take that into account, and move on to the next one. There are numerous online medical dictionaries. We often refer to them when reading studies, so don't feel bad if you have to do the same.

Our primary message in this book is that you must take responsibility for your health and your families' health in order to survive in our current medical system. If there is one "action item" to take with you after reading this book, let it be a renewed effort to find a caregiver who understands and embraces comprehensive medicine and also shares your vision to live a healthy life and enjoy everything this wonderful life has to offer. We are here to help and guide you, but in the end, you are and always will be the final arbiter of your healthcare and your future. **Never let that right be taken from you.** Once it is gone, it will never return, and you will be left with a government that will decide what is "best" for you and to whom you must go for medical care, regardless of your knowledge and desire. Be bold and willing to be public in your fight for truth about the current state of medicine and never settle for less than you deserve.

On a more personal note, if you are a physician that is interested in comprehensive care, please realize that you are not alone. Our dream for many years has been to find a state that would welcome a true integrative medical center – a place near a medical school so we could take new physicians from the school and have them work alongside other specialists and learn exactly what the oath they took was about – a place where the patients have the opportunity to interact with their doctors and learn from them at the same time the doctors learn from the patients – a place where the quest to learn is paramount and the patient is the center of the circle of care.

Already there is a small group of extraordinary doctors comprised of an orthopedic surgeon, an oncological surgeon, a periodontist, a cardiologist, a naturopath, and a family practitioner that are all ready to begin. We need more providers and we need the magic state that still gives the primary caregiver the right to choose what is best for the patient. We also need patients willing to be active and educated participants in the art of healthcare. Please let us know if you are interested in joining our quest.

Thank you for reading this book. We sincerely hope that it has given you both ammunition and hope. God willing, the day will come when the general public has free access to any and all comprehensive medical treatment options. But until then, perhaps this book will be a source of information for you and your loved ones who desperately need assistance in comprehensively treating your illness and working with your doctor to accomplish this goal.

All our best!

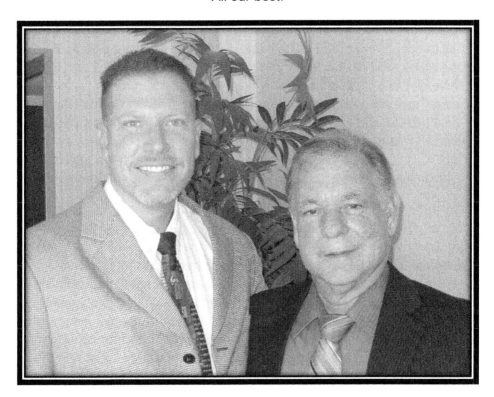

Ty M. Bollinger   Dr. Michael Farley, NMD

ty@medicaldreamteam.com   mike@medicaldreamteam.com

GLOSSARY

ACE Inhibitor – ("angiotensin-converting-enzyme" inhibitor) – a pharmaceutical drug used primarily for the treatment of hypertension (high blood pressure).

Acetogenins – long chains of carbon atoms which reduce the growth of blood vessels that nourish cancer cells and inhibit the growth of MDR cells.

Acidic – having a low pH.

Acrylamides – carcinogenic chemical formed by the heating of starches.

Adaptogenic – a substance that demonstrates a nonspecific enhancement of the body's ability to resist a stressors.

Adenosine Triphosphate (ATP) – the "energy currency" of cells.

Adrenal Glands – a pair of glands located above the kidneys; produce hormones such as epinephrine, corticosteroids, and androgens.

Aerobic – "with oxygen" (contrasted with anaerobic – "without oxygen").

Alkaline – having a high pH.

Allicin – organosulfur compound obtained from garlic.

AMAS Test – ("Anti Malignin Antibody in Serum" test) – the most accurate diagnostic test to detect and monitor cancer, when used correctly.

Amino Acids – building blocks of proteins and intermediates in metabolism.

Amylase – digestive enzyme that breaks down carbohydrates.

Anaerobic – means "without oxygen."

Anemia – a condition in which a decreased number of red blood cells that may cause symptoms including tiredness, shortness of breath, and weakness.

Angina – chest pain or discomfort resulting from lack of blood to the heart.

Angiogenesis – the physiological process involving the growth of new blood vessels from pre-existing vessels.

Antibiotics – drugs that fight bacterial infections.

Antibody – a Y-shaped protein on the surface of B-cells that is secreted into the blood or lymph in response to an antigenic stimulus

Antihistamine – a drug used to counteract the physiological effects of histamine production in allergic reactions and colds.

Antioxidants – chemical compounds or substances that inhibit oxidation.

Antineoplastic – preventing the growth or development of abnormal or cancer cells.

Apoptosis – programmed cell death.

Arachnodactyly – ("spider fingers") – a condition in which the fingers are abnormally long and slender in comparison to the palm of the hand; characteristic of Marfan Syndrome.

Aromatase – an enzyme responsible for a key step in the biosynthesis of estrogens.

Autoimmune Response – a condition in which a person's immune system produces antibodies that attack the body's own tissues.

Bacterium (plural Bacteria) – single-celled microorganisms that can exist either as independent (free-living) organisms or as parasites that may be found individually or in chains and come in various forms and species that may be either benign of pathogenic.

Benign – a non-cancerous tumor or growth; antonym of malignant.

Beta-Blockers – drugs that treat angina and other heart rhythm disorders, migraines, high blood pressure, panic attacks, and tremors; (aka beta-adrenergic blocking agents, beta-adrenergic antagonists, beta-adrenoreceptor antagonists, or beta antagonists).

Beta Carotene – precursor to vitamin A; the most well-known carotenoid.

Bile – a yellowish-green fluid produced by the liver that aids in digestion of fats and the excretion of toxins.

Biopsy – the surgical removal of tissue for microscopic examination.

Blood Cells – minute structures produced in the bone marrow and spleen that consist of erythrocytes (red blood cells), leukocytes (white blood cells), and platelets and blood corpuscle circulating in the blood.

Blood Pressure – the pressure exerted by circulating blood upon the walls of blood vessels.
> *Diastolic* – the bottom number in a blood pressure reading; when your heart is resting.
> *Systolic* – the top number in a blood pressure reading; the force of blood in the arteries as the heart beats.

Bone Marrow – soft, fatty, vascular tissue that fills most bone cavities and is the source of red blood cells and many white blood cells.

Capillaries – the smallest blood vessels that function to distribute oxygenated blood from arteries to the tissues of the body and to feed deoxygenated blood from the tissues back into the veins.

Carcinogen – a cancer-causing substance or agent.

Carcinoma – cancer that starts in the skin or tissue that line or cover body organs.

CAT scan – a test using x-rays and sometimes contrast media to create images of various body parts.

CEA (Carcino Embryonic Antigen) – a blood tumor marker.

Cell Fibers – fibers made up of cylindrical, multinucleate cells composed of numerous myofibrils that contracts when stimulated.

Cell Membrane – the "outer skin or membrane" of our cells.

Chelation – the process of removing a heavy metal from the bloodstream by means of a chelating agent.

Chlorophyll – a group of related green pigments that convert light energy into ATP and other forms of energy needed for biochemical processes; found in green plants, brown and red algae, and certain aerobic and anaerobic bacteria.

Cirrhosis – a type of liver damage in which normal liver cells are replaced with nonfunctioning fibrous scar tissue.

Co-Enzyme – an organic substance that usually contains a vitamin or mineral that combines with a specific protein to form an active enzyme system.

Collagen – the fibrous protein "cement" that holds our bones, cartilage, tendons, connective tissue, and cells together.

Conjugated Linoleic Acid (CLA) – naturally occurring free fatty acid found mainly in grass-fed meats and dairy products; builds muscle and reduces body fat; classified as an omega-6 fatty acid.

Corticosteroids – a class of chemicals that includes steroid hormones naturally produced in the adrenal cortex of vertebrates.

Cyanosis – the appearance of a blue or purple coloration of the skin or mucous membranes due to the tissues near the skin surface being low on oxygen.

Cytokines – "messenger cells" such as interferons and interleukins which set off a cascade reaction of positive changes throughout the immune system.

Cytopenia – low levels of blood cells.

Cytoplasm – the jelly-like part of a cell.

Deoxyribonucleic Acid (DNA) – carries the cell's genetic information and hereditary characteristics via its nucleotides and their sequence; capable of self-replication and RNA synthesis.

DHEA – (dehydroepiandrosterone) – an important endogenous steroid hormone occurring naturally in the body.

Dimethyl sulfoxide (DMSO) – an organosulfur compound, non-toxic and 100% natural that comes from the wood pulp industry.

Disaccharide – a chain of two sugar molecules (like lactose which is composed of glucose and galactose).

Dysbiosis – the condition when good bacteria in the gut flora (required for immune system function and proper digestion) are overrun by pathogenic bacteria (which cause harm).

Dyskinesia – distortion or impairment of voluntary movement.

EDTA Chelation – a therapy by which repeated administrations of a weak synthetic amino acid (EDTA, ethylenediamine tetra-acetic acid) gradually reduce heavy metal deposits throughout the cardiovascular system by attaching to them and taking them out with urine, solid waste and sweat.

Electron – an elementary particle with a negative charge.

Electron Transport Chain – the final stage of the Krebs Cycle.

Endothelium – the thin layer of cells that lines the interior surface of blood vessels and lymphatic vessels.

Enzymes – any of numerous proteins produced by living organisms and functioning as biochemical catalysts.

Epidermis –the outer layer of skin.

Erythrocytes – see "Red Blood Cells."

Eukaryotic Cell – a cell with a nucleus and organelles.

Excitotoxins – substances, usually amino acids, that damage neurons through paroxysmal over activity.

Free Radical – an atom or group of atoms that has at least one unpaired electron and is, therefore, unstable and highly reactive; damages cells and accelerates the progression of cancer and other diseases.

Gliadin – a protein found within wheat gluten.

Glioblastoma Multiforme – the most common and most aggressive type of primary brain tumor in humans, involving glial cells.

Gluconeogenesis – the formation of glucose, especially by the liver, from non-carbohydrate sources, such as amino acids, lactic acid and the glycerol portion of fats.

Glucose – a monosaccharide sugar the blood that serves as the major energy source of the body; it occurs in most plant and animal tissue and is also called blood sugar.

Glucosuria – the excretion of glucose into the urine; aka glycosuria.

492

Glycan – a chain of saccharides.

Glyconutrients – approximately 200 naturally occurring biologically active plant monosaccharide sugars.

Golgi Body – a net-like structure in the cell's cytoplasm which stores ATP.

Glycogen – a polysaccharide that is the main form of carbohydrate storage in animals and occurs mainly in liver and muscle tissue; it is readily converted to glucose; also called animal starch.

Gram-positive Bacteria – those bacteria that are stained dark blue or violet by Gram staining; contrasted with Gram-negative bacteria, which cannot retain the crystal violet stain.

Granulocytes – white blood cells filled with granules of toxic chemicals that enable them to digest microbes by a process called phagocytosis (literally "cell-eating"). Three types of granulocytes are neutrophils (which kill bacteria), eosinophils (which kill parasites), and basophils, which release histamine and other enzymes that can lead to inflammation, bronchoconstriction, and asthma symptoms.

Hemoglobin – the protein pigment in red blood cells that contains iron and transports oxygen to the tissues and carbon dioxide from them.

Homocysteine – a naturally occurring amino acid found in blood plasma.

Human chronic gonadotropin (HCG) – a hormone produced by the placenta that maintains the corpus luteum during pregnancy.

Hydrogen – the most abundant chemical element; constitutes 75% of the universe.

Hydrogenation – the addition of hydrogen to a compound, especially to solidify an unsaturated fat or fatty acid.

Hydrolysis – the decomposition of a chemical compound by reaction with water.

Hypertension – high blood pressure.

Hypochloridic – low stomach acid.

Hypoxia – lack of oxygen.

Iatrogenic – resulting from the activity of physicians.

Immune System – the bodily system that protects the body from foreign substances, cells, and tissues by producing the immune response and that includes the thymus, spleen, lymph nodes, lymphocytes, and antibodies.

Insulin – a hormone secreted by the pancreas which regulates the metabolism of carbohydrates and fats, especially the conversion of glucose to glycogen, which lowers the blood glucose level.

Interferon – any of various proteins that are produced by virus-infected cells that inhibit reproduction of the invading virus and induce resistance to further infection.

Interleukin – a naturally produced chemical released by the body extracted from white blood cells that stimulates their activity against infection and may be used to combat some forms of cancer.

Jejunum – the middle section of the small intestine.

Krebs Cycle – A series of enzymatic reactions occurring in aerobic organisms that involves oxidative metabolism of acetyl units and producing high-energy phosphate.

Lauric Acid –a fatty acid obtained chiefly from coconut oil.

Leukemia – a cancer of the lymphatic system which may include any of the cancers of the bone marrow that prevent the normal manufacture of red and white blood cells and platelets

Leukocytes – see "White Blood Cells."

Lewy Bodies – abnormal aggregates of protein that develop inside nerve cells in Parkinson's disease.

Lymphocytes – small white blood cell (leukocyte) that plays a large role in defending the body against disease which includes T-cells, B-cells, and NK cells.

Lymphoma – cancer of the lymphatic system which originates in the lymphocytes; two types are Hodgkin's (includes the presence of a Reed-Sternberg cell) and non-Hodgkin's (Reed-Sternberg cell is not present).

Lipids – group of molecules including fats, oils, and cholesterol.

Lipase – digestive enzyme that breaks down lipids.

Macrophage – literally "big eater" – a type of white blood cell that ingests foreign material.

Malignancy – a cancer, neoplasm, or tumor that grows in an uncontrolled manner, and may invade nearby tissue and metastasize (spread) to other areas of the body.

Melanocytes – cells that produce the pigment melanin that colors our skin, hair, and eyes and is heavily concentrated in most moles.

Melanoma – the most serious form of skin cancer; a malignant tumor that originates in melanocytes.

Melatonin – a hormone produced from the amino acid tryptophan by the pineal gland that holds a primary function of regulating the sleep, wake cycle of the brain.

Microbe – a microorganism, especially a bacterium that causes disease.

Mineral – an inorganic element that promotes chemical reactions within the body and is necessary for proper cellular metabolism.

Mitochondria – "cellular power plant"; an organelle in the cytoplasm of nearly all eukaryotic cells containing genetic material.

Monosaccharide – any of several carbohydrates that cannot be broken down to simpler sugars.

Monocytes – white blood cells that ingest dead or damaged cells and provide immunological defenses against many infectious organisms; eventually develop into macrophages.

Monosodium glutamate (MSG) – food additive made from glutamic acid which acts as an excitotoxin.

Monounsaturated – containing only one double or triple bond per molecule; monounsaturated fats decrease the amount of LDL cholesterol in the blood and include olive and avocado oils.

Myelin – an insulating layer that forms around nerves, including those in the brain and spinal cord; made up of protein and fatty substances.

Myeloma – tumor of antibody-producing cells, called plasma cells, which are normally found in the bone marrow.

Neoplasm – any new or abnormal growth in which cell multiplication is uncontrolled and progressive.

Neurons – nerve cells; conduct electrical impulses.

Nucleotide – the basic component of DNA and RNA.

Nucleus – the "control center" of the cell; includes the DNA of the cell.

Oligosaccharide – a carbohydrate that consists of a relatively small number of monosaccharides and consists of a chain of sugars that is from 3 to 20 molecules long.

Omega-3 fatty acids – polyunsaturated fatty acids that are found especially in fish, fish oils, vegetable oils, and green leafy vegetables; omega-3 fats include alpha-linolenic acid (ALA), eicosapentaenoic acid (EPA), docosahexaenoic acid (DHA), and docosapentaenoic acid (DPA).

Omega-6 fatty acids – polyunsaturated fatty acids that are found especially in nuts and grains;omega-6 fats include linoleic acid (LA), conjugated linoleic acid (CLA), gamma linolenic acid (GLA), dihomo-gamma linolenic acid (DGLA), and arachidonic acid(AA).

Omega-9 fatty acids – essential fatty acids found in olive oil and avocados; also known as oleic acid.

Organelle – a differentiated structure within a cell that performs a specific function.

Orthomolecular – the theory that diseases can be cured by restoring the optimum amounts of substances normally present in the body.

Osteosarcoma – most common type of bone cancer which presents as a cancerous tumor that occurs in the bone

Otitis Externa – inflammation of the canal between the ear canal and external opening of the ear.

Otitis Interna – inflammation of the inner ear.

Otitis Media – inflammation of the middle ear.

Oxidation – the addition of oxygen to a compound with a loss of electrons, the process when oxygen combines with an element

P53 – a protein that is the product of a tumor suppressor gene, regulates cell growth and proliferation, and prevents unrestrained cell division after chromosomal damage.

Pathogenic – capable of causing disease.

pH Balance – the acid/alkaline balance in our body; pH = potential hydrogen.

Phagocytosis – the process the human body uses to destroy bacteria by surrounding and digesting them with digestive enzymes and consuming them with macrophages that are the scavenger cells that are part of this process; literally "cell eating."

Pituitary Gland – a pea-sized gland located at the base of the skull between the optic nerves which secretes hormones.

Plasma – clear, yellowish fluid portion of blood, lymph, or intramuscular fluid in which cells are suspended and an important part of our immune system

Platelets – the smallest of the three types of blood cells; also called thrombocytes; principal function is to prevent abnormal or excessive bleeding.

Pleomorphic – having many forms.

Polydipsia – excessive thirst.

Polysaccharide – any of a class of carbohydrates whose molecules contain chains of 10 or more monosaccharaides.

Polyuria – excessive urination.

Probiotics – "good bacteria;" live microbial supplements which improve intestinal balance, complete digestion and actively increase our immune systems function.

Prokaryotic cell – a cell (such as bacteria) which lacks a nucleus.

Protease – digestive enzyme that breaks down proteins.

Proteinuria – excess protein in the urine.

Proton – an elementary particle with a positive charge.

Protoplasm – the complex substance that constitutes the living matter of plant and animal cells; composed of proteins and fats; includes the nucleus and cytoplasm within the cell wall.

PSA (Prostate Specific Antigen) – test used to diagnose prostate cancer; though it has been found to increase in many breast cancer cases and is not prostate specific. It has been losing favor as a cancer diagnostic tool.

Pyloric Valve – the sphincter muscle of the pylorus that separates the stomach from the duodenum.

Red blood cells (Erythrocytes) – blood cells that deliver oxygen to tissues and remove carbon dioxide from them.

Resveratrol – a compound found in grapes, red wine and purple grape juice which inhibits the growth of cancer cells.

Rhinorrhea – a condition where the nasal cavity is filled with a significant amount of mucus.

Ribonucleic acid (RNA) – transmits genetic information from DNA to the cytoplasm and controls certain chemical processes in the cell.

Saccharide – a sugar molecule.

Sarcoma – malignant tumor of the muscles or connective tissue such as bone and cartilage.

Seizure – a burst of abnormal electrical activity in the brain.

Selenium – trace mineral that acts as an antioxidant.

Staphylococcus – a genus of Gram-positive bacteria which causes staph infections.

Streptococcus – a genus of spherical Gram-positive bacteria which causes strep throat.

Stroke – interruption of the normal flow of blood to the brain due to a blood clot or hemorrhage.

Superoxide Dismutase (SOD) – enzyme that destroys free radicals.

Thrombopoietin (TPO) – cytokine that stimulates production of platelets.

Thrombosis – development of abnormal blood clots within blood vessels, lungs or heart.

Thyroid Gland – organ at the base of the neck that produces thyroxin and other hormones involved in regulating metabolism.

Tinnitus – ringing in the ears.

Triglycerides – a type of fat in the bloodstream and fat tissue derived from glycerol and three fatty acids.

Toxin – harmful or poisonous agent.

Trans-Fats – "pseudo-fats" produced by the partial hydrogenation of vegetable oils; present in hardened vegetable oils, most margarines, commercial baked foods, and fried foods; increase the risk of cancer.

Trophoblasts – cells that attach the fertilized ovum to the uterine wall and serve as a nutritive pathway for the embryo.

Tumor – abnormal uncontrolled growth of cells.

Uric Acid – a chemical created when the body breaks down substances called purines.

Villi (singular Villus) – tiny, finger-like projections that protrude from the epithelial lining of the intestinal wall.

Virus – a small infectious agent that can replicate only inside the living cells of an organism.

Vitamin – an organic substance that acts as a co-enzyme or regulator of metabolic processes.

White blood cells (Leukocytes) – blood cells that engulf and digest bacteria and fungi; an important part of the body's immune system; specific white blood cells include lymphocytes, granulocytes, and monocytes.

Xenoestrogens – "foreign" estrogen like substances that have been "altered "and act like free radicals in the body; shown to cause various types of cancer, especially estradiol receptor positive cancers.

X-ray – electromagnetic radiation used to diagnose disease and view bone.

Yersinia Pestis – a Gram-negative rod-shaped bacterium responsible for the plague.

Yunan Pao – (a traditional chinese medicine) for hemorrhage; aka tienchi.

INDEX

499

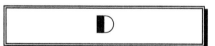

D

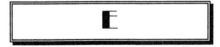
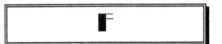

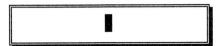

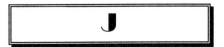

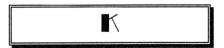

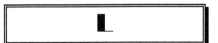

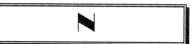

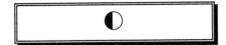

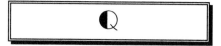

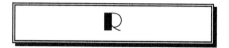

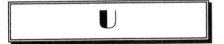
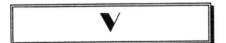
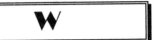
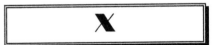
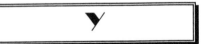
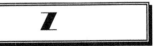

Other books that may be of interest:

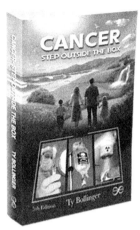

Cancer – Step Outside the Box
www.CancerTruth.net

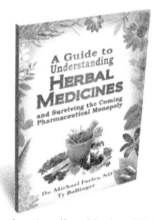

*A Guide to Understanding Herbal Medicines and
Surviving the Coming Pharmaceutical Monopoly*
www.SurvivalHerbs.com

Or visit **www.Infinity510Partners.com**

CPSIA information can be obtained at www.ICGtesting.com
Printed in the USA
LVOW04s1501251015

459661LV00026B/976/P